Healthy Ageing in Asia

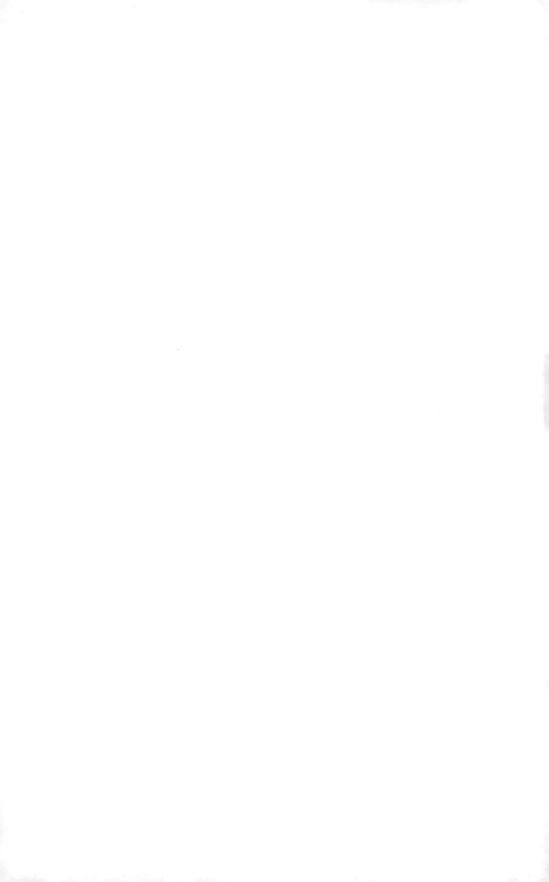

Healthy Ageing in Asia
Culture, Prevention and Wellness

Edited by
Goh Cheng Soon
Traditional and Complementary Medicine (T&CM) Division,
Ministry of Health (MOH), Kuala Lumpur, Malaysia

Gerard Bodeker
Green Templeton College, University of Oxford

Kishan Kariippanon
University of Wollongong, Australia

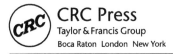

CRC Press is an imprint of the
Taylor & Francis Group, an **informa** business

First edition published 2022
by CRC Press
6000 Broken Sound Parkway NW, Suite 300, Boca Raton, FL 33487-2742

and by CRC Press
4 Park Square, Milton Park, Abingdon, Oxon, OX14 4RN

© 2022 Taylor & Francis Group, LLC

CRC Press is an imprint of Taylor & Francis Group, LLC

Reasonable efforts have been made to publish reliable data and information, but the author and publisher cannot assume responsibility for the validity of all materials or the consequences of their use. The authors and publishers have attempted to trace the copyright holders of all material reproduced in this publication and apologize to copyright holders if permission to publish in this form has not been obtained. If any copyright material has not been acknowledged please write and let us know so we may rectify in any future reprint.

Except as permitted under U.S. Copyright Law, no part of this book may be reprinted, reproduced, transmitted, or utilized in any form by any electronic, mechanical, or other means, now known or hereafter invented, including photocopying, microfilming, and recording, or in any information storage or retrieval system, without written permission from the publishers.

For permission to photocopy or use material electronically from this work, access www.copyright. com or contact the Copyright Clearance Center, Inc. (CCC), 222 Rosewood Drive, Danvers, MA 01923, 978-750-8400. For works that are not available on CCC please contact mpkbookspermissions@ tandf.co.uk

Trademark notice: Product or corporate names may be trademarks or registered trademarks and are used only for identification and explanation without intent to infringe.

Library of Congress Cataloging-in-Publication Data
Names: Goh, Cheng Soon, editor. | Bodeker, Gerard, editor. | Kariippanon, Kishan, editor.
Title: Healthy ageing in Asia : culture and tradition in prevention and wellness /
edited by Goh Cheng Soon, Gerard Bodeker, Kishan Kariippanon.
Other titles: Healthy aging in Asia
Description: First edition. | Boca Raton, FL : CRC Press, 2022. |
Includes bibliographical references and index.
Identifiers: LCCN 2021049186 (print) | LCCN 2021049187 (ebook) |
ISBN 9780367488741 (hardback) | ISBN 9780367473884 (paperback) |
ISBN 9781003043270 (ebook)
Subjects: LCSH: Aging–Health aspects–Asia. | Older people–Health and hygiene–Asia. |
Older people–Medical care–Asia. | Well-being–Age factors–Asia. | Health behavior–Age factors–Asia.
Classification: LCC RA564.8 .H4558 2022 (print) | LCC RA564.8 (ebook) |
DDC 362.6095–dc23/eng/20211029
LC record available at https://lccn.loc.gov/2021049186
LC ebook record available at https://lccn.loc.gov/2021049187

ISBN: 9780367488741 (hbk)
ISBN: 9780367473884 (pbk)
ISBN: 9781003043270 (ebk)

DOI: 10.1201/9781003043270

Typeset in Times
by codeMantra

Contents

Foreword ix

Acknowledgement xi

Editors xiii

Contributors xv

Chapter 1   Healthy Ageing in Asia during the COVID Pandemic 1

                  Goh Cheng Soon and Gerard Bodeker

Chapter 2   An Integrated Approach to Creating Healthy Ageing in the
                  Nation: A Malaysian Perspective 11

                  Noor Hisham Abdullah, Goh Cheng Soon,
                  Noraliza binti Noordin Merican, and
                  Sheleaswani binti Inche Zainal Abidin

Chapter 3   Challenges of Holistic Healthcare System for Ageing
                  Population in Malaysia 21

                  Lee Fatt Soon

Chapter 4   Policy Development on Ageing in Malaysia: Issues and
                  Challenges 25

                  Tengku Aizan Hamid, Wan Alia Wan Sulaiman,
                  Mohamad Fazdillah Bagat, and Sen Tyng Chai

Chapter 5   Enriching the Lives of Seniors in Japan
                  (Ikigai Healthy Ageing Policy in Japan) 63

                  Tomonori Maruyama

Chapter 6   South Korea's Prospect for Aging and Preparation for the
                  Future: Focusing on the Korean Traditional Medicine in
                  the National Health Insurance 73

                  Kim Hyung-Ho

Chapter 7   The Triple Response to Population Ageing: Systems, Networks
                  and Culture Change Perspectives from the UK and Europe 81

                  Muir Gray

Chapter 8 The Health and Well-Being of the Left-Behind Elderly in Rural China 89

Paul Kadetz

Chapter 9 The Definition of TM: Perspectives from WHO and Countries across Asia 109

Goh Cheng Soon

Chapter 10 Traditional Malay Ulam for Healthy Ageing 135

Jamia Azdina Jamal and Khairana Husain

Chapter 11 The Value of TCM in Health Preservation in Healthy Ageing 151

Zhang Qin

Chapter 12 The Value of Disease Prevention and Health Promotion of Hua Tuo Five-Animal Play with Traditional Chinese Medicine 157

Yang Yu

Chapter 13 An Ayurvedic Approach for Healthy Ageing 163

Gopesh Mangal

Chapter 14 Principles and Practice of Yoga for Rejuvenation 171

Gunjan Garg

Chapter 15 Rapid Ageing in Thailand and Implications for Thai Traditional Medicine 179

Anchalee Chuthaputti and Khwanchai Wisithanon

Chapter 16 Health Benefits of Exercise for Older People: The Research Evidence and Approaches to Maximize Participation 189

Keith Hill

Chapter 17 Discussion on Principles and Methods of Tai Chi Qigong in Preventing Falling Among the Elderly 197

Xie Yuhong

Contents

Chapter 18 Integrated Management in Elderly 205

Liu Xiao Hang

Chapter 19 Mental Health and Healthy Aging – Prevention and Management 209

Gerard Bodeker

Chapter 20 Laughter Is the Best Therapy for Happiness and
Healthy Life Expectancy 229

Tetsuya Ohira and Masahiko Ichiki

Chapter 21 Impact of Music Therapy on Complicated Grief Reactions in
Elderly Persons 241

Ranka Radulovic

Chapter 22 Empowering the Community in Healthy Ageing............................253

Goh Cheng Beh and Aaron K.T. Ang

Chapter 23 Aging in Place: Beyond the Home 265

Jean Woo

Chapter 24 Mapping Healthy Ageing Start-ups: The Role of Accelerators
and Incubators in Supporting Innovation for Prevention and
Wellness in Southeast Asia 271

Kishan Kariippanon

Chapter 25 Translational Research: A Novel Yam Protein with
Tremendous Potential for Menopausal Syndrome 289

Stephen Cho Wing Sze

Chapter 26 Conclusion – The Way Forward 299

Goh Cheng Soon, Gerard Bodeker, and Kishan Kariippanon

Index of Countries 301
Index of Policies & Legislation 305
Index of Herbal Plants...309
Index of Practices..311
Subject Index 313
Index of Name 321

Foreword

DEVELOPING A SYSTEM AND A CULTURE FOR LIVING LONGER BETTER

Population ageing is one of the most complex challenges facing every society on earth, but the responses have often focused on bureaucratic changes such as the development of new departments focused on ageing or the integration of health and social care. However, a complex challenge, which by definition is beyond the capability of structural solution, requires the development of a system and the creation of a new culture.

A system is a set of activities and a common aim, clarified by a set of objectives defining the outcomes to be achieved, and here is a set of objectives to achieve the aim of living longer better or, to use other language, increasing healthspan:

- To prevent and mitigate isolation
- To increase physical ability, fitness and healthspan and decrease the risk of frailty
- To promote knowledge and understanding about living longer better among older people and the wider population to counteract the detrimental effects of ageism
- To create an environment in which people can fulfil their potential
- To enable strengthening of purpose
- To support carers better
- To minimize and mitigate the effects of deprivation
- To reduce the risk of and delay or prevent dementia
- To prevent and minimize the effects of disease and multimorbidity
- To reduce the risk of a bad death

For each objective, criteria that can be used to measure progress or the lack of it need to be measured. To achieve the objectives requires the development of networks, not the reorganization of structures with every network pursuing the same objectives and using the same criteria so that they can learn from one another as a community of practice and this requires a collaborative culture.

There is general agreement that the key feature distinguishes leadership from management is that the former is responsible for changing culture whereas the function of management is to work within the culture and as well as creating a culture of collaboration, the system has to create a new culture for living longer with a better quality of life.

The science is now clear. It is now known that what happens to us after the age of 60 should not be assumed to be caused solely by the ageing process. The ageing process affects everyone and from about forty on but by itself does not cause major problems until after ninety. There are three interrelated and modifiable causes of the problems that occur more frequently as people live longer:

- Loss of fitness
- Disease, much of which is preventable, complicated by accelerated loss of fitness, and
- Pessimistic and negative beliefs and attitudes

What is required is a new culture based on the science in which older people are expected to remain, or become increasingly, active, physically, cognitively and emotionally maintaining or strengthening a strong sense of purpose.

This new approach requires a new set of activities to make healthcare sustainable:

1. a change in culture;
2. training in new skills and concepts;
3. the development of population-based systems.

Europe is looking to Asia because this culture is more prevalent there than in Europe. The core theme is not one of 'caring' for a passive subset of the population but of promoting lifelong learning because knowledge is the elixir of life. The chapters in this book go a long way to creating the foundations of this approach within an Asian context, and this book will stand as a seminal reference for policy makers, planners, public health professionals and elder care providers for the future.

Professor Sir Muir Gray
Founding Director, The Optimal Ageing Programme
& Professor in the Nuffield Department of Surgery, University of Oxford
www.livelongerbetter.uk
59 Lakeside; Oxford OX2 8JQ, UK

Acknowledgement

The idea for this book took shape during the planning for an international conference in Kuala Lumpur on the theme of Healthy Ageing in the Context of Traditional and Complementary Medicine. Hosted in early August 2019 by the Division of Traditional and Complementary Medicine (T&CM) of the Malaysian Ministry of Health, the conference (INTRACOM-9) showcased the work of experts from across Asia–Pacific and beyond.

It has taken a further 2.5 years for the book to come to fruition, drawing on the presentations made by contributors at INTRACOM-9 and additional invited chapters. The COVID-19 pandemic has caused delays for all concerned, and the additional workload associated with the pandemic has meant that the chapters were produced under conditions of significant professional and personal challenge. For this, we would like to express our most sincere appreciation to all chapter authors for staying the course and making significant contributions to the understanding and promotion of healthy ageing in Asia.

We would also like to thank all of those involved in making INTRACOM-9 a highly successful knowledge exchange and opportunity for networking and for new friendships to form. This includes the organizing team, INTRACOM-9 sponsors, presenters, distinguished speakers and guests and media who covered much of the content of INTRACOM-9 as it unfolded. INTRACOM-9 laid the foundation for developing the collection of perspectives and strategies contained in this book, which we hope will serve as a useful reference resource for all involved in the field of healthy ageing in the region.

We are especially grateful to Professor Sir Muir Gray (University of Oxford, UK), a leading authority in the field of healthy ageing and policy, for his foreword and chapter.

We also wish to express sincere thanks to Tan Sri Dato' Seri Dr. Noor Hisham Bin Abdullah, Director General of Health, MOH, Malaysia, for his continuous encouragement and support; and our sincere appreciation to Associate Professor Dr. Te Kian Keong (University of Tunku Abdul Rahman, Malaysia) for reviewing the translated chapter.

Our special thanks to Ms. Randy Brehm, Senior Editor, Life Sciences and Nutrition, CRC Press/Taylor and Francis Group LLC, our publisher, for her initial and enthusiastic receptivity to the book proposal and her patience with the continually extended deadline due to the challenges of the COVID-19 pandemic.

On a personal level, we would like to thank our family members and colleagues. Their love and support have sustained us through these challenging times.

It is our hope that this book will make a difference to lives, economies and generations across Asia, and we would like recognition to be shared by all of those who have supported the collective efforts leading to this publication.

Goh Cheng Soon, Gerard Bodeker, Kishan Kariippanon

Editors

Dr. Goh Cheng Soon is currently the Director of the Traditional and Complementary Medicine (T&CM) Division in the Ministry of Health (MOH), Malaysia. After completing her MBBS from Kasturba Medical College, Manipal, she undertook the Master of Medical Law (LLM) and Doctor of Philosophy in Law (PhD) from England. She began her career at Queen Elizabeth Hospital, Kota Kinabalu, Sabah, in 1993. After amassing 14 years of experience in allopathic clinical medicine, she embarked into the T&CM world after realizing the great potential of integrating healthcare in this borderless world having more than 10 years' involvement in the field of T&CM.

She has received the Excellent Service Award for her work from MOH, Malaysia. She has been conferred a Public Health Specialist due to her dedicated participation and expert contribution to Malaysia's public health. Holding the post of the Director of T&CM Division, she has represented MOH at international as well as national level. She is a consultant for the World Health Organization in T&CM policies and regulations of practice. Currently, being one of the Standing Committee in the Crisis Preparedness and Response Centre (Hospital Services), she participates in policy-making and administrative support to fight against COVID-19.

Professor Gerard Bodeker, an Australian, completed his doctoral studies at Harvard. He has held research and teaching appointments in the Division of Medical Sciences at the University of Oxford for two decades and is a member of Oxford's Green Templeton College.

An Adjunct Professor of Epidemiology at Columbia University, New York, and in integrative medicine at the University of Western Sydney, Prof. Bodeker has worked with several UN agencies, including the WHO, World Bank, UNDP. He served as Editor-in-Chief of the World Health Organization Global Atlas of Traditional, Complementary and Alternative Medicine. He has served as an advisor to National Geographic magazine and to CNN.

Prof. Bodeker co-produced with the Asian Development Bank a 2020 white paper on Wellness in Asia and a 2021 book on perspectives and policy frameworks for Wellness in Asia. He is a fellow of the International Union of Pure and Applied Chemistry and is the Chair of the Mental Wellness Initiative of the Global Wellness Institute.

Dr Kishan Kariippanon researches in healthy ageing combining public health, design and innovation to promote well-being. He was born in Malaysia, received his Doctorate in Medicine from Russia and worked in Timor-Leste as a doctor during the 2006 civil crises. He earned his Master's in Public Health with a focus on global public health from Monash University, Australia, in 2007 and worked in the Aboriginal lands of the Northern Territory. His doctoral studies at the University of Wollongong focused on an interdisciplinary study of remote Aboriginal youth and their use of technology to promote health and maintain well-being. He is a co-author in the Oxford Research Encyclopaedia for Global Public Health on *Traditional Medicine: Indigenous health in Indigenous hands*, and *Wellbeing & Mental Wellness*.

Kariippanon and colleagues from the University of Wollongong and TAFE New South Wales won the first prize in interior design and innovation with the *Desert Rose Dementia-Friendly House* at the Solar Decathlon Middle East 2018. His poster presentation on the use of collective reflexivity in working with people living with dementia, their carers and designers was awarded first prize in the *International Conference on Healthy Ageing and Traditional and Complementary Medicine* in 2019. He completed the MIT and Harvard Centre for Primary Care Health Technology Innovation Course in 2020.

Contributors

Noor Hisham Bin Abdullah
General of Health
Ministry of Health
Putrajaya, Malaysia

Aaron K.T. Ang
Putra Polyclinic
Nilai, Malaysia

Mohamad Fazdillah Bagat
Malaysian Research Institute on Ageing
University Putra Malaysia
Serdang, Malaysia

Goh Cheng Beh
Hospital Tuanku Ja'afar Seremban
Seremban, Negeri Sembilan, Malaysia

Gerard Bodeker
Mental Wellness Initiative, Global
    Wellness Institute; & Green
    Templeton College
University of Oxford
Oxford, United Kingdom

Anchalee Chuthaputti
Department of Thai Traditional and
    Alternative Medicine
Ministry of Public Health
Nonthaburi, Thailand

Gunjan Garg
Department of Swasthavritta & Yoga
Mahatma Jyotiba Fule Ayurveda
    Mahavidhayala
India

Muir Gray
Nuffield Department of Surgical
    Sciences
Green Templeton College
University of Oxford
Oxford, United Kingdom

Tengku Aizan Hamid
Malaysian Research Institute on Ageing
University Putra Malaysia
Serdang, Malaysia

Liu Xiao Hang
Internal Medicine
Tung Shin Hospital
Kuala Lumpur, Malaysia

Keith Hill
Ageing and Independent Living
    Research Centre, School of Primary
    Care and Allied Health
Monash University
Melbourne, Australia

Khairana Husain
Faculty of Pharmacy
National University of Malaysia (UKM)
Bangi, Malaysia

Kim Hyung-Ho
Health Insurance Review and
    Assessment Service (HIRA)
Korea

Masahiko Ichiki
Department of Psychiatry
Tokyo Medical University
Shinjuku-ku, Japan

Jamia Azdina Jamal
Faculty of Pharmacy
National University of Malaysia (UKM)
Bangi, Malaysia

Paul Kadetz
Institute for Global Health and
  Development, Queen Margaret
  University
United Kingdom

and

Shiley-Marcos School of Engineering
University of San Diego
United States

Kishan Kariippanon
School of Health & Society
University of Wollongong
Wollongong, Australia

Gopesh Mangal
PG Department of Panchkarma
National Institute of Ayurveda
Jaipur, India

Tomonori Maruyama
The Japan Mibyou Institute United
Setagaya-ku, Japan

Noraliza binti Noordin Merican
Family Health Development Division
Ministry of Health
Putrajaya, Malaysia

Tetsuya Ohira
Dept of Epidemiology, School of
  Medicine
Fukushima Medical University
Fukushima, Japan

Zhang Qin
National Key Research Institute of
  Daoism and Religious Studies,
Sichuan University
Chengdu, Sichuan Province
P.R. China

Ranka Radulovic
Clinic for Psychiatry, Clinical Centre of
  Serbia
Serbia & Centre for Education and
  Counselling in Music Therapy
Serbia

and

Hatorum – Centre for Education and
  Counselling in Music Therapy
Belgrade, Serbia

Goh Cheng Soon
Traditional & Complementary Medicine
  Division
Ministry of Health
Kuala Lumpur, Malaysia

Lee Fatt Soon
Geriatric Physician
Ministry of Health Malaysia
Kuala Lumpur, Malaysia

Wan Alia Wan Sulaiman
Faculty of Medicine and Health
  Sciences
University Putra Malaysia
Serdang, Malaysia

Stephen Cho Wing Sze
Department of Biology, Faculty of
  Science
The Golden Meditech Centre for
  NeuroRegeneration Sciences
Hong Kong Baptist University
Hong Kong, China

Contributors

Sen Tyng Chai
Malaysian Research Institute on Ageing
University Putra Malaysia
Serdang, Malaysia

Khwanchai Wisithanon
Department of Thai Traditional and
Alternative Medicine
Ministry of Public Health
Nonthaburi, Thailand

Jean Woo
Department of Medicine &
Therapeutics
Chinese University of Hong Kong
Hong Kong, China

Yang Yu
First Affiliated Hospital of Guangxi
University of Chinese Medicine
China

Xie Yuhong
Chinese Doctor Clinic, Llandudno
United Kingdom

**Sheleaswani binti Inche Zainal
Abidin**
Family Health Development Division
Ministry of Health
Malaysia

1 Healthy Ageing in Asia during the COVID Pandemic

Goh Cheng Soon
T&CM Division, Ministry of Health (MOH) Malaysia

Gerard Bodeker
Chair, Mental Wellness Initiative, Global
Wellness Institute, & Green Templeton College,
University of Oxford, United Kingdom

CONTENTS

COVID Pandemic in the Elderly...2
The Chapters of the Book 4
Conclusion 8
References..8

Don't let your age control your life. Let your life control your age.

Anthony Douglas Williams

The ageing of the world's population is rapidly increasing primarily due to increasing life expectancy and declining fertility rate. The 2016 Population Data Sheet by United Nations Economic and Social Commission for Asia and the Pacific (ESCAP) disclosed that approximately 16% (1.3 billion) of the population in the Asia-Pacific region will be of 60 years or older by 2050 (United Nations, 2016). On the other hand, the fertility rate in many countries in Asia had fallen by 50% within 40 years. All countries, especially countries in Asia, are facing major challenges in social, economic and political arenas, associated with the rapid demographic transition in particular. Prior to the COVID-19 pandemic, this had been due to a decrease in infectious and acute diseases, accompanied by a surge in non-communicable and degenerative diseases. Healthcare costs are expected to rise with the demand for care for the ageing population and have nearly doubled in most countries.

Currently, most national healthcare systems focus on disease-based management, particularly in the acute stage. Following the rapid changes in disease epidemiology and demographic transition, a paradigm shift towards health promotion and disease prevention could favour more universal health and well-being across the lifespan.

DOI: 10.1201/9781003043270-1

1

Looking ahead to the post-COVID era, this will strengthen preparation for the future of rapid ageing and associated diseases in Asia and globally.

While the shift of a country's population towards an increasingly older age could not be avoided without a major growth in the national birth rate, with the right policies and services put in place, population ageing can be viewed as providing new opportunities for the older population, policymakers, healthcare providers, and for societies as a whole. Successful ageing is more than just the absence of diseases. It is actually a lifespan approach to well-being, embracing the maintenance of functional ability and well-being of pre-elderly and elderly people, despite various morbidities or health problems encountered.

In responding to rapid ageing and its challenges, this book is written to share the relevant health policies and integrated approach for the ageing populations as well as the experiences of community empowerment in several countries across Asia. Healthy ageing in Asia is largely promoted in a number of ways: through traditional forms of exercises (yoga, tai chi and martial arts), psychological enrichment via meditation and qigong, healthy diet complemented with supplements along with social laughter. Walking, jogging, dance, regular social contact, having a purpose in life and being in Nature are also very widespread means of enhancing healthy ageing.

There is a need for community education that ageing does not necessarily imply a gradual decrease in physical and mental capacity and ultimately dependence and death. Elders can have great health if they can live in a supportive environment, remain active and socially engaged, and have the freedom to do the things they most value.

When preparing this book, the authors have considered the social, cultural, political and economic contexts relevant to rapid ageing and have focussed particularly on the contribution of integrated medicine to healthcare systems in the Asian region. Potential readers of this book can be policymakers, healthcare providers, academicians, researchers, entrepreneurs and the public as a whole. The book is designed to provide insight, models of relevance, inspiration and guidance pertaining to ageing and the optimal handling of its challenges.

Although begun before the onset of COVID, this book has been compiled and developed during the COVID-19 pandemic period. Accordingly, it is important that we address the implications for and impact of COVID on elderly populations in this introductory chapter, with a particular focus on the role and potential of traditional healthcare practices in the management of COVID-19. Following this, the key content for each chapter in the book will be summarized in brief.

COVID PANDEMIC IN THE ELDERLY

COVID-19 is an infectious viral disease caused by a newly discovered coronavirus called SARS-CoV-2 that can lead to a pandemic of respiratory illness (Crunfli et al., 2021). Older people are more likely to develop serious illness. At the time of writing, viz. the second half of 2021, it has been well established that older people, especially those with advanced frailty, are highly vulnerable to coronavirus disease (COVID-19) infection and its adverse effects. The World Health Organization's COVID-19 Strategy Update in April 2020 reported that fatality increases with increasing age, rising to approximately 15% or higher in patients over 80 years of age (World Health Organization, 2020a).

In view of the high morbidity and mortality risk of vulnerable and neglected elderly people, extra effort is needed for their care to ensure that they stay safe and healthy during this pandemic period. This could be implemented through four key priority actions indicated in the Impact of COVID-19 on Older Persons, namely (i) to preserve their rights and dignity at all times, (ii) to strengthen social inclusion and solidarity during physical distancing, (iii) to provide financial support to those in socio-economic and humanitarian crisis and (iv) to encourage their participation and sharing of good practices and knowledge or data (United Nations, 2020). Moreover, identification and recognition of their contribution to the crisis response could be an additional encouragement for their active participation and to further foster healthy ageing.

In Asia, the literature on ancient wisdom and accumulated clinical experiences of traditional healthcare approaches has been drawn on and evaluated to combat the COVID pandemic – this along with conventional medicine. For many years, an approach that has integrated traditional Chinese medicine (TCM) and conventional medicine has been employed in combatting epidemic infection and preventing infected patients from escalating to severe cases. This was very much the case in the battle against the "severe acute respiratory syndrome" (SARS) in 2003.

So, when the coronavirus outbreak was reported in China's Wuhan, the capital of China's Hubei Province in early January 2020, traditional Chinese herbal medicine with the evidence of antiviral activity was used immediately to treat COVID-19 infection. This TCM treatment was reported to have more than 90% efficacy (Lee et al., 2021). Moreover, a meta-analysis subsequently reported that the integration of TCM and Western medicine had better efficacy than Western medicine alone in shortening the length of hospital stay, defervescence time, cough resolution rate, fatigue resolution rate and tachypnoea resolution rate (Pang et al., 2020). As for safety, there was no significant difference between two groups.

In order to address this global public health crisis, the National Health Commission of the People's Republic of China has developed treatment guidelines with appropriate prescriptions for patients individually based on Chinese medicine principles of syndrome differentiation.

"Three TCM prescriptions and three medicines" were recommended by the Chinese authorities during the pandemic for preventing and treating COVID patients (Luo et al., 2020). Three TCM prescriptions including Huashi Baidu Formula (化濕敗毒方), Xuanfei Baidu Formula (宣肺敗毒方) and Qingfei Paidu Decoction (清肺排毒湯) are used to remove dampness, expel phlegm and arrest coughing. On the other hand, three medicines, namely Jinhua Qinggan Granule (金花清感顆粒) and Lianhua Qingwen Capsule (連花清瘟膠囊) for reducing fever, and Xuebijing Injection (血必淨注射液), are used for preventing blood stasis in patients in moderate and critical stages. Early intervention of TCM in COVID management is reported to improve the cure rate, shorten the course of the disease, delay disease progression and reduce the mortality rate.

Clinically, Qingfei Paidu Decoction has been used together with Western medicine to treat COVID-19, such as lopinavir and ritonavir tablets, methylprednisolone sodium succinate injection, moxifloxacin hydrochloride, and sodium chloride injection, interferon α-2b injection especially for severe cases of COVID-19 (Zhang, 2020). Qingfei Paidu Decoction composes of 21 herbs and possesses anti-inflammatory and antiviral effects (Li et al., 2020). When isolated, several molecules from a wide variety of herbs in Qingfei Paidu Decoction have demonstrated potent antiviral and immune-modulating properties. However, the possibilities of these properties remaining after integrating with Western medicine have yet to be determined. This is due to the fact that examining the effect of specific components of TCM herbal formula and eluci-dating the biologic mechanisms underlying the therapeutic effects of formula in the treatment of COVID-19 is a great challenge in the clinical study of TCM. Moreover, when conducting a randomized clinical trial in TCM, some of the challenges faced are ensuring that TCM-treated patients, healthcare providers, outcome assessors and a feasible analyst are kept unaware of the treatment condition of each group in order to ensure no other variables are introduced into the trial (Shi et al., 2021). The treatment of TCM is personalized, and its efficacy may vary with severity of symptoms. In response to these idiosyncratic characteristics of TCM treatment, Dr. Andre Kalil proposed the utilization of an adaptive clinical trial design, which is "able to rapidly accept or reject multiple experimental therapies throughout the trial, while being adequately powered for meaningful clinical outcomes", during a pandemic (Kalil, 2020). This may allow a TCM herbal formula to be included as a potential therapy to be tested.

At the same time, India's classical system of health care, Ayurveda, has been applied to the management of COVID cases across India since early 2020. A special online COVID research issue of the *Journal of Ayurveda and Integrative Medicine (J-AIM),* published by Elsevier Press, has presented the "COVID-19 Collection", a series of peer-reviewed studies on multiple approaches of Ayurveda in treating patients with COVID-19 (*Journal of Ayurveda and Integrative Medicine | COVID-19 Collection | ScienceDirect.com by Elsevier).*

The published studies range from hypothesis-generating case reports, to clinical trials, and policy and public health analyses that are being updated and added to on a continuous basis. A biochemical paper (*https://doi.org/10.1016/j.jaim.2021.05.003*) reported on the evaluation of the efficacy of 15 bioactive compounds from Indian medicinal plants with known antiviral properties as potential inhibitors of SARS-CoV-2 M^{pro}. Ursolic acid (DrugBank ID DB15588), compound of the Ayurvedic plant tulsi, which has known antiviral activity, had the highest docking score −8.7 (kcal/mol) and has been flagged as a promising candidate for an herbal medicine to be tested for use in integrative COVID-19 case management.

Across Asia, traditional practices have been shown to be useful to help elderly people during the period of lockdowns to cope with stress, fear, anxiety and depres-sion – for example music therapy (Zhao et al., 2016), yoga and meditation practices (Mohanty, Sharma and Sharma, 2020). Traditional medicine (TM) practices could offer a holistic preventive and rehabilitative measure for the elderly.

THE CHAPTERS OF THE BOOK

The book touches on policy related to ageing, traditional Asian approaches to ageing, an integrated medical systems approach to ageing, ageing in place, and community empowerment.

Policies provide guidance for decision-making, streamlining internal processes, and ensuring compliance with laws and regulations. In Chapter 2, Dr. Noor Hisham, Director-General of the Malaysian Ministry of Health, indicates that ageing is strongly influenced by the environment and behaviours of an individual. He also mentions that an integrated healthcare policy based on older people's needs and preferences will further strengthen people-centred health services and allow older people to live freely and independently with greater dignity. Malaysia is experiencing rapid demographical and epidemiological transitions and will become an aged nation prior to its readiness. Dr. Lee, a senior geriatrician, further emphasizes in the following chapter that the lack of resources and provision of individualizing care in a busy overcrowded acute care environment is one of the greatest challenges of the healthcare system for the ageing population in Malaysia.

The other challenges are that the older person was not seen as a whole and receives "recipe-like" prescriptions, which will result in polypharmacy and fragmentation of care. This in turn affects their activities of daily living and consequently their quality of life. In responding to a growing emphasis on old age and ageing issues in national development plans in Malaysia, Dato' Dr. Tengku Aizan Hamid in her chapter had proposed policy review considerations and linkages to broader initiatives in the region as well as to the UN Sustainable Development Goals (SDG).

Then, we look at Japan, a country with a rapidly ageing population and more than 80,000 citizens aged 100 years or above. Mr. Maruyama Tomonori in his chapter has stated the challenges for creating a healthy ageing society. In order to ensure the accessibility and sustainability of the healthcare system, Japan's government has promoted the "100-Year Life Society", a societal model in which all citizens are dynamically engaged and productive. This could be done by having a scheme on educating and updating the knowledge and skill of elderly, and promoting elderly employment by subsiding those who employ people over 65 years old. Moreover, holding the principle of "ikigai" (a purpose in life) priority is given to practising a healthy lifestyle and engaging in social contributions to live with happiness and to extend a healthy lifespan.

The integrated approach for this public health aspect should include medical health insurance in order to move towards a universal national health care for all. Here, we learn of the Korean medical health insurance for Korea's older population. Based on policy analysis and research data on TM, medical health insurance is applied to both Western and traditional Korean medicine systems. Challenges of health insurance to traditional Korean medicine pertaining to ageing have been identified by Kim Hyung-Ho, and measures have been proposed for the sustainability of national health insurance in Chapter 6.

An ideal policy for the elderly should be benefiting all the older people in every part of a country with no one left behind. Hence, policy to protect the health and well-being of the rural "left-behind" elderly in China is essential to look into and ameliorate the impacts of years of policies that have exacerbated the vulnerability of the rural "left-behind" elderly. Chapter 7 by Professor Paul Kadetz indicates that the overwhelming number of "left-behind" elderly in rural China is an outcome of a government-instituted confluence of social and demographic changes.

The practice of TM and its recognition can vary from country to country and from region to region. Generally, TM practice in a particular country has a close linkage with their historical and cultural heritage, including the influence of religion. Yet, TM practices in certain countries may not be derived from the country's own traditions. After exploring the historical and cultural linkage of TM in the Asian countries, Chapter 8 (by Dr. Goh Cheng Soon) also provides several examples of the usage of TM in older population, namely traditional Malay medicine, TCM, traditional Indian medicine and traditional Thai medicine (TTM). Following this, several chapters have demonstrated the complementary or synergistic effects in terms of treatment options in integrating TM with conventional medicine.

Until today, traditional herbs and vegetables (ulam) have been used by the Malay community in Malaysia for healthy ageing. They include jering, papaya, pegaga (Asiatic pennywort), ulam raja, turmeric, sambung nyawa (longevity spinach), cekur (sand ginger), tenggek burung, peria katak (bitter melon), curry leaves and petai (stink bean) (it would be good if we could provide a botanical species name for each of these plants). These are either eaten raw like salads or blanched. Professor Dr Jamia also shares scientific information on the benefits of ulam consumption which promotes healthy dietary habit for improving and maintaining health and wellness across the lifespan.

In accordance with Daoism's cultivation of TCM, Professor Zhang has mentioned in Chapter 10 that health promotion needs begin from an early stage and are followed across the lifespan by health maintenance in old age. Several Chinese Daoist practices that help one to live healthily into old age include having adequate and good-quality sleep, the timely consumption of local and seasonal food, and good conjugal love. Subsequently, regular physical exercise, consistent meditation, continuity of learning and the making of informed choices are good practices for health promotion and maintenance in old people. Regarding physical exercise, Hua Tuo Wu Qin Xi (five-animal play) provides an example of physical and breathing exercise for health preservation in China. Professor Yong in Chapter 11 elaborates on how the five-animal play system would help prevent and cure diseases, along with its relationship to yin yang, five elements and zang xiang theories. It is a step-by-step exercise and a personalized exercise plan that could be developed for different diseases.

Chapter 12 is about one of the ancient Indian medical systems for healthy ageing. Ayurveda is the science of life with a concept of Vayasthapana which deals with conserving the youthfulness of the body from the conception and continues for a lifetime. For longevity and a healthy life, Ayurveda emphasizes waking up pre-dawn, drinking water, regular exercise, bathing with warm water, adequate sleep, and proper diet and to not withhold natural urges. Moreover, Panchakarma is employed to eliminate toxic elements from the body prior to the administration of Rasayana, which is a rejuvenation therapy designed to delay the ageing process and is upheld as a treasure of Ayurveda in sustaining healthy ageing. In particular, yoga is a great measure to create rejuvenation due to its capability of uniting an individual's body, mind and soul for healthy living. Dr. Gunjan elaborates further on the Ashtanga yoga (the eightfold practice of yoga) in her chapter (Chapter 13).

Thailand is expected to become aged society in 2021, and an integrated approach, including the usage of TTM in the public health service system, has been promoted

Healthy Ageing in Asia during the COVID Pandemic

for health maintenance, disease treatment and rehabilitation of elderly patients. In her chapter (Chapter 14), Dr. Anchalee Chuthaputti has noted that Thai people are advised to practise "Dhammanamai" in TTM manner for healthy body, mind and lifestyle and behaviours. By correcting and balancing the four dhatu (earth, wind, water and fire), TTM is deployed as treatment for common and minor diseases, for example "Nuad Thai" (traditional Thai massage) and "Luk Pra Kob" (hot herbal compress) for the relief of pain in certain conditions.

In Chapter 15, Dr. Xie demonstrates that one key evidence-based approach to ageing well is exercise. Evidence is reviewed from the research relating to exercise benefits for older people, with a particular emphasis on exercise approaches that can reduce the risk of falling. These include tai chi programmes, the Otago programme for balance dysfunction, as well as some less widely recognized programmes that can achieve benefits such as reducing the risk of falling. Tai chi is an excellent form of exercise to enhance balance and confidence, ameliorate cardiovascular risk factors, and has been shown to improve strength, balance, and function of the elderly. Dr. Xie has proposed a set of twelve movements of tai chi and qigong in his chapter for reducing the risk of falling in amongst the elderly people. He elaborates that tai chi and qigong are for strengthening the bone, muscle and sinew in accordance with Chinese medicine's fundamental principles. Applying the similar Chinese medicine principle of syndrome differentiation to regulate the body's constitution, Dr. Liu has shared examples of using integrated Chinese and Western medication for treating non-communicable diseases. The advantages of integrating two medical systems have been indicated, specifically to cut down on polypharmacy and dosage of Western medicine, along with enhancing immunity and improving the quality of life.

In addition to the research evidence relating to exercise benefits for older people, Dr. Ohira (in Chapter 19) has presented several published studies on laughter which has been found to help in preventing and managing functional disabilities and various diseases, including stress- and lifestyle-related diseases. The frequency of laughter has been found to decrease with age and is considered as an indicator of ageing. Laughter can contribute to health promotion, and hence, it is an excellent therapy for happiness and healthy life expectancy.

Moreover, music therapy has been proven as a diagnostic and supportive tool for complicated grief reactions in elderly people, especially those with dementia and other health problems in Chapter 20. The study reported by Dr. Radulovic shows that prevalence of complicated grief is highest among women who are older than 60 years of age. Listening to music or singing in choirs contributes to reducing complicated grief reactions and enabling elderly people to cope with death of their loved ones in a less sorrowful manner. Music therapy also facilitates communication and maximizes learning while making a connection to the premorbid person and their previous coping styles.

Subsequently, in the chapter on empowerment, Dr Goh Cheng Beh, a geriatrician from Ministry of Health Malaysia explains that older people could participate and make informed choices about their health-related activities after realizing their role with sufficient and accurate information through engaging with their healthcare provider. Moreover, the presence of a facilitating environment could further empower the individual to perform a task. Professor Jean Woo of the Chinese University of

Hong Kong has indicated that identifying the unmet needs and common geriatric syndromes through assessments is vital to help in designing a personalized, safe and enabling home with an age-friendly environment, especially for those with declining physical and cognitive function, to achieve healthy ageing.

Presently, there have been endeavours to create innovative businesses and technologies in the process of solving health issues in regard to ageing population to support the healthy ageing life. Dr Kishan Kariippanon's chapter has shared innovative healthcare activities in the Asian region. These include innovation and commercialization approaches for healthy ageing which are technologically savvy and culturally sensitive, while promoting local practices. Particularly, the "Desert Rose House" presented at the Solar Decathlon in the Middle East (University of Wollongong, Australia and Dubai) is an innovative residential construction that enables an ageing-friendly atmosphere and was built on the dementia-friendly environmental design framework. The collaboration in this innovative business between Dubai's government and the University of Wollongong in Australia aims to improve the quality of life of older people and their carers. This greater innovation has supported the promotion of a healthy ageing lifestyle in the Middle East.

In his concluding chapter, Professor Gerard Bodeker addresses the mental health and well-being dimensions of ageing in Asia, with particular consideration of the impact of COVID on elderly people and their families and communities. Traditional wellness practices, including meditation, integrative movements such as yoga, tai chi and qigong, healthy ageing TM approaches, and a loving and supportive living environment based on deep Asian values of compassion and kindness, are addressed.

CONCLUSION

The expression "It is the life in your years that count rather than the years in your life" is underpinned by evidence that emphasizes the importance of a comprehensive lifespan approach to wellness and healthy ageing.

This includes maintaining good health from young, optimal nutrition, regular movement and physical activity, ways of reducing and managing stress and of promoting rest and peace of mind, and active participation in social activities well into old age to enjoy an independent and a high quality of life.

The current pandemic presents an opportunity not only for culturally based Asian healthcare traditions to play a role in addressing the behavioural, emotional and spiritual dimensions of poor health, but also for integrated medicine to provide preventive and therapeutic options for strengthening the physical, mental and emotional dimensions of the older population. Most importantly, the perspectives and lived experiences of elders need to guide policy and new directions in the evolution of healthy ageing and elder care in the direction of living the hundred-year life.

REFERENCES

Crunfli, F. et al. (2021) 'SARS-CoV-2 infects brain astrocytes of COVID-19 patients and impairs neuronal viability', *medRxiv*, p. 2020. doi: 10.1101/2020.10.09.20207464.

Kalil, A. (2020) 'Treating COVID-19 Off-label drug use, compassionate use, and randomized clinical trials during pandemics', *Journal of the* American Medical Association, 323(19), pp. 1897–1898.

Lee, D. Y. W. et al. (2021) 'Traditional Chinese herbal medicine at the forefront battle against COVID-19: Clinical experience and scientific basis', *Phytomedicine*, 80(September 2020), p. 153337. doi: 10.1016/j.phymed.2020.153337.

Li, C. et al. (2020) 'Discussion on TCM theory and modern pharmacological mechanism of Qinfei Paidu decoction in the treatment of COVID-19', *Journal of Traditional Chinese Medicine*, pp. 1–4.

Luo, H. et al. (2020) 'Reflections on treatment of COVID-19 with traditional Chinese medicine', *Chinese Medicine (United Kingdom)*, 15(1), pp. 1–14. doi: 10.1186/s13020-020-00375-1.

Mohanty, S., Sharma, P. and Sharma, G. (2020) 'Yoga for infirmity in geriatric population amidst COVID-19 pandemic': Comment on "Age and Ageism in COVID-19: Elderly mental health-care vulnerabilities and needs", *Asian Journal of Psychiatry*, 53, p. 102199.

Pang, W. et al. (2020) 'Chinese herbal medicine for coronavirus disease 2019: A systematic review and meta-analysis', *Integrative Medicine Research*, 9(160), p. 100477. doi: 10.1016/j.phrs.2020.105056.

Shi, N. et al. (2021) 'Efficacy and safety of Chinese herbal medicine versus Lopinavir-Ritonavir in adult patients with coronavirus disease 2019: A non-randomized controlled trial', *Phytomedicine*, 81(January). doi: 10.1016/j.phymed.2020.153367.

United Nations (2016) *ESCAP Population Data sheet Population and Development Indicators for Asia and the Pacific, 2012.* Available at: https://www.unescap.org/sites/default/d8files/knowledge-products/SPPS PS data sheet 2016 v15-2.pdf.

United Nations (2020) *Policy Brief: The Impact of COVID-19 on Older Person, Online2.* Available at: https://www.un.org/development/desa/ageing/wp-content/uploads/sites/24/2020/05/COVID-Older-persons.pdf (Accessed: 5 June 2021).

World Health Organization (2020) *COVID-19 Strategy Update*, Online.

Zhang, Y. (2020) 'A case of severe COVID19 cured by Qinfei Paide decoction combined with Western Medicine', *Tianjin Journal of Traditional Chinese Medicine*, pp. 1–4.

Zhao, K. et al. (2016) 'A systematic review and meta-analysis of music therapy for the older adults with depression', *International Journal of Geriatric Psychiatry*, 31(11), pp. 1188–1198. doi: 10.1002/gps.4494.

2 An Integrated Approach to Creating Healthy Ageing in the Nation
A Malaysian Perspective

Noor Hisham Abdullah
Ministry of Health Malaysia

Goh Cheng Soon
Ministry of Health Malaysia

Noraliza binti Noordin Merican and
Sheleaswani binti Inche Zainal Abidin
Ministry of Health Malaysia

CONTENTS

Introduction 11
Health Challenges of Ageing 12
Healthy Ageing 14
Integration Approach 15
Conclusion 17
References 18

INTRODUCTION

Ageing population is a global phenomenon. As reported in the World Population Prospects 2019, the number of persons aged 65 and above globally is projected to be more than double between 2019 and 2050 (Department of Economic & Social Affairs, 2019). Particularly in Japan with the high rate of economic growth, it has led the list of aged nation and has experienced a rapid ageing process. 28% of Japan's population is over 65 years old, thus facing a 'super-ageing' society (Muramatsu and Akiyama, 2011). It is expected to increase to 38% by 2050 (Walia, 2019). Hong Kong and Macao Special Administrative Regions of China come next to Japan. According to the World Population Prospects 2019, Malaysia was ranked 45th place with the greatest number of older people in the world (United Nations Population Division, 2019), and we are expected to reach ageing nation status by the year 2030.

DOI: 10.1201/9781003043270-2

Despite the international census classifying elders as those aged 65 and above, Malaysia classifies elders as any person aged 60 years and above for its policy development in relation to older persons (Malaysian Government, 2020). This is to ensure that the planning and development of policies and programmes for older persons are in line among the ministries and agencies in the country. Currently, an estimated 10.7% or 3.5 million from the 32.7 million Malaysians are aged 60 years and above in 2020 (Department of Statistics, 2020b). Life expectancy in Malaysia has increased considerably from an average of 55.8 years in 1957 to 74.9 years in 2020 (72.6 years for males and 77.6 years for females) (Department of Statistics, 2020a). Conversely, over the last three decades, the total fertility rate in Malaysia has declined dramatically from 4.9 children per woman of childbearing age in 1970 to 1.8 children per woman of childbearing age in 2019. With increasing life expectancy and declining fertility rate, Malaysia is moving towards an aged nation.

The population doubling rate is a crucial factor to consider when formulating a national policy. Malaysia is expected to double its elderly population within 23 years. The expected rate of elderly population doubling in Malaysia is comparatively similar to countries such as Brazil, China, India and Japan, which required 25 years (Department of Economic & Social Affairs, 2016). In contrast, France recorded the slowest rate of elderly population doubling (138 years). Interestingly, other Caucasian developed countries also recorded a slow rate of elderly population doublings, such as Sweden (85 years), Australia (73 years) and United States of America (69 years). This finding may be attributable to the earlier decline in fertility rate secondary to the high cost of living and other social factors. The objective of this chapter is to explore the fundamental principle of 'healthy ageing' and formulate an integrated approach to optimize functional ability of older people in Malaysia so as to address the corresponding increase in the dependency ratio. There is a projected increase in the total dependency ratio from 47.8 in 2010 to 49.5 in 2040 in part due to a rise in the old-age dependency ratio from 7.4 in 2010 to 21.7 in 2040, which is almost threefold increase (Department of Statistics, 2016).

HEALTH CHALLENGES OF AGEING

The accelerated speed of rapid ageing will have a profound effect on the social, cultural, economic as well as the health delivery system of the country in which we need to anticipate and prepare for. The World Health Organization (WHO) has identified that ageing presents both challenges and opportunities. These include an increase in demand for primary and long-term health care and a larger and better-trained workforce and intensify the need for a more age-friendly environment to be made (World Health Organization, 2018).

The change in the socio-demographic in Malaysia caused by the rapidly ageing population is expected to increase the incidence of chronic and non-communicable diseases (NCD). The 2018 National Health and Morbidity Survey (NHMS), indicated that 27.7% of the self-reported NCDs, such as diabetes mellitus is among the elderly. Moreover, the percentage of hypertension and hypercholesterolemia in the elderly population is 51.1% and 41.8% respectively (Ministry of Health Malaysia, 2018). This could be directly or indirectly due to the fact that nearly one in five elderly people have limitations in carrying out activities of daily living (ADL). Lack of physical activities is a leading risk factor for NCD and death worldwide.

The NHMS 20–18 survey also revealed that 6% of elderly are living alone, 8.5% have probable dementia, 5.3% with depression, 5% vision disability, 6% hearing disability, 2.9% stress urinary incontinence, 3.4% urge urinary incontinence and 14.1% have experienced a fall. Multiple symptoms along with acute and chronic diseases are a common phenomenon in the older adults. Moreover, approximately one-third of the elderly have poor quality of life, poor social support and malnutrition due to changes in dietary habits, poor dentition and food insecurity. The worst scenario is one-tenth of them have experienced some form of abuse.

With regard to poor oral health, a survey in 2018 indicated that 20% of the elderly people need dental treatment. As being reported in the *Annual Report of the Oral Health Programme*, approximately 41.6% of Malaysians aged 60 and above have 20 or more teeth in 2018 (Ministry of Health Malaysia, 2019). Majority of them have an average of 16.2 teeth. Due to the fact that there are less than 60% of 60-year-olds who have at least 20 or more teeth by 2020, the oral health status of Malaysian elderly is still far below the targeted goal of the National Oral Health Plan 2011-2020 (Ministry of Health Malaysia, 2011).

Understandably, an increase in an aged population could link to many global public health problems. Without addressing the health and well-being of ageing population, the attainment of Sustainable Development Goals and Universal Health Coverage in a country is almost impossible.

The United Nations World Assembly on Ageing was held in Vienna in 1982 in response to the growing portion of the world's ageing population. Following this, the Vienna International Plan of Action on Ageing was developed providing a basis for the formulation of policies and programmes on ageing (United Nations, 1982). It included health and nutrition, protection of elderly consumers, housing and environment, family, social welfare, income security and employment, and education.

Malaysia is guided by the National Policy for Older Persons in 1995 (amended 2011) under the Ministry of Women, Family and Community Development, and implemented via the Plan of Action for Older Persons 1998. For more than a decade, our ageing population has been a cornerstone of the Ministry of Health's policy agenda. However, I must emphasize that this will be an even more important issue to be addressed now, and also in future. Recognizing this reality, in 1997, the Ministry of Health (MOH) Malaysia developed the National Plan of Action for Health Care of Older Person (revised in 2008), followed by establishment of the National Health Policy for Older Persons in 2008.

The policy aims 'to ensure healthy, active and productive ageing by empowering the older persons, family and community with knowledge, skills, an enabling environment, and the provision of optimal healthcare services at all levels and by all sectors.' (Ministry of Health Malaysia, 2008). The policy was implemented under the guiding principles of maintaining autonomy and self-reliance, recognizing the distinctive needs, supporting caregivers of older person, and promoting healthy ageing as well as providing continuity of care. The goal is to achieve optimal health for older persons through integrated and comprehensive health and health-related services using multifaceted approach.

HEALTHY AGEING

A longer and high-quality lifespan provides opportunities, not only for older people and their families, but also for societies as a whole (World Health Organization, 2018). Therefore, promoting healthy ageing is one of the principles of healthcare service provision outlined in our *National Health Policy of Older Person*. All services for older person should optimize their opportunities for healthy ageing through the life course perspective on ageing.

Living longer is indeed an achievement, which may be attributed to high-quality health care and an improved standard of living in our country. However, the important question is: Does living longer equate to living healthily and productively? There may be 80-year-olds having physical and mental capacities similar to many 20-year-olds, whereas other people experience significant declines in physical and mental capacities at much younger ages.

As cited by the WHO, healthy ageing has been the focus of WHO's work on ageing between 2015 and 2030 since it is one of the public health priorities. Healthy ageing replaces the concept of 'Active Ageing' in the *WHO Policy Framework on Active Ageing 2002* which focuses on promoting healthy and active ageing to enhance quality of life as individual ages (World Health Organization, 2002). Healthy ageing, like active ageing, emphasizes the need for action across multiple sectors and enables older people to remain evaluable to their families, communities and economies.

WHO defines healthy ageing as 'the process of developing and maintaining the **functional ability** that enables **wellbeing** in older age' (World Health Organization, 2015, p. 28). The goal is to have elderly with high functional ability and stable capacity. This will further lengthen healthy life expectancy (HALE). Functional ability is about having the capabilities that enable all people to be and do what they have reason to value. This includes a person's ability to meet their basic needs; to learn, grow and make decisions; to be mobile; to build and maintain relationships; and to contribute to society. Functional ability contributes to the intrinsic capacity of the individual. It comprises all the mental and physical capacities that a person can draw on and includes their ability to walk, think, see, hear and remember; relevant environmental characteristics and the interaction between them. In addition to the ability to move around, older people would prefer to have the ability to build and maintain relationships; meet their own basic needs; learn, grow and make decisions; and contribute to the society.

As reported by WHO in 2020, the HALE of a Malaysian at birth is 69.1 years for women and 69 years for men (World Health Organization, 2020). When comparing this with life expectancy, it equates to women only living healthily until 69.1 years of age and men until 69. As being mentioned earlier in this chapter, life expectancy in Malaysia in 2020 is 77.6 years for women and 72.6 years for men. An inference to the above data may suggest that the elderly population in Malaysia will have some form of illness with declining health status for the significant remaining years of life. The healthy life expectancy may worsen as the current situation of NCD prevalence in Malaysia continues to increase.

INTEGRATION APPROACH

Many shreds of evidence suggest that the best way to design health systems to meet the needs of older people is by placing them at the centre of service delivery. Hence, integration between primary health care and all other levels and settings of care are crucial. With these considerations in mind, the Ministry of Health strives to promote healthy ageing via integrated approaches and holistic health. Hopefully, these approaches will empower the nation and community to take a more proactive role in healthy ageing. With the commitment in harmonizing the coexistence of traditional and complementary medicine (T&CM) with modern medicine, the Ministry has to look into its most significant challenge to ensure quality and safe T&CM services to the public, plus incorporating evidence-based medicine into T&CM practices.

As being stated in the National Health Policy for Older Persons, the strategy on addressing public health challenges on ageing should begin from prevention through building personal skills and knowledge to maintain the intrinsic capacity and healthy behaviours while moving away from disease risk factors. In other words, the inclusion of a continuity of healthy lifestyle promotion and practices from young adult to aged people could facilitate healthy ageing with an example like altering their eating habits. By encouraging the consumption of fresh and appropriate amount of 'ulam' (salad) comprising of herbs, vegetables, ferns and some part of big tree (fruits or leaves), they could establish health beneficial properties due to its antioxidant activity (Mohd Nor et al., 2020). Moreover, T&CM could complement the inadequacy of the current conventional healthcare system by improving physical health and subsequently preventing falls. Particularly, a combination of the tai chi and Otago exercise programmes could improve the older people's gait, velocity and mobility thereby reducing the risk of falling (Son et al., 2016). Otago exercise improves the lower limb strength, and tai chi helps in balance which indirectly reduces the burden on hospitalization and other chronic care due to falls or poor mobility.

Furthermore, health and nutrition programmes must be organized regularly. This is particularly so to install into their mindset that ageing is not a disease and early intervention can prevent them from frailty and disability. Aside from improving mental health amongst the elderly population, health education by using 'laughter' is a behavioural therapy for psychological stress or depression and can further lower the risk of NCD (Yim, 2016).

Health education programmes include one-to-one hands-on guidance on the use of new technology such as smartphone home systems which will enable them to enjoy their rights and freedom. The new technology-assistive devices provide them access to their distant family, virtual health services (home doctor services through apps, teleconsultation and Internet pharmacy) and online learning, especially so during the COVID-19 pandemic period of lockdown.

On the other hand, healthcare system for them has to be geared towards long-term care apart from short-term care and hospitalization. A sufficient quantity of effective healthcare facilities including oral health care, goods and services (both conventional medicine and T&CM) need to be established to meet the health needs of older people who have diseases. In order to provide seamless care for the ageing population, the Ministry of Health Malaysia has formulated a strategic plan on facilitating the accessibility for elderly in MOH hospitals by increasing number of hospitals providing geriatric services such as cognitive stimulation therapy, geriatric rehabilitation and skill mix of oral healthcare services together with the management of fall- or osteoporotic-related injuries. The development of the National Action Plan for Ageing Population 2021–2025 aims to strengthen post-hospitalization care for elderly through collaboration with primary care services including T&CM (Ministry of Health Malaysia, 2020).

Furthermore, for those who have declined in functional ability, apart from adapting to their current residence, they could be relocated to a more supportive environment which allows them to remain with their community and family. Relocation to a more supportive environment in the same age groups may be beneficial to their social wellbeing by having common communication topics. A supportive environment with major structural features will encourage healthy behaviours of older people to live safely and independently and ultimately reduce their risk of diseases. The brainchild of this built environment was known to be an 'ageing in place' to enable the older people to live in a place safely, independently and comfortably, regardless of age, income or level of intrinsic capacity (Centres for Disease Control and Prevention, 2009). Ageing in place can be further strengthened by having an age-friendly environment with appropriate medical care, recreational activities and other community facilities. Nevertheless, creating an environment that is truly age-friendly requires a close interagency and inter-sectoral collaboration, especially so among the Ministry of Health, Ministry of Transport, Ministry of Housing & Local Government, Ministry of Human Resources, Ministry of Women, Family & Community Development, and Ministry of Communications & Multimedia. As a matter of fact, these collaborations could bridge new ties among all relevant ministries. An integrated care by roping in non-governmental organizations (NGOs) and private medical professions could create an integrated continuum and comprehensive care for delivering health care and social care to older people (Dunér, Blomberg and Hasson, 2011).

The government plays an important role in the long-term plan for the healthy ageing of its nation. It must ensure a fair distribution of society's resources (access to healthy food or information) and healthcare service provision to all. The apparent insufficiency of a trained health workforce comprising geriatricians, gerontologists and caregivers to older people must be resolved by increasing the workforce capacity and training more personnel to meet the nation's growing demand. Integration of trained T&CM practitioners could effectively improve the health workforce and provide a myriad of treatment options.

Moreover, participation of family members to encourage older people to be more active and ensure a nutritious diet for them will slow down the loss of capacity and ability. In the later stages of debility, essential support such as washing, using toilet and bathing may be required. Participation and commitment from family members will be higher, especially for those older people who are incapable to exercise choice independently, and yet, 'supported decision-making' is required (United Nations, 2006).

Focusing beyond the improvement in human resources and facilities, the policy for the long-term care insurance for the elderly could be formulated to provide sustainable reform. For example, the Law on Long-Term Care Insurance for the Senior

An Integrated Approach to Creating Healthy Ageing in the Nation 17

Citizens in Korea was passed in the Assembly's plenary session in 2007 and implemented in 2008 to support senior citizens who cannot maintain a healthy living due to ageing or geriatric diseases (Won, 2013). This policy provides the benefits pertaining to ensuring equity and access for the elderly to the residential facility care and home care (home nursing and home bathing). It is different from the National Health Insurance in Korea which ensures the services provided by clinics, hospitals and pharmacies in disease diagnosis, outpatient or inpatient treatment, and rehabilitation (Kwon, Lee and Kim, 2015). This long-term care insurance for the elderly will also benefit those who are responsible for taking care and nursing their elderly by allowing the carer to participate in economic sectors and contribute to the country's productivity.

Last but not least, one of the proposed strategies of the National Health Policy for Older Persons is 'to advocate the development of new legislation and review the existing legislation' (Ministry of Health Malaysia, 2008). Our current legal framework, for example, the Penal Code, Care Centre Act 1993 and Pensions Act 1980, offers piecemeal protection and is insufficient in addressing the needs of the elderly these days. The proposed new legislation is to ensure the preservation of the dignity and autonomy of older persons, accessibility to the quality and standards of service provision in their golden years, prevention of age discrimination and protection of the welfare of older persons. It will be great if the new legislation could also benefit families who require help in caring for their aged loved ones.

Malaysia is a multi-ethnic and multicultural nation with a society of strong tradition. Concerning the older persons particularly those with limited access to adequate health care and social care, the healthcare services should be age-friendly and responsive to their needs of various health risks.

CONCLUSION

Population ageing is largely attributed to longer life expectancy and lower fertility rates but not without challenges in which the increasing prevalence of chronic health conditions manifests commonly as multi-morbidities in older people (Afshar et al., 2015). The urgency is on the health and social services which requires a sharing of responsibilities between the government, private sector, non-governmental agencies and the community.

Comprehensive public health action (social strategies, policies and legislation) on ageing is urgently needed. Population ageing requires a transformation of health system that moves away from disease-based curative models towards the provision of older person-centred and integrated care. It will require a coordinated effort from many other sectors and multiple levels of the government agencies. Healthy ageing depends on promotion of health and prevention of disease and injury. Hence, it is inherent to formulate a national public health response to support healthy ageing in all policies and at all levels of the government.

The 1978 Declaration of Alma Ata advocated strengthening primary health care, including the role of traditional medicine practitioners, to attain acceptable levels of health for all. Integration of T&CM may offer alternative pathways in achieving Universal Health Coverage through many levels such as health system, service delivery and consumer levels. Quality of healthcare services can be improved through regulation of T&CM products, practitioners and services used by the community.

Malaysia has established and implemented T&CM regulatory system (T&CM Act 2016 and T&CM Regulation 2021) into its national healthcare system. The goal is to improve or maintain the quality and safety of practitioners and practices. Qualified and competent T&CM practitioners are an essential requirement to support inter-professional collaboration, and to provide integrated, people-centred healthcare services that meet individual and population's health needs.

With ageing populations and increasing number of older persons with chronic disease, healthcare system's effectiveness and efficiency can be improved through the integration of T&CM practitioners which effectively increase the health workforce. Programmes/activities can be designed to promote well-being and disease prevention towards healthy ageing. This is to ensure that older people are not left behind.

To conclude, health is crucial and elderly needs are different and cannot be 'one size fits all'. Hence, an integrated approach to healthy ageing is required to help in addressing the legal, social and structural barriers to good health for ageing population. Moreover, emphasis on having a long-term and person-centred approach to look after the older people who face an increased risk of losing their functional ability is crucial. The healthcare reform to address healthy ageing is an emergent public health issue. After all, we would wake up one day and realize that we are also in the elderly category too!

REFERENCES

Afshar, S. et al. (2015) 'Multi-morbidity and the inequalities of global ageing: A cross-sectional study of 28 countries using the World Health Surveys', *BMC Public Health*, 15, 776. doi: 10.1186/s12889- 015–2008–7.

Byun, S.-J. and Hwang, N.-H. (2018) 'The major contents and future tasks of the basic plan for low birthrate and aging society', *Health and Welfare Forum*, 258, pp. 41–61.

Centres for Disease Control and Prevention (2009) *Healthy Aging & The Built Environment, Online*. Available at: https://www.cdc.gov/healthyplaces/healthtopics/healthyaging.htm (Accessed: 2 April 2021).

Chae, J.-M., Choi, Y.-J. and Choi, Y.-M. (2015) *A study on the rationalization of insurance benefits for Korean medicine services, HIRA Research Institution*.

Cho, J. K. (2010) 'Changes in health care environment and medical integration of Korean medicine and western medicine', *Health and Welfare Issues & Focus*, 27, pp. 1–8.

Cho, K.-S. (2001) Difference in the Behavior of Oriental Medicine, *Yonsei University*.

Department of Economic & Social Affairs (2016) *World Population Ageing 2015*.

Department of Economic & Social Affairs (2019) *World Population Prospects 2019, Geneva, Switzerland*.

Department of Statistics (2016) *Population Projection (Revised) Malaysia, 2010–2040*, Online. Available at: https://www.dosm.gov.my/v1/index.php?r=column/pdfPrev&id=Y3kwU2tSNVFDOWp1YmtZYnhUeVBEdz09 (Accessed: 26 February 2021).

Department of Statistics (2020a) *Abridged Life Tables, Malaysia, 2018–2020*, Online. Available at: https://www.dosm.gov.my/v1/index.php?r=column/pdfPrev&id=R0VPdE1mNEdRQms2S0M4M1ZsSlVEdz09 (Accessed: 22 February 2021).

Department of Statistics (2020b) *Current Population Estimates, Malaysia*, Online. Available at: https://www.dosm.gov.my/v1/index.php?r=column/cthemeByCat&cat=155&bul_id=OVByWjg5YkQ3MWFZRTN5bDJiaEVhZz09&menu_id=L0pheU43NWJwRWVSZklWdzQ4TlhUUT09 (Accessed: 22 February 2021).

Do, S.-R. (2009) 'Medical use status and policy tasks of the elderly', *Health and Welfare Forum*, 11, pp. 66–79.

Dunér, A., Blomberg, S. and Hasson, H. (2011) 'Implementing a continuum of care model for older people - results from a Swedish case study', *International Journal of Integrated Care*, 11, e136.

Jeon, H. S. and Kan, S. K. (2012) 'Age differences in the predictors of medical service use between young-old and old-old: implications for medical service in aging society', *Health and Social Studies*, 1, pp. 28–57.

Jeong, H.S., Lee, K.S. and Song, Y.M. (2007) 'Population aging and medical expenses', *Journal of Health and Social Affairs*, 15(1), pp. 3–36.

Kang, E.-J., Seol, H.-H. and Choo, W.-J. (2005) 'A study for integrated traditioanal Korean/Western medicine to reform public medicine', *Journal of Health and Social Affairs*, 25(1), pp. 3–36.

Kang, S. M. et al. (2009) 'The future projection of public medical expenses considering population aging', *Health and Policy Studies*, 15(2), pp. 1–20.

Kim, J. S. et al. (1998) 'Unification of Oriental and Western medicine wtih study on Oriental and Western medicine', *Korean Journal of Medical History*, 7(1), pp. 47–60.

Kim, K. (2004) *A Study on the Status of Physicians Collaborating with Oriental Medicine Hospital, Medical Policy Institute of Korean Medical Association*.

Kim, Y. J. et al. (2018) *Oriental Medicine Utilization and Oriental Medicine Consumption Survey*.

Kim, Y. J. (2019) 'A study on the establishment of patient-oriented medical delivery system-oriented to the European union's examples of primary care reinforcement', *Medical Law*, 20(3), pp. 235–262.

Kwon, S., Lee, T. J. and Kim, C. Y. (2015) *Republic of Korea Health System Review: Health Systems in Transition*. Geneva, Switzerland.

Lee, H. J. et al. (2019) 'The present state of long-term planning for domestic health and welfare', *Journal of Health and Administration*, 29(3), pp. 368–373.

Lee, H. S. (2004) 'A study on factors related to elderly health and medical expenditure', *Korean Elderly Studies*, 24(2), pp. 163–179.

Lee, M. S. and Kwon, Y. K. (2009) 'Reviewing the legal basis of oriental medicine through case analysis', *Journal of the Korea Institute of Oriental Medicine*, 15(3), pp. 19–28.

Lee, P. S. (2015) 'The Contents and Challenges of medical integration of Korean medicine and western medicine', *Medical Policy Forum*, 13(4), pp. 39–46.

Lee, S. Y. (2004) 'Policy direction for vitalization of the cooperative medical system between Korean medicines and western medicines', *Health and Welfare Forum*, 97, pp. 66–70.

Malaysian Government (2020) *Bahagian Pasca Perkhidmatan, Jabatan Perkhidmatan Awam*, Available at: http://www.jpapencen.gov.my/english/senior_citizen.html (Accessed: 22 February 2021).

Ministry of Health Malaysia (2008) *National Health Policy for Older Persons 2008*.

Ministry of Health Malaysia (2011) *National Oral Health Plan for Malaysia 2011–2020*.

Ministry of Health Malaysia (2018) *National Health and Morbidity Survey 2018: Elderly Health*.

Ministry of Health Malaysia (2019) *Oral Health Program Annual Report 2018*.

Ministry of Health Malaysia (2020) *Strategic Framework of the Medical Program 2021–2025*.

Mohd Nor, H. S. et al. (2020) 'Phytochemical Content and Anti-Oxidant Activity of Selected Wild Ulam/Vegetables Consumed by Indigenous Jakun Community in Taman Negara, Endan Rompin, Johor', *Food Research*, 4(1), pp. 28–33.

Moon, K. H. (2017) *The Analysis of Trends and Determinants of Korean Medical Service Utilization in Outpatients. Kyung Hee University*.

Muramatsu, N. and Akiyama, H. (2011) 'Japan: super-aging society preparing for the future', *The Gerontologist*, 51(4), pp. 425–432.

Oh, Y. H. (2011) 'The problems adn improvement plans of medical staff supply and demand', *HIRA Policy Trend*, 5(6), pp. 12–20.

Son, N. K. et al. (2016) 'Comparison of 2 different exercise approaches: Tai Chi versus Otago, in community dwelling older women. *Journal of Geriatric Physical Therapy*, 39(2), pp. 51–57.

The Korean Institute for Oriental Medicine (2014) *Trends and Environmental Analysis of Korean Medicine Standards at home and abroad.*

United Nations (1982) *Report of the World Assembly on Aging.* Available at: https://www.un.org/esa/socdev/ageing/documents/Resources/VIPEE-English.pdf.

United Nations (2006) *Conventions on the Rights of Persons with Disabilities and Optional Protocol (CRPD), Online.* Available at: https://www.un.org/development/desa/disabilities/convention-on-the-rights-of-persons-with-disabilities.html.

United Nations Population Division (2019) *World Population Prospects 2019.* Geneva, Switzerland. Available at: https://population.un.org/wpp/Download/Standard/Population.

Walia, S. (2019) 'The economic challenge of Japan's aging crisis', *Online.* Available at: https://www.japantimes.co.jp/opinion/2019/11/19/commentary/japan-commentary/economic-challenge-japans-aging-crisis/.

Won, C. W. (2013) 'Elderly long-term care in Korea', *Journal of Clinical Gerontology and Geriatrics*, 4(1), pp. 4–6.

World Health Organization (2002) *Active Ageing: A Policy Framework.*

World Health Organization (2015) *World Report on Ageing and Health.*

World Health Organization (2018) *Ageing and Health*, Online. Available at: https://www.who.int/news-room/fact-sheets/detail/ageing-and-health (Accessed: 23 February 2021).

World Health Organization (2020) *Life expectancy and Healthy life expectancy Data by Country*, Online.

Yim, J. (2016) 'Therapeutic benefits of laughter in mental health: a theoretical review'. *The Tohoku Journal of Experimental Medicine*, 293(3), pp. 243–249.

Yoon, K. J. (2012) 'The utilization and recognition of oriental medicine by the Korean people', *Health and Welfare Issues & Focus*, 140, pp. 1–8.

3 Challenges of Holistic Healthcare System for Ageing Population in Malaysia

Lee Fatt Soon
Ministry of Health Malaysia

CONTENTS

Demography...21
How We Are Meeting the Needs..22
Challenges to Our System...22
References...22

DEMOGRAPHY

Malaysia has been witnessing a major demographic transformation. The average life expectancy has risen rapidly from 57 years in 1957 to 75 years in 2018, and the population of this cohort is expected to double in the next 20 years. Even though the majority of this population is expected to be healthy, there will be increasing numbers of a subpopulation of this older generation who are unwell. Therein lies the challenge in preparing for this population explosion.

The World Health Organization looks into healthy ageing in an all-inclusive manner. The issues affecting the health of the older person are variable and multiple, but they can be broadly divided into individual and environmental factors. Individual factors would include behaviour, genetics and disease attributes, while environmental factors would include housing, transport, social facilities and assistive technologies (World Health Organization, 2018). (i) Hence, being holistic is the essential principle in the management of older persons. In the medical context, the older person has to be seen as a whole, influenced by factors arising from physical health, mental health and socio-environmental domains rather than being managed as a diseased organ.

In addition, "recipe-like" prescriptions will not be ideal as the older population is very heterogeneous in nature. This is because, it is not just ageing alone which influence the phenotype of the older patient but comorbidities, disabilities and frailty (Morley et al., 2013) (ii) interplay in various combinations to generate a profoundly diverse population. Lately, frailty has come to the forefront with growing data providing evidence of poor outcome in its presence alone or when coexisting with other

DOI: 10.1201/9781003043270-3

medical conditions. As a consequence of all these factors, the needs of the older population will be very varied and require individualized care and support services.

HOW WE ARE MEETING THE NEEDS

In my old days in medical school, we were taught medicine according to organ or disease states. There was no exposure to geriatrics then. The approach to illness was, and maybe still is, for a major portion, based on evidence-based care for an organ system. Unfortunately for the older person with frailty, comorbidities and disabilities, this model of care will lead to multiple uncoordinated interventions which may result in polypharmacy and fragmentation of care. This will result in increased cost and gap in medical care (Frandsen et al., 2015). (iii) In our quest for excellent care of disease and "treatment to target", we sometimes lose sight of the concerns of the patient. As an example, the treatment of hypertension and diabetes is driven by targets to reduce complications which sometimes lead to postural hypotension and hypoglycaemia, respectively. These adverse effects may be non-existent to mild for some, but for the frail individual, these events lead to giddiness making mobility difficult which in turn affects their activities of daily living and consequently their quality of life.

CHALLENGES TO OUR SYSTEM

In Malaysia, health service provision is a dichotomy of government funded or privately owned. As expected, the older population mainly accesses public health facilities (IV) by virtue of their poorer income (Yunus et al., 2017). The public health facilities are in need of a comprehensive seamless system to address the needs of the older population at all levels of care.

The history of geriatric services in Malaysia is fraught with many challenges. Our most dire need is to develop resources, not only of doctors, but the full complement of trained, dedicated interdisciplinary team so as to function in facilities throughout the country.

The local training programme has got off the ground, but the issue arising is if we are able to train enough, soon enough. Apart from this, other issues that need to be addressed include the challenges of individualizing care in a busy overcrowded acute care environment, which is the scenario in many secondary and tertiary care set-ups, improving on the nihilistic perception that there is nothing much that can be done for older people, and attracting trainees at all levels and categories as they will be the future professional care providers for this country.

The challenge then is matching resource to the demand, developing downstream support for overcrowded care facilities while managing cost constraints and integrating different agencies to provide person-centred care to the older individuals.

REFERENCES

Frandsen, B. et al. (2015) 'Care fragmentation, quality, and costs among chronically ill patients', *American Journal of Managed Care*, 21 (5 May 2015), pp. 355–362. Available at: http://www.ajmc.com/journals/issue/2015/2015-vol21-n5/Care-Fragmentation-Quality-Costs-Among-Chronically-Ill-Patients.

Morley, J. et al. (2013) 'Frailty consensus: a call to action', *Journal of the American Medical Directors Association*, 14(6), pp. 392–397.

World Health Organization (2018) *Ageing and Health*, Online. Available at: https://www.who.int/news-room/fact-sheets/detail/ageing-and-health (Accessed: 23 February 2021).

Yunus, N. M. et al. (2017) 'Determinants of healthcare utilisation among the elderly in Malaysia', *Institutions and Economies*, 9(3), pp. 117–142.

4 Policy Development on Ageing in Malaysia
Issues and Challenges

Tengku Aizan Hamid, Wan Alia Wan Sulaiman,
Mohamad Fazdillah Bagat, and Sen Tyng Chai
Universiti Putra Malaysia

CONTENTS

Introduction 25
Demography of Ageing 26
Policies and Programmes on Ageing 31
    Pre-Independence to 1994 32
    1995–2010 34
    2011 to Present 36
    Overview of Major Programmes and Services for Older Persons 40
        Health 40
        Finance 42
        Housing 45
        Social Participation 48
        Transport and Others 50
Policy Issues, Challenges and Recommendations 50
    Health Care, Social Care and Long-Term Care for Older Persons 50
    Income Security and Financing Old Age 53
    Assistive Technology, Built and Social Environments 54
Conclusion 56
References 57

INTRODUCTION

Malaya is a federation of nine Malay states (Johor, Kedah, Kelantan, Negeri Sembilan, Perak, Perlis, Pahang, Selangor and Terengganu) and two Straits Settlements (Melaka and Pulau Pinang) that became independent from British colonial rule on 31 August 1957. Malaysia came into being on 16 September 1963 when North Borneo (Sabah) and Sarawak joined the Federation of Malaya via the Malaysia Agreement. A Federal constitutional elective monarchy and Westminster parliamentary democracy, the country's Head of State or *Yang di-Pertuan Agong* is elected from among nine hereditary rulers of the Malay States. A bicameral Federal parliament of the House

DOI: 10.1201/9781003043270-4

of Representatives and the Senate holds legislative power, while each of the thirteen states has a unicameral State Legislative Assembly. The three Federal Territories of Kuala Lumpur 1974, Labuan 1984 and Putrajaya 2001 were formed in successive years. Executive power is vested in the Cabinet, led by the Prime Minister as the Head of Government. Malaysia is a newly industrialized, export-oriented economy with a total GDP of US$364.7 billion in 2019 and is officially recognized as an upper middle-income country with a GNI per capita (Atlas method) of US$11,230 (World Bank, 2020).

This chapter briefly describes Malaysia's demographic and epidemiological transitions since Independence as context for related policies and programmes development to address the emerging issues and challenges of population ageing. It traces the development and implementation of national ageing policies in the early years from a health and social welfare perspective until the turn of the new millennium. With growing recognition of the rising demands for products and services that can improve the lives of the elderly and their families, there is a critical need to examine the impact of past and current policies on ageing in Malaysia to inform future actions in a post-pandemic world.

DEMOGRAPHY OF AGEING

The Peninsular of Malaysia had a total population of 2.9 million in 1921. A decade prior to Independence, the Malayan population numbered 4.9 million in 1947. Between 1957 till 1970, the total population grew from 6.3 to 8.8 million (Chander, 1975; Hirschman, 1980). After the Population and Housing Census in 1980, it was estimated that Sabah and Sarawak added about 1.6 million persons to the Federation in 1970 (Leete and Kwok, 1986). The total population of Malaysia has grown from 10.9 million in 1970 to 23.5 million in 2000, and it was expected to reach 32.7 million in 2020 and 41.5 million in 2040 (Department of Statistics Malaysia, 2001a; 2016a).

Population growth has slowed considerably since the 1970s as death rates bottomed out while birth rates continue to drop. Malaysia is currently in the late or third stage of demographic transition where fertility has fallen below replacement levels in 2010 and mortality rate is rising again (Figure 4.1). Although life expectancy at birth has increased from 61.6 years for males and 65.6 for females in 1970 to 72.6 years and 77.6 years, respectively, in 2020, Malaysia is ageing from the bottom due to a steady decline in the share of younger population.

Malaysia uses the age 60 years and over as the cut-off point in deliberating ageing trends since the first World Assembly on Ageing in 1982 (Pala, 1998; 2005). In developed countries, the age of 65 is used instead. Demographers have long used the proportion or percentage of older population to signify different levels of ageing in a society. Chen and Jones (1989) adapted the categorization developed by Cowgill and Holmes (1972) and defined a society as "aged" when its older population aged 60 years and above reaches 15% or more. Coulmas (2007) proposed that population ageing levels are determined by the proportion of those aged 65 years or over in "ageing" (7%–14%), "aged" (14%–21%) and "hyper-aged" (21% or more) societies.

Population ageing in Malaysia is happening much more rapidly than in other developed countries and at a lower level of development. It took France 115 years for

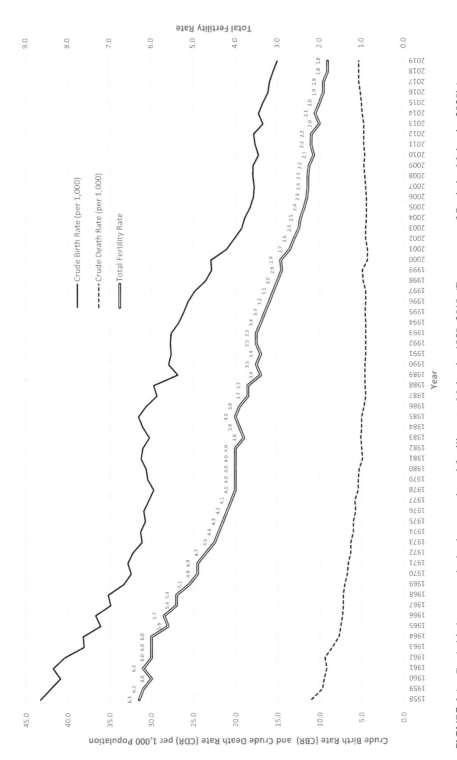

FIGURE 4.1 Crude birth rate, crude death rate and total fertility rate, Malaysia, 1958–2019. (Department of Statistics Malaysia, 2020b.)

its 65 years or over population to double from 7% to 14% (Kinsella and He, 2009), but it will take Malaysia just 24 years to do the same (Figure 4.2). According to medium-variant projections by the United Nations, Malaysia's 65 years or over population will reach 14% in 2044 and 21% in 2059. This means that the right policies and programmes catering to the needs of current and future generations of older persons must be in place over the next few decades. A whole-of-society and whole-of-government approach is needed as Malaysia is becoming old before becoming rich. Shrestha (2000) noted that the growth of the aged population in developing countries is much faster than in developed nations due to rapid fertility decline and advancements in medical technology as well as public health improvements. The expansion of the old-old (75–84) and oldest-old (85+) populations as more and more Malaysians survive into later ages has implications on the demand of health and social care services, long-term care, housing as well as transportation, just to name a few. The demographic transition is happening rather rapidly, and not in sync with the development and reforms in related social institutions.

Table 4.1 shows the distribution of older persons by State in Malaysia in past census years and projections for 2020 and 2040. A casual glance confirms the increasing number and proportion of the population aged 60 years or over in all Malaysian States and Federal Territories. Selangor, together with Kuala Lumpur that encompasses the greater Klang Valley area, has the largest population of older persons, but it remains a relatively young State in 2020. Compared to Perak, which has the highest percentage of older persons at 14.9%, the local situation of population ageing varies due to a complex interplay of fertility, mortality and inter-state migration patterns. By 2040, nearly all the States' older population would have crossed the 15% mark. The variations in rates of ageing in the respective States can be attributed largely to internal migration, where younger population leaves the rural area for towns and cities seeking better employment opportunities (Hamid, 2017).

The number of older persons aged 60 years and over in Malaysia has shown a steady upward trend. The older population doubled in the last two decades from 1.45 million in 2000 to 3.44 million in 2020. Today, one out of every 10 persons in Malaysia is an older person and share of the aged population is expected to reach 16.3% in 2040, numbering nearly 6.3 million. Nevertheless, the older population in Malaysia has some notable characteristics due to its unique past. Malaysia is a multiracial country consisting of the Malays and Bumiputeras (including the indigenous and native peoples in Peninsular Malaysia, Sabah and Sarawak), Chinese and Indians as the three main ethnic categories, with smaller minorities such as the Sikhs and Eurasians. Historically, the older sex ratio has an excess of males due to the waves of Chinese and Indian male labour immigration in colonial Malaya up till the post-Depression era of the 1930s, before World War Two. After the 1980s, the older male surplus disappeared, and the number of older women began to rise in tandem with the increase in average life expectancy of females. The differences in fertility levels, life expectancy and socio-economic status especially among the Malaysian Chinese have resulted into a scenario where the various communities are experiencing population ageing very differently. As seen in Table 4.2, nearly 17% of the total Malaysian Chinese population in 2020 are older persons and this is expected to increase to 26% in 2040. The ethnic Chinese population has registered the fastest rate of ageing since

Policy Development on Ageing in Malaysia

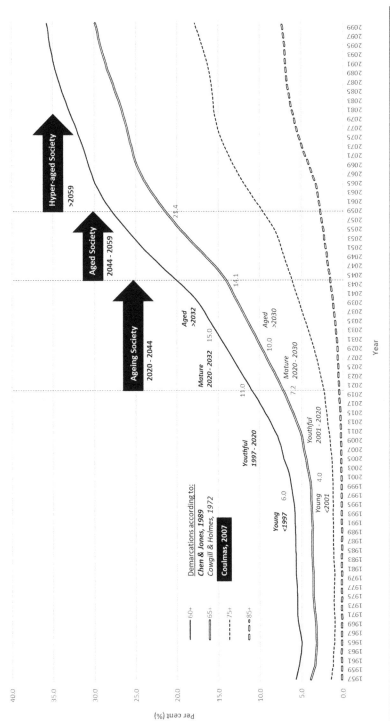

FIGURE 4.2 Increase of older populations and speed of ageing, Malaysia, 1957–2100. (United Nations, 2019a.)

TABLE 4.1
Distribution of Older Persons (60+) by State, Malaysia, 1980–2040

	1980		2000		2020		2040	
State	N ('000)	%	N ('000)	%	N ('000)	%	N ('000)	%
Johor	89.6	5.4	167.1	6.4	418.7	11.2	755.4	18.0
Kedah	68.4	6.1	129.8	7.9	259.8	11.8	401.7	15.1
Kelantan	55.2	6.2	94	7.0	187.1	10.1	261.0	10.4
Melaka	30.7	6.6	50.4	8.1	113.6	12.2	183.3	16.5
Negeri Sembilan	37.0	6.4	61.9	7.4	148.5	12.6	242.7	17.0
Pahang	37.5	4.7	69.9	5.7	183.2	10.4	300.6	13.1
Penang	63.1	6.6	100.7	7.9	242.4	13.9	436.6	22.6
Perak	111.1	6.1	186.6	9.1	385.8	14.9	507.9	17.1
Perlis	10.7	7.2	18.5	9.1	30.2	11.6	35.9	11.2
Selangor	73.0	4.8	89.3	4.5	553.7	8.9	1,309.1	19.1
Terengganu	31.4	5.8	131.5	6.5	115.9	9.1	191.7	10.5
Sarawak	74.1	5.5	184.1	4.6	317.4	11.4	570.5	17.5
Sabah	33.4	3.2	54.4	6.1	261.3	6.8	617.0	12.5
F. T. Kuala Lumpur	44.4	4.5	70.7	5.4	212.0	11.5	444.6	22.5
F. T. Labuan	–	–	2.1	3.5	7.6	7.2	21.8	16.3
F. T. Putrajaya	–	–	–	–	3.7	3.7	15.2	12.1
Malaysia	759.6	5.5	1,410.9	6.4	3,440.9	10.6	6,295.3	16.3

Source: Department of Statistics Malaysia, 2007; 2016b [unpublished data].

TABLE 4.2
Distribution of Older Persons (60+) by Ethnicity, Malaysia, 1980–2040

	Number in Thousands (N '000)				Percentage of 60+ (%)			
Year	Malay and Bumi.	Chinese	Indian	Others	Malay and Bumi.	Chinese	Indian	Others
1980	379.8	311.7	60.1	8.1	4.8	7.0	5.1	2.7
1990	562.9	359.2	77.0	16.4	5.0	7.2	5.5	3.1
2000	803.8	501.0	94.0	12.4	5.6	8.7	5.5	4.5
2010	1,242.8	778.0	150.4	11.4	7.0	12.1	7.8	4.9
2020	1,889.3	1,153.8	254.7	21.1	9.1	16.9	12.1	4.9
2030	2,709.1	1,540.3	373.5	33.9	11.4	21.9	16.8	8.7
2040	3,504.3	1,854.6	473.9	47.0	13.5	26.1	21.0	9.8

Source: Department of Statistics Malaysia, 2007; 2016 [unpublished data].
Note: Figures exclude non-Malaysians.

Independence and their extremely low levels of fertility and international migration trends have indicated that this situation will likely persist (Tey and Lai, 2018).

With increasing longevity and feminization of old age in Malaysia, there is another major trend with significant impact on the development of ageing-related policies

TABLE 4.3
Distribution of Older Persons (60+) by Stratum in Past Censuses, Malaysia, 1970–2010

	Urban			Rural		
Year	*N* ('000)	%	% 60+ in Urban	*N* ('000)	%	% 60+ in Rural
1970	146.9	26.9	5.2	399.2	73.1	5.2
1980	245.2	32.9	5.5	500.0	87.1	5.8
1991	470.7	45.6	5.3	561.6	54.4	6.5
2000	785.3	54.1	5.4	686.4	45.9	7.5
2010	1,478.1	65.7	7.3	773.2	34.3	9.4

Source: Department of Statistics Malaysia, 1998; 2001; 2011.

and programmes. Prior to the 2000s, most of the older population are found in rural areas but more and more older persons are now living in urban cities and towns. Nevertheless, the rate of ageing is much higher in the rural areas due to a steady outmigration of the younger population in search for economic and tertiary education opportunities. According to the 2010 Census, 9.4% of the rural population are made up of older persons aged 60 years or over (Table 4.3). The outmigration of the younger population created naturally occurring retirement communities (NORC) in pockets of rural areas. After the 2000 Census, more older persons are found in urban areas, but this shift can also be in part explained by the rapid rate of urbanization or urban growth in Malaysia. Since 1991, urban areas were defined as gazetted areas, alongside adjoining built-up areas, that had a combined population of 10,000 or more. The proportion of urban population in Malaysia has increased from 28.4% in 1970 to 71% in 2010 (Yaakob et al., 2011; Department of Statistics Malaysia, 2011a). Urban ageing is now an emerging phenomenon that requires due consideration and planning, while the growing urban-rural ageing gaps must be addressed.

In summary, demographic ageing in Malaysia is happening rapidly with differing rates among ethnic groups, gender and geography in Malaysia. In addition to the macro-level differences in ageing experiences, the heterogeneity of individuals makes it even more challenging for any Government to address. Rapid ageing, in tandem with urbanization, modernization and digitization, represents one of the megatrends faced by our country now. The lags in development as well as reforms in healthcare, economic and social protection systems will lead to gaps in supply and demand for needed products and services by the new and successive cohort of older persons in Malaysia. In the following section, we shall trace the development of related policies and programmes on ageing in Malaysia since Independence and highlight the issues and challenges faced from a multidisciplinary perspective.

POLICIES AND PROGRAMMES ON AGEING

Policy development in Malaysia is largely a top-down affair, and central planning is directed by the Federal Government. As noted by Lee and Lee (2017), the 5-year development plans in Malaysia have been driven by "both domestic needs and external developments" and are usually "structured into sectoral chapters" where each chapter is often aligned to a distinct Federal ministry, mirroring the manner in which the plans are formulated and put together. Working groups formed by the Economic Planning Unit (EPU) will collate and coordinate planning activities, which usually involve consultations with private and civil society sectors. It is at these consultative sessions, broadly considered a token bottom-up approach where specific projects or ideas are presented for adoption, the achievements of past programmes are highlighted for continuation or expansion, with the use of shared audit or research findings to support innovations or improvements.

As such, it is important to note that policies and programmes on ageing are driven primarily by the Ministry of Women, Family and Community Development (MWFCD), or before this, the Ministry of Unity and Social Development (MUSD). The Department of Social Welfare (DSW) has remained the focal point for older persons and ageing issues since Independence. When we examine the National Social Welfare Policy 1990, National Social Policy 2003 and even the National Family Policy 2010, the policymaking narratives of old age and ageing issues in Malaysia are set within a social development context. Malaysia advocates the concept of familial well-being based on values such as love, caring, justice and equity, putting family development as the central pillar in achieving the objective of creating a caring society – one of the seven goals for Vision 2020. For this section, we will trace origins of the welfare-centric concerns for the aged, the formulation of the first National Policy for the Elderly (NPE), subsequent policy and legal developments, as well as the prevailing programmes and services for older Malaysians.

Pre-Independence to 1994

One of the earliest records of the Parliament or Hansard indicated the concerns of the MP of Damansara regarding "the conditions in old-age homes" in December 1959, specifically the one at Serdang and the fact that many are waiting to be taken in into such welfare institutions. The then Minister for Health and Social Welfare acknowledged that the Government "cannot unfortunately cater for every old person who needs a place in the home" (Hansard, 1959). In reality, old people's homes (*rumah orang tua*) are well established even before Malaya's Independence for a very specific group of people – unmarried and childless elderly, especially ageing Chinese and Indian male labourers or post-war survivors without next of kin to support them in later life. Most of these charitable old folks' homes are known to us today as *Rumah Sejahtera*s, and they are usually set up in new villages with historical links to the Central Welfare Council (CWC)[1] that was established in 1946. After the dissolution of the Social and Welfare Services Lotteries Board in 1991, the old folks' homes under the Central Welfare Council Malaysia (later renamed as *Majlis Pusat Kebajikan Se-Malaysia* or MPKSM) continue to receive funding from the Department of Social Welfare as well as public donations to sustain its operations.

---

[1] The CWC received funding via the Social Welfare Lottery regulated through the Lotteries Act 1953.

Policy Development on Ageing in Malaysia

This welfare-centric approach to elderly matters is typical of public policy thinking in the years before and after Independence (Sushama, 1985). In these early days under the Second Malaya Plan (1961–1965), as well as the First (1966–1970) and Second (1971–1975) Malaysia Plans, the Government began to build or take over the operations of several Federal-funded old folks' homes (*Rumah Seri Kenangans*), as well as providing financial assistance for the elderly through the Older Person Assistance Scheme (*Skim Bantuan Orang Tua* or BOT) (Hansard, 1973). Institutionalization (shelter) and financial assistance would remain the mainstay ageing policy response for the next 30 years after Independence. When the pro-natalist policy of 70 million population by 2100 was officially introduced in 1984 and included in the Fifth Malaysia Plan (1986–1990) – an administrative reaction to falling fertility rates to boost the size of the domestic market, few economists and demographers considered it practical or realistic (Jones and Tan, 1985; Dwyer, 1987; Abdullah, 1993).

By the 6th Development Plan (1991–1995), the policy situation on ageing is clearly changing and this is evident from several successive developments. The UN General Assembly organized a World Assembly on Ageing in Vienna in 1982, and the Vienna Plan of Action on Ageing (VIPAA) was endorsed and adopted in the same year (UNGA Resolution 37/51). Chief among its recommendations, VIPAA called for action addressing research, data collection and analysis, training and education on ageing as well as its sectoral areas (health and nutrition, protection of elderly consumers, housing and environment, family, social welfare, income security and employment, and education). Malaysia was part of a World Health Organization (WHO)-sponsored four-country study on Health Care of the Elderly[2] and the report "Health and Aging in Malaysia" was duly published in 1986 (Chen et al., 1986). Another survey report under the ASEAN-Australian Population Programme on "Socio-economic Consequences of Ageing of the Population" was published by the National Population and Family Development Board Malaysia in 1988 (Mohd. Yatim et al., 1988).

On 14 December 1990, the United Nations General Assembly designated October 1 as the International Day of Older Persons (UNGA Resolution 45/106). The General Assembly also adopted the United Nations Principles for Older Persons (UNGA Resolution 46/91) in 1991. Malaysia started celebrating its own **National Day of Older Persons** on 1 October 1992. The early 1990s also saw a flurry of civil society movement with the official establishment of the National Council of Senior Citizens Organizations Malaysia (NACSCOM, 1990), the Gerontological Association of Malaysia (GeM, 1991) and the Golden Age Foundation (USIAMAS, 1991). Until then, most of the older people associations (OPAs) in Malaysia consisted primarily of senior citizens clubs for retiree recreational activities, and NGOs on ageing are usually clan-based or faith-based welfare charities. It was clear that by the mid-1990s, the growing activism and advocacy movement sustained by a combined critical mass of physicians, demographers, academicians, policymakers, social workers and older persons culminated in the formulation of the first **National Policy for the Elderly** (NPE) in 1995.

---

[2] The other three countries are Fiji, the Republic of Korea and the Philippines.

1995–2010

Details on the implementation and achievements of the NPE have been discussed at length by other authors (Ong, 2002; Hamid and Yahaya, 2008). It was broadly inspired by the UN Principles for Older Persons 1991, with similar themes on independence, care, participation, self-fulfilment, and dignity in old age. The NPE's Plan of Action (1997–2005) would arrive 2 years later and officially adopted in 1998. Critically, the NPE and its Plan of Action established two enduring features, namely 1. the National Advisory and Consultative Council for the Elderly (NACCE) first convened in 1996, chaired by the Minister of Unity and Social Development (later the Minister of Women, Family and Community Development), and 2. the set-up of six sub-committees[3] chaired by different departments or ministries under the overall coordination of the Department of Social Welfare (DSW) as the agency responsible for its implementation. Notably, the Ministry of Health formed a National Council of Health for the Elderly in 1997 and implemented an elderly healthcare programme that included the training of geriatricians and nurses, set-up of geriatric wards/units as well as other preparations towards a comprehensive healthcare service for the elderly. In 2000, Malaysia's first geriatric ward at a public hospital was opened in Seremban, Negeri Sembilan.

It is important to point out that actual changes came at a much slower pace despite the initial fanfare surrounding the NPE, partially due to the 1997 Asian financial crisis. While the first national policy on ageing also heralded a departure from the welfarist point of view where older persons are treated exclusively as passive recipients of care and support, there have been few new programmes and services in the beginning. As an example, in the 7th Malaysia Plan (1996–2000), the elderly were mentioned within the ambit of "Family Development", under "Other Social Services" for the chapter on Housing and Other Social Services (Chapter 18, Economic Planning Unit, 1995). It stated that:

> Planning for the elderly will take cognizance of changes in the characteristics and expectations of the elderly such as the need for greater financial and personal independence as well as developing relationships of mutual reliance rather than dependency.

> *– Economic Planning Unit, 1995, p. 584*

The plan went on to reiterate that "the family will continue to be encouraged to take care of the elderly" (Economic Planning Unit, 1995). Nevertheless, two important pieces of legislation that were put in place in the 1990s have impacted the regulation of non-government or private aged care facilities, namely the Care Centre Act 1993 (Act 506) and the Private Healthcare Facilities and Services Act 1998 (Act 586) that replaced the Destitute Persons (Welfare Homes) Rules 1981 and the Private Hospitals Act 1971 (Act 43), respectively. Government-operated facilities by DSW remain under the Rules for the Management of Old Folks Homes 1983. The beginnings of the residential aged care industry, especially monthly fee-based private care centres and nursing homes, could trace its beginnings to this period, spurred by increasing

---

[3] Social and Recreation (Department of Social Welfare); Health (Ministry of Health); Education, Religion and Training (Ministry of Education); Housing (Ministry of Housing and Local Government); Research (National Population and Family Development Board); Liaison (Ministry of Information).

Policy Development on Ageing in Malaysia

demands from smaller, wealthier families and dual-income households as well as the liberalization of the private healthcare sector (Barraclough, 2000; Ong, 2007).

When the 8th Malaysia Plan (2001–2005) came round, the immediate influence of NPE and its Plan of Action could be felt as the elderly were highlighted in two separate paragraphs (18.52 and 18.53), calling for the "participation of older persons in society" (p. 516) and to ensure "that the caring for older persons remained with the family", day care centres[4] were to be established by the Government for the community care for older persons (p. 517) (Economic Planning Unit, 2000). In paragraph 18.107, "adequate housing, educational and recreational facilities, as well as amenities for the disabled and the elderly" were promised. In comparison, both the youth and women got their own dedicated chapters in the 7th and 8th Malaysia Plans, but older persons are relegated under "Other social services".

Throughout most of the first 10 years of the National Day of Older Persons celebrations, variants of the chosen theme had always been about loving and caring families. It was only at the turn of the millennium that active and productive ageing would enter the lexicon. When the Second World Assembly on Ageing was held in 2002 approximately 20 years later, the Madrid International Plan of Action on Ageing (MIPAA, 2002) outlined a focus on three priority areas, 1. older persons and development; 2. advancing health and well-being into old age; and 3) ensuring enabling and supportive environments. In the 9th Malaysia Plan (2006–2010), "Older Persons" was placed under a separate sub-header apart from "Family Development" (Economic Planning Unit, 2005). It comes under Chapter 15 on Fostering Family and Community Development, and the section noted the progress achieved that highlighted a shift of programmes "from a welfare approach to a development approach to ensure active and productive ageing", where phrases such as lifelong learning and ICT were first associated with older persons (p. 311). The plan promised to undertake measures "to provide for an environment for the elderly to remain healthy, active and secure while being able to age with dignity and respect as well as leading independent and fulfilling lives as integral members of their families, communities and country" (pp. 316–317). Home help and family support, including mobile welfare units, were to be made available[5]. A total of eight paragraphs (15.17–15.20 and 15.39–15.41) were dedicated to the matter of older persons who are now no longer viewed as frail and passive care recipients. There was even a mention of developing mental health services "for specific target groups such as adolescents and older persons" (para. 20.50, p. 427, Economic Planning Unit, 2005). The Alzheimer's Disease Foundation Malaysia (ADFM), officially registered in 1997, would begin operating its dementia day care centre at Petaling Jaya in 2002.

---

[4] The senior day care centres or Pusat Jagaan Harian Warga Emas (PJHWE) would be operated by MPKSM with DSW funding support, with the first of such facilities operational in 2002 at Cheras Baru (Berita Harian, 4 October 2002).

[5] Both MPKSM and USIAMAS have embarked on home-help services as well as home visits for the elderly since the early 1990s with funding support by the DSW. In 2005, HelpAge Korea supported a home-help pilot project by USIAMAS and it has significantly influenced the present Khidmat Bantuan di Rumah (KBDR) programme. MPKSM remains the only voluntary welfare organization partner to the DSW for the Unit Khidmat Penyayang initiative that provided van transportation for the elderly since 2006.

36   Healthy Ageing in Asia

The early 2000s also heralded the arrival of other new actors with the establishment of the Institute of Gerontology (IG) at Universiti Putra Malaysia and the founding of the Malaysian Healthy Ageing Society (MHAS). The former is the first research institute of its kind in the country dedicated to the study of old age and ageing, and IG would be rebranded into the Malaysian Research Institute on Ageing in 2015.

Under the administration of the new fifth Prime Minister, several notable developments in social welfare would result in lasting impact on the elderly. The development of the National Poverty Data Bank or eKasih in 2007 by the Implementation Coordination Unit (ICU), as well as the proactive measures of *Program Cari* (Hansard, 2009) would later pave the way for the massive national social allowance scheme now known to us as Household Living Aid (*Bantuan Sara Hidup*, previously *Bantuan 1Rakyat Malaysia*), which was first disbursed in 2012. The immediate impact of *Program Cari*, of course, was a massive surge in the number of welfare recipients including the financial assistance for the elderly. The Older Persons' Aid (BOT) scheme benefits were increased from RM135 per month to RM200 in 2006 and would be increased again to RM300 in 2008. The number of BOT recipients jumped from 27,636 older persons in 2007 to 111,791 older persons in 2009, an increase of more than 304.5% although it was also partially attributed to Federal-State welfare realignments for Sabah and Sarawak (Hamid and Chai, 2013).

In 2008, the Ministry of Health (MOH) developed and adopted its own **National Health Policy for Older Persons** and action plan after more than a decade of building up geriatric services and training of health personnel in the care of older patients under the elderly healthcare programme (NHPOP, 2008). The NHPOP runs concurrently with the existing policies and programmes under the MWFCD. Like its DSW counterpart for the NPE, the Family Health Development Division under the MOH is responsible for NHPOP's implementation. At the time, the NPE itself was overdue for a renewal. The Institute of Gerontology, UPM, was commissioned in 2009 to conduct a study to assess the impact of the NPE and its plan of action as well as to propose a new national policy on ageing.

2011 TO PRESENT

In the 10th Malaysia Plan (2011–2015), the concerns of older persons received nearly equal attention as women's empowerment. In Chapter 4: Moving Towards Inclusive Socio-economic Development, the sub-header reads "Supporting Older Persons to Lead Productive and Fulfilling Societal Roles" (Economic Planning Unit, 2010), promising "to provide a conducive environment for older persons to remain healthy, active and secure", with programmes that "will focus on enhancing elderly-friendly infrastructure, improving access to affordable healthcare, ensuring adequate provision of shelters and improving financial security and opportunities for employment" (p. 185). This will be the first time old-age employment is explicitly referenced in the national development plans, marking a huge departure from the past where older persons are considered retired or past the age for work.

In 2011, the Cabinet approved a new **National Policy for Older Persons** (*Dasar Warga Emas Negara*, NPOP) and its Action Plan (2010–2020) to replace the NPE. The revised policy adopts a lifespan perspective, with a goal of empowering the individual,

Policy Development on Ageing in Malaysia

the family and the community, making provisions for age-friendly services as well the development of enabling and supportive environment towards the well-being of older Malaysians. It highlighted the need for continued initiatives for the protection of vulnerable older persons, but at the same time calling for more old-age employment opportunities. The DSW under the Ministry of Women, Family and Community Development (MWFCD) retains its original role as custodian of the NPOP, and the renamed National Advisory and Consultative Council for Older Persons (NACCOP) continues to be chaired by its Minister. Members of the council consist of representatives from various government agencies, GLCs, as well as NGOs on ageing. For the NPOP, seven sub-committees are tasked to implement the policy initiatives, namely 1. Health (MOH), 2. Social and Recreation (DSW), 3. Education and Spirituality (Ministry of Education), 4. Housing and Environment (Ministry of Housing and Local Government), 5. Economy (EPU), 6. Employment (Ministry of Human Resources), and 7. Research and Development (Ministry of Science, Technology and Innovation) (Figure 4.3).

With a renewed attention and focus on older persons, and because of earlier efforts, 2012 turned out to be a significant year for policy development on ageing. The mandatory retirement age for civil servants has been increased from 55 to 56 in 2001 before being revised to 58 in 2008 and 60 in 2012. With the passing of the Minimum Retirement Age Act 2012 (Act 756), private sector workers now enjoy the same right to work up to at least the age of 60. Together with the National Wages Consultative

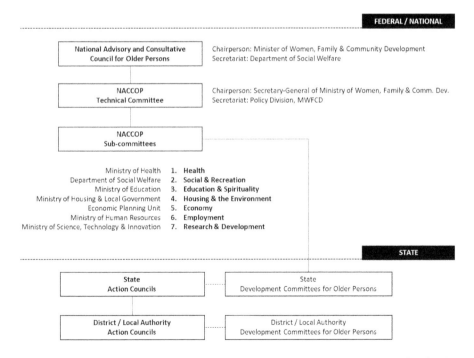

FIGURE 4.3 Implementation and coordination of the national policy and plan of action for older persons, Malaysia, 2011. (Ministry of Women, Family and Community Development, 2011.)

Council Act 2011 (Act 732) passed a year ago, the extended period of employment and guaranteed minimum wages are expected to improve the retirement savings of working Malaysians. The Private Retirement Schemes (PRS), a voluntary long-term savings and investment plan, was also launched in July 2012. The PRS regulatory framework was established under the Capital Markets and Services Act (CMSA) 2007 and is regulated and supervised by the Securities Commission Malaysia (SC) with the Private Pension Administrator (PPA) Malaysia providing central administration and industry support. In 2012, the DSW also converted all 22 senior day care centres (*Pusat Jagaan Harian Warga Emas*, PJHWE) into Senior Citizen Activity Centres (*Pusat Aktiviti Warga Emas*, PAWE). From this point onwards, PAWE would get its own guideline and funding through the Department of Social Welfare, swelling rapidly in numbers to 143 in late 2020 (Department of Social Welfare, 2021).

Another notable development in 2012 was the identification of Seniors' Living as a Business Opportunity under the National Key Economic Area (NKEA) for Healthcare. PEMANDU, through the Economic Transformation Programme (ETP), believed that the long-term care industry, especially retirement villages (RV), and the care economy could be a potential engine of growth in a greying society. This attracted the interest of Australian aged care and retirement village players[6] with active efforts of the Australian Trade and Investment Commission (Austrade). Initial work for the Private Aged Healthcare Facilities and Services Act 2018 (Act 802) could trace its origins to this period. At about the same time, a National Occupational Skills Standard (NOSS) for Elderly Care Centre Operations (Levels 3, 4 and 5) was being developed and published in 2013. PLANMalaysia under the Ministry of Housing and Local Government published a Physical Planning Guideline for the Elderly (GP031) in 2013 that specified parameters for optimal build-up and design of physical spaces for older persons living at home or in institutions. This document would be updated again in 2018 (GP031-A).

When the 11th Malaysia Plan (2016–2020) arrived, older persons are already one of the targeted population segments alongside youth, women, children, the family, persons with disabilities, Bumiputeras, rural communities, as well as B40 and M40 households (Economic Planning Unit, 2015). Under "Focus area B: Empowering communities for a productive and prosperous society", one of the six strategies outlined is on "Enhancing the living environment for the elderly" (Strategy B5). It aims to improve supportive environment for the elderly and promote active ageing. Apart from providing "elderly-friendly infrastructure and improving care services", the plan hopes to streamline and integrate "social protection for the elderly poor" to ensure better quality of life (pp. 3–27). Volunteerism was also promoted as a way for the elderly to continue contributing to national development.

In the academia, gerontology and geriatrics are growing in stature as a field of study. The Social Security Research Centre (now the Social Well-being Research Centre, SWRC) was established at University of Malaya in 2011 with support from the Employees' Provident Fund (EPF). The Community Rehabilitation and Ageing Research Centre (H-CARE) was set up at Universiti Kebangsaan Malaysia in 2012.

---

[6] Flex Health, Jeta Care and Eden on the Park were among the early Australian players that set up shop here in Malaysia.

In the same year, the Malaysian Society of Geriatric Medicine (MSGM) was also founded. Older persons and ageing issues have become a major regional issue so much so that when the Kuala Lumpur Declaration on Ageing: Empowering Older Persons in ASEAN was made in 2015, it was already the second of such documents[7] There had been many major studies on older persons in recent years, as well as the inclusion of older persons as a focus in national statistics. For example, the 5th Malaysian Population and Family Survey (MPFS-5) in 2014 included a submodule for older respondents (NPFDB, 2015). Similarly, additional questions for the elderly were included in the 2020 Census. The National Health and Morbidity Survey (NHMS) in 2018 focused on Elderly Health (Ministry of Health, 2019), and the Ministry of Human Resources commissioned a study on the employment of older persons (ILMIA, 2019). In 2017, two DSW consultancies on the effectiveness of financial assistance programmes, as well as meeting the facilities and services needs of older persons were completed (Universiti Putra Malaysia, 2017a; 2017b). Long-term Research Grants (LRGS) on ageing have been awarded by the Ministry of Higher Education (MOHE) to Universiti Kebangsaan Malaysia 2013, University of Malaya 2019 and Sunway University 2019. The Malaysian Ageing Research Network (MARN) was launched in 2017 to provide a platform to foster scientific development in gerontology and bridging gaps between policy, research and practice.

In 2019, amidst preparations for the 12th Malaysian Plan, the administration under the 7th Prime Minister launched the Shared Prosperity Vision 2030 (SPV2030) blueprint. With three core objectives,[8] fifteen guiding principles, seven strategic thrusts and eight enablers, the blueprint was intended to steer Malaysia on a path of sustainable development and prosperity for all over the next 10 years. Senior citizens were included under the nine target groups (others are the B40 group, communities in economic transition, indigenous communities, Bumiputeras in Sabah and Sarawak, people with disabilities, youths, women, and children). The SPV2030 blueprint was considered the sister blueprint of Vision 2020, but a new administration under the 8th Prime Minister sworn-in on the 1st of March 2020 resulted in some fresh uncertainties as the rapid political successions led to probable recalibrations. Tabling of the 12th Malaysia Plan has also been postponed due to a suspension of the Parliament under a COVID-19-related Emergency Proclamation in February 2021.

The national development plan is one of the most important and oft-referenced documents by government ministries and departments. In the past two decades, the matter of older persons in Malaysia has shifted considerably from a social service issue to one of active development. An unmistakable ideological shift has occurred, and the situation of older persons is no longer looked upon from a quintessentially welfare perspective. The number of government agencies involved in old age and ageing issues has also increased, involving others such as the Ministry of Housing and Local Government, Ministry of Human Resources, Ministry of Finance, Ministry of Science, Technology and Innovations as well as the Ministry of Transport. The

---

[7] The Brunei Darussalam Declaration on Strengthening Family Institution: Caring for the Elderly (2010) was adopted five years ago.

[8] 1. Development for all, 2. addressing wealth and income disparities and 3. establishing a united, prosperous and dignified nation.

Income Tax (Deduction for Employment of Senior Citizen, Ex-Convict, Parolee, Supervised Person and Ex-Drug Dependant) Rules 2019 is an example of government efforts to promote old-age employment. New actors such as the Association for Residential Aged Care Operators of Malaysia (AgeCOpe) were established in 2018, and the market is now expanding with many mobile care or home care service providers, some utilizing a social enterprise model. It is evident that a silver-hair industry is emerging, and policy developments must consider the needs of current and future generations of older persons who are more educated, healthier, wealthier and have higher expectations for retirement living.

OVERVIEW OF MAJOR PROGRAMMES AND SERVICES FOR OLDER PERSONS

In this sub-section, a brief overview of current programmes and services for older persons in Malaysia is presented according to five different domains, namely a. Health, b. Finance, c. Housing, d. Social Participation, as well as e. Transport and others.

Health

Older persons have many healthcare needs, ranging from the management of chronic illnesses, coping with physical and mental impairments, to minimizing the mortality risks of communicable diseases. As shown in Table 4.4, the NHMS 2018 survey reported high prevalence of hypertension (51.1%), hypercholesterolaemia (41.8%) and diabetes (27.7%) among older Malaysians, with 17% reporting difficulties in performing some basic activities of daily living. The NHMS 2018 also recorded a prevalence of 9% for self-reported elder abuse (7.5% is neglect). The estimated prevalence of probable dementia and depressive symptoms is 8.5% and 5.3%, respectively. The survey results have been consistent with past studies, indicating increasing need and demand for healthcare services by ageing populations, especially among older women (Ho et al., 2014; Vanoh et al., 2016; Ho et al., 2020). As non-communicable diseases dominate the causes of death in Malaysia's epidemiological transition away from infectious diseases, lifestyle diseases such as heart disease, obesity and diabetes due to smoking, unhealthy diet and lack of physical activity become more commonplace like in other developing countries (Shrestha, 2000).

As medical and health matters fall under the Federal List in the Malaysian Constitution,[9] the massive network of Federal government hospitals and health clinics are the major providers of health care, treatment and medicine for older patients. In 2019, there are 154 government hospitals and 3,171 government medical clinics (health clinics = 1,114; rural clinics = 1,771; community clinics = 286) (Department of Statistics Malaysia, 2020c). Older persons in Malaysia have been paying nominal or token fees for outpatient and hospitalization services at government facilities. In 2011, the Ministry of Health even issued a circular announcing the waiver of the RM1 registration fee for all elderly outpatients at government hospitals and clinics. Government hospitals and clinics under the Ministry of Health provide free medicine to patients and only collect ward charges for hospitalization (RM3-RM80 per

---

[9] Social and welfare services come under the Concurrent List (shared Federal and State list).

Policy Development on Ageing in Malaysia

TABLE 4.4

Health Status of Older Malaysians ($n = 3,977$), 2018

Variable	Prevalence (%)				
	Malaysia	Urban	Rural	Male	Female
Self-reported Hypertension ($n = 3,966$)	51.1	50.5	52.6	46.9	55.1
Self-reported Diabetes ($n = 3,966$)	27.7	29.0	24.0	26.5	28.8
Self-reported Hypercholesterolaemia ($n = 3,966$)	41.8	43.3	37.8	37.8	45.7
Self-reported Cancer ($n = 3.945$)	1.6	1.8	1.1	2.1	1.2
Current Smoker ($n = 3,968$)	13.3	11.5	18.3	25.6	1.6
Former Smoker ($n = 3,968$)	12.5	12.1	13.7	23.3	2.1
Obese (BMI $\geq$ 30kg/m^2)	17.6	18.1	16.4	13.5	21.7
Underweight (BMI < 18.5kg/m^2)	5.2	4.4	7.5	4.8	5.6
Hearing Disability ($n = 3,965$)	6.4	6.2	7.0	6.3	6.6
Use of Hearing Aid ($n = 3,961$)	1.5	1.9	0.5	1.1	1.9
Vision Disability ($n = 3,968$)	4.5	3.8	6.5	4.4	4.6
Stress Urinary Incontinence ($n = 3,716$)	2.9	2.7	3.5	1.4	4.4
Urge Urinary Incontinence ($n = 3,716$)	3.4	3.3	3.9	2.8	4.1
Falls in past 12 months ($n = 3,969$)	14.1	14.1	13.9	13.4	14.7
Functional Limitations (ADL) ($n = 3,965$)	17.0	16.7	17.9	12.7	21.2
Dependency in IADL($n = 3,967$)	42.9	38.7	54.3	36.2	49.4
Probable Dementia ($n = 3,774$)	8.5	6.8	12.9	7.1	9.7
Depressive Symptoms ($n = 3,772$)	11.2	10.1	14.4	10.7	11.7
Self-reported Elder Abuse ($n = 3,466$)	9.0	8.3	10.7	9.9	8.1

Source: Institute for Public Health, 2019.

day, depending on ward class). Older persons aged 60 years or over receive a reduction of 50% if they are hospitalized and total payment is capped at a maximum of RM250 (Ministry of Health, 2016). Since 1997, the Elderly Health Services programme under the Family Health Development Division tracked older patients' data at government health clinics, provided health screening services, as well as aged care training for healthcare personnel and caregivers. To promote community outreach and health education, older person health clubs were set up and there are 284 such senior citizen clubs under their respective health clinics as of December 2019 (Ministry of Health, 2020).

Past studies have shown that most older Malaysians, especially of lower income and those living in rural areas, are dependent of public healthcare services (Chai and Hamid, 2015; Koris et al., 2019). The expansion in geriatric services has been well elaborated by Tan and her colleagues (2018), where the number of practising geriatricians (public and private) has increased from 14 in 2011 to 39 in 2018, with geriatric ward services in public hospitals, including teaching hospitals, in at least 11 States. Unfortunately, the small number of available geriatric services is mostly located in Selangor and Kuala Lumpur, thus unable to meet "even a fraction of the needs of the existing older population" throughout the country (Tan et al., 2018).

Finance

Older persons in Malaysia are asset rich, income poor. More than half (54.7%) of the older respondents in a 2016 survey reported receiving cash transfers from their children, although the average monthly value is lower than that of other sources such as wages, businesses, rental or pensions (Table 4.5). Nearly two-thirds or 71.4% of the respondents possess at least a house, while 52.6% own land. While property ownership is high among the current cohort of older persons, this is likely to change for future generations of the elderly. In addition, older women have lower income and are more dependent on transfers from adult children.

Many authors have discussed at length the many provisions that make up the old-age pensions system in Malaysia (Abdul Khalid, 2016; Holzmann, 2015; Hamid and Chai, 2013; Mat Zin, 2012; Ong and Hamid, 2010). Apart from the financial assistance schemes under DSW mentioned earlier, there are also State Islamic authorities that disburse Zakat alms for qualified recipients[10]. Civil servants are covered under the Public Service Pension scheme (Act 227, 1980), while private sector workers (11%) and their employers (13%) contribute to the EPF (EPF Act 452, 1991). About half of the active labour force is covered under the EPF scheme where lump sum withdrawals can be made at the age of 55 years old. Government pensioners, on the other hand, receive a monthly pension worth about one-third of their last take-home pay, with an annual 2% pension increment since 2013. Private sector workers (0.5%) earning less than RM4,000 a month (previously RM3,000 before 1 June 2016) and their employers (1.75%) also jointly contribute to a Social Security Organization (SOCSO) fund (Employees' Social Security Act 4, 1969) to cover for injuries and health problems arising from work (see Figure 4.4). Starting from 2018, SOCSO is also responsible for the Employment Insurance System (EIS) that provided unemployment benefits. An employer and employee each contribute about 0.2% of a worker's monthly salary (capped at RM4,000) to the protection plan. In 2021, the monthly value of the Senior Citizens' Aid (BOT) under DSW was increased from RM350 to RM500, benefitting an expected 142,325 recipients (Department of Statistics Malaysia, 2020c). Many older persons also receive financial assistance via General Aid (Bantuan Am) under the respective State welfare provisions as well as the Federal B40 household cash allowance programme known as Bantuan Sara Hidup (BSH).

In Malaysia, the care of the elderly falls on adult children or close family members. The personal income tax structure reflects these broad expectations as an individual is entitled to an automatic tax relief of RM1,500 for each parent[11] in a given assessment year. If more than one adult child claims for this deduction, the amount must be divided equally according to the number of claimants for this tax relief.

---

[10] 1. *Fakir* – those who does not have material possessions or means of livelihood; 2. *Miskin* – those with insufficient means of livelihood to meet basic needs/necessities; 3. *Amil* – those who are involved in the collection and distribution of Zakat; 4. *Muallaf* – those who are new converts to the faith of Islam; 5. *Al-riqab* – those who wish to seek independence from control (i.e. slavery or military occupation); 6. *Al-gharimin* – those who are in debt to meet basic needs/necessities for themselves and/or their dependents; 7. *Fisabilillah* – those who are involved in activities in the cause of Allah s.w.t; and 8. *Ibnu Sabil* – those who are stranded during a journey.

[11] Include legally adoptive parents but not step-parents, aged 60 years and above, with each parent's annual income must not exceed RM24,000 a year.

TABLE 4.5

Sources of Income for Older Malaysians, 2016

Sources of Income/Asset	Near Elderly (55–59) ($N_e = 687$)			Older Persons (60+)								
				Total ($N_{op} = 612$)			Male ($n = 314$)			Female ($n = 298$)		
	n	%	M	n	%	M	n	%	M	n	%	M
Salary/Wages	331	48.2	2,675.09	78	12.7	1,142.12	60	19.1	1,264.33	18	6.0	734.72
Business	118	17.2	2,095.68	60	9.8	1,720.83	38	12.1	1,936.84	22	7.4	1,347.73
Rental	29	4.2	844.90	16	2.6	934.38	11	3.5	1,050.00	5	1.7	680.00
Interest/Dividend	4	0.6	2,905.00	3	0.5	1,900.00	2	0.6	2,750.00	1	0.3	200.00
Welfare	29	4.2	296.03	76	12.4	309.01	36	11.5	306.53	40	13.4	311.25
Pension	35	5.1	1,241.60	109	17.8	1,406.20	80	25.5	1,421.45	29	9.7	1,364.14
Agriculture	71	10.3	540.56	65	10.6	679.85	41	13.1	871.46	24	8.1	352.50
Child(ren)	224	32.6	420.98	335	54.7	448.06	168	53.5	438.93	167	56.0	457.25
Other Sources	48	7.0	854.58	34	5.6	652.35	21	6.7	755.24	13	4.4	486.15
Personal Income/month	629	91.6	2,232.19	535	87.4	1,141.53	287	91.4	1,463.73	248	83.2	768.65
Household Income/month	675	98.3	4,202.74	560	91.5	2,449.42	294	93.6	2,680.98	266	89.3	2,193.48
Own House	480	69.9		437	71.4		260	82.8		177	59.4	
Own Land	303	44.1		322	52.6		188	59.9		134	45.0	
Have Life Insurance	138	20.1		31	5.1		25	8.0		6	2.0	
Have Medical Insurance	117	17.0		31	5.1		20	6.4		11	3.7	

Source: Universiti Putra Malaysia, 2017 [unpublished data].

Pension Pillars	Name of Programme Institution	Benefit Type	Financing Type
Pillar 0: Basic benefits through social pensions or at least social assistance	Department of Social Welfare (DSW) - Financial assistance (*Bantuan Orang Tua, Bantuan Am*, etc.) - Old folks' home (*Rumah Seri Kenangan*)	Cash benefit (up to RM500/mth) In-kind benefit	General revenue General revenue
Pillar 1: Mandated, unfunded, defined benefit or contribution schemes	Public Service Department & Retirement Fund (Incorporated) - Civil service pension fund Social Security Organization (SOCSO) - Employment Injury Scheme - Employment Insurance System	Old-age, disability, survivorship Work injury, disability, survivorship, unemployment benefits (18-60 y.o.)	General revenue Employer contribution; Employer and employee contribution
Pillar 2: Mandated, fully funded, occupational or personal schemes	Armed Forces Fund Board Employee's Provident Fund (EPF) - Private sector worker compulsory savings plan	All benefits Lump sum / phased withdrawal	Employer and employee contribution Employer and employee contribution; Voluntary contribution (self-employed)
Pillar 3: Voluntary, fully funded, occupational or personal schemes	Private Pension Administrator (PPA) - Private Retirement Scheme (PRS) Permodalan Nasional Berhad (PNB) - Government-owned investment company	Lump sum, fixed term / annuity Fixed term (interest / dividend)	Voluntary premium, tax incentives Voluntary savings / investment
Pillar 4: Access to informal and other formal provisions, and personal assets	Family Basic health care Public housing	Cash and in-kind benefits	Family members Budget financed; Budget support

FIGURE 4.4 Mapping of Malaysia's pension programmes. (Adapted with updated modifications from Holzmann, 2015.)

Policy Development on Ageing in Malaysia

Expenses on medical treatment, special needs or carer expenses for parents as evidenced by medical certification can also be deducted up to a limit of RM5,000. In the 2021 Budget speech, this figure for medical expenses was increased to RM8,000, including a RM1,000 tax relief for vaccinations. Individuals are also allowed deductions up to a maximum of RM6,000 if they purchase basic supporting equipment such as wheelchair, hearing aids or limb prostheses for themselves, spouse, children or parents. As of 2020, total deductibles allowed for life insurance and EPF contributions are capped at RM7,000 while an additional relief of RM3,000 is provided for private retirement and deferred annuity schemes. Nevertheless, it must be pointed out that low-income households or families[12] might not benefit from all these tax reliefs as they are only applicable for individuals with a taxable income of at least RM34,000 a year (after EPF deductions) or those earning over RM2,833 a month.

The rapid modernization and industrialization of the economy have resulted in fewer agriculture and informal sector work. Increasingly, formal sector workers, whether in blue- or white-collar jobs, are officially retired at the age of 55 or 60 years old. Labour force participation rate for older persons (aged 60–64 years) has steadily declined from 47.7% in 1980 to 39.2% in 2020 (Pala, 1998; Department of Statistics Malaysia, 2021). As shown in Figure 4.5, the changes in labour force participation rates are affected by broader social forces. As more younger adults receive tertiary education, their entry into the labour force was delayed. With the increase of mandatory and minimum retirement ages to 60 years old in 2012, the labour force participation rate (LFPR) of workers aged between 55 and 59 years old increased in tandem. The gap in labour force participation between males and females, however, has remained at 80.6% for men and 55.3% for women in 2020 (Department of Statistics Malaysia, 2021). While more and more women have joined the workforce over the years, increasing commodification of care for the young and the old has underscored the true value of unpaid care work traditionally performed, and still being provided, by our wives and daughters.

Housing

Like many Asian countries, the responsibility of caring for the elderly in Malaysia tends to fall on the family. Older Malaysians are more likely to co-reside with their adult children, and only an estimated 1% of the elderly live in residential aged care facilities (United Nations, 2017; Hasmuk et al., 2020). An analysis of the Household Expenditure Survey microdata showed that while family sizes are shrinking, households with older persons have increased from 23.2% in 1998/99 to 36.8% in 2019 (Table 4.6). Using the HES microdata and reconfiguring the data by individuals, 6.3% of the older persons in the sample are living alone, while 19.1% live with other older persons, and the remaining 74.5% live in households with at least a non-elderly. Patterns of living arrangement have a direct impact on the availability of child support for older persons, and the data suggest a growing need for ageing-in-place solutions. Helping families to care for ageing family members should be a policy priority, especially for poor and low-income households.

---

[12] Mean B40 household income increased from RM2,848 in 2016 to RM3,152 in 2019 (DOSM, 2020a).

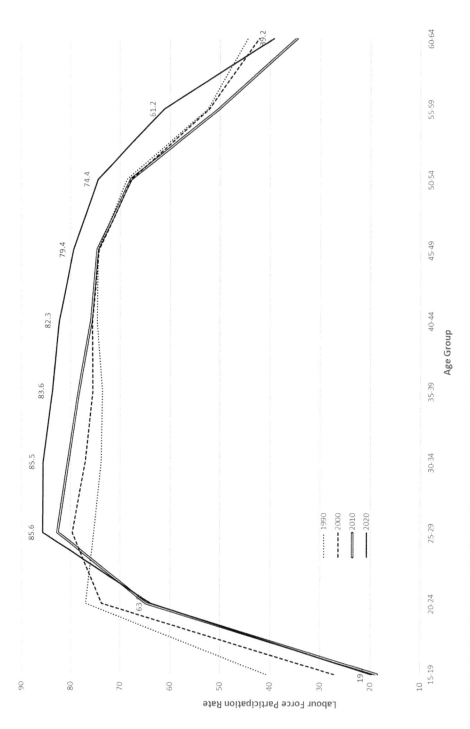

FIGURE 4.5 Labour force participation rate by age group, Malaysia, 1990–2020. Department of Statistics Malaysia, 1991; 2001b; 2011b; 2021

Policy Development on Ageing in Malaysia

TABLE 4.6

Households With and Without Older Persons, Malaysia, 1998/99–2019

Household Composition	1998/99			2009			2019		
	n	%	Hh Size	*n*	%	Hh Size	*n*	%	Hh Size
One-Person Households									
Non-older Persons Living Alone	259	9.4	1.0	436	6.7	1.0	809	4.9	1.0
Older Persons Living Alone	77	2.8	1.0	159	2.4	1.0	540	3.3	1.0
Multi-person Households									
Households without Older Persons	1,861	67.4	4.8	4,350	67.0	4.6	9,530	58.3	4.3
Households with Older Persons and Non-older Persons	516	18.7	4.9	1,373	21.1	4.7	4,678	28.6	4.4
Households with only Older Persons	48	1.7	2.0	177	2.7	2.0	797	4.9	2.0
Households in Microdata Sample (30%)	**2,761**	**100.0**	**4.3**	6,495	100.0	4.2	16,354	100.0	**3.9**
Total Households (in Thousands)		**5,047.0**			6,557.9			8,001.7	

Source: Author tabulated from HES Microdata from the Department of Statistics Malaysia, 2012; 2020.

The history of old folks' homes in Malaysia can be traced to charity homes and shelters for unmarried and childless elderly in pre-Independence days (Ibrahim et al., 2018). Many of these institutions, including the Federal-funded *Rumah Seri Kenangan* ($n = 10$) and various State-supported facilities, provide an option of last resort for older persons without dependents in terms of board and lodging. In the 1990s, with the liberalization of the private healthcare sector, nursing homes and care centres began to proliferate, providing middle-class families with an alternative for paid assisted living services. The residential aged care facilities are regulated under the Care Centres Act 1993 (Act 506) and the Private Healthcare Facilities and Services Act 1998 (Act 586). According to the data released by the Department of Social Welfare, there are 358 registered care centres under Act 506 in 2019 with 1,758 care workers caring for 7,440 older residents (Department of Social Welfare, 2020). This does not include the 1,405 older residents in the nine Federal-funded old folks' homes in the same year, as well as the 826 beds at the 21 MOH-registered private nursing facilities under Act 586. Alternative housing such as the recent mushrooming of retirement villages and traditional Islamic elder hostels (*pondok warga emas*) are emerging senior living trends that have often been overlooked. Past studies at the Malaysian Research Institute on Ageing, UPM, have estimated about two-thirds of the residential aged care facilities remain unregistered or unlicensed and this is a major challenge for the newly established Association for Residential

48 Healthy Ageing in Asia

Aged Care Operators of Malaysia (AgeCOpe). While the latest Physical Planning Guideline for Older Persons (GP031-A) had been published by PLANMalaysia since 2018, its adoption is still limited to a few States. Policies, rules and regulations on aged care are sometimes interpreted and enforced differently by local government authorities, district welfare offices and public health/safety regulators (Haron et al., 2019).

Social Participation

Social programmes refer to the participation of older persons in organized sociocultural and political activities. There are limited nationwide data on volunteer activities as well as the participation of seniors in civil society organizations. A cursory search of the Registrar of Societies using keywords such as senior citizens, pensioners, retirees, elderly and older persons yielded over 548 active associations in mid-2019.

Senior citizens clubs or senior centres are the oldest and perhaps the most popular form of recreational entity that attracts the elderly. The non-profit National Council of Senior Citizens Organizations Malaysia, or NACSCOM was established in 1990, and it is an umbrella body with 40 affiliates and over 20,000 members throughout the country. Since its inception, NACSCOM has been an active advocate of elder rights and senior voice in promoting the welfare and well-being of the older population. Under the National Policy for the Elderly (NPE), the Ministry of Health also actively helps establish senior citizen health clubs that are linked to the respective public primary health clinics all over Malaysia. There are about 284 active senior health clubs in Malaysia with 14,115 members (Family Health Development Division, 2020 [personal communication]). Most carry out learning activities related to health and fitness as well as social programmes among its members. The Senior Citizen Activity Centres or PAWE with annual grant support from the Department of Social Welfare grew quickly, and presently, there are about 143 PAWEs throughout Malaysia, and many have registered themselves with the ROS. MyAgeing™, UPM, introduced a self-help lifelong learning initiative under the University of the Third Age (U3A) programme in 2008, and there are now three independent U3As in Kuala Lumpur and Selangor, Bandar Utama and Petaling Jaya (Hamid et al., 2019). All the 102 community colleges in Malaysia also offer free short-term courses for senior citizens and persons with disabilities, as the Department of Community Colleges under the Ministry of Higher Education actively targets older persons through their in-house programmes and activities. Neighbourhood watch programmes (Komuniti Rukun Tetangga, KRT) under the Department of National Unity and Integrity also support a Senior Neighbour (Jiran Warga Emas) initiative to engage older persons living in the community as mentors and advisors.

The World Values Survey has regularly collected information on social participation and activism in many countries around the globe, and Malaysia has been involved in three waves (5, 6 and 7) since 2006. Using the latest publicly available microdata for 2018, it is evident that older persons, despite the small survey sample, are more active in religious organizations and in getting out to vote (Table 4.7). Social engagement is important for seniors as those who are socially active can benefit from the sense of belonging and fellowship that can boost their self-esteem, sense of self-worth as well as reducing loneliness. Today, there are many civil society

TABLE 4.7
Social Participation of Malaysians by Age Group, 2018

	Young Adult ($n_{18-29} = 419$)		Adult ($n_{30-44} = 471$)		Middle-aged Adult ($n_{45-59} = 339$)		Older Person ($n_{60+} = 84$)	
	n.	%	*n.*	%	*n.*	%	*n.*	%
Membership in Religious Organization	202	48.2	204	43.3	159	46.9	43	51.2
Membership in Sports or Recreational Organization	180	43.0	178	37.8	106	31.3	15	17.9
Membership in Arts, Music or Educational Organization	152	36.3	135	28.7	86	25.4	18	21.4
Membership in Political Party	114	27.2	135	28.7	88	26.0	20	23.8
Membership in Environmental Organization	135	32.2	112	23.8	86	25.4	12	14.3
Membership in Professional Organization	131	31.3	147	31.2	104	30.7	23	27.4
Membership in Charitable or Humanitarian Organization	148	35.3	138	29.3	110	32.4	13	15.5
Membership in Self-help or Mutual Aid Group	136	32.5	118	25.1	93	27.4	16	19.0
Social Activism: Donated to a Group or Campaign	181	43.2	196	41.6	148	43.7	35	41.7
Social Activism: Contacted a Government Official	117	27.9	138	29.3	75	22.1	17	20.2
Social Activism: Encouraged Others to Vote	139	33.2	184	39.1	167	49.3	39	46.4
Always Vote in Elections: Local Level	118	28.2	254	53.9	206	60.8	59	70.2
Always Vote in Elections: National Level	107	25.5	239	50.7	199	58.7	59	70.2

Source: Author Tabulated from World Values Survey, Malaysia (Haerpfer et. al., 2020).

organizations (CSO) and non-governmental organizations (NGO) championing the rights of and opportunities for older persons. Many social enterprises as well as businesses are carving out new markets for old-age employment, senior housing, third age education, media and recreation, including mobile healthcare services and social care services tailored to the needs of the elderly and their families. What was once a target group dominated by welfare-centric and end-of-life issues and concerns, many stakeholders today are slowly recognizing older consumers as a viable market segment in an emerging silver-hair economy.

Transport and Others

Older persons have always enjoyed discounts and concession fare for rail, bus and even some flight services. The MyRapid Senior Citizen Concession Card, for example, allows individuals aged 60 years or over to enjoy a 50% discount on all travels via Rapid KL Bus, Bus Rapid Transit (BRT), Light Rapid Transit (LRT), Monorail and Mass Rapid Transit (MRT) services that are found in the greater Klang Valley area. Similarly, for a small yearly fee of RM10, older persons can get a KTM Commuter Link Senior Citizen Card to be eligible for 50% discounts on travels between KTM commuter stations under the Malayan Railways Berhad (KTMB).

Older persons also can use their Identity Card to be entitled for express bus interstate travel discounts offered by private operators. The same works for other promotional offers by private businesses and corporations, including hotel accommodation, dining and retail. The Kenyalang Gold Card, for example, is a Sarawak State Government initiative that enables senior citizens to enjoy essential products and services with instant discounts and rebates. The Selangor State Government's Elderly-friendly Scheme (*Skim Mesra Usia Emas*) provides a RM100 shopping voucher and RM500 death benefits for senior citizens through the respective State Assembly person's service centres. The Penang State Government, on the other hand, runs a Senior Citizen Appreciation Programme that gives RM130 to registered voters aged 60 years or over. Some State religious authorities operate Islamic care homes, and Zakat welfare relief recipients include the elderly poor and destitute.

Much infrastructure and system improvement are needed apart from rebates, concessionaries and discounts. Age-friendly physical and social environments are critical to encourage healthy, active and productive ageing by enhancing opportunities for security, participation and better quality of life. In the following section, we will deliberate on key policy issues, challenges and recommendations to address the different stages of ageing across the life course.

POLICY ISSUES, CHALLENGES AND RECOMMENDATIONS

Policies on ageing and older persons in Malaysia have been put in place since the NPE in 1995. As a rapidly ageing middle-income country, Malaysia is greying at lower levels of development with little time to put in place proper administrative responses to the changing population dynamics as a result of intertwined economic, public health and social developments.

HEALTH CARE, SOCIAL CARE AND LONG-TERM CARE FOR OLDER PERSONS

The most critical issue about health care for older persons in Malaysia is intrinsically tied to our two-tier public health system. The older population is highly dependent on the heavily subsidized services provided by government hospitals and health clinics. Yet, the rising private household out-of-pocket (OOP) health expenditure suggests new dynamics at play. The Malaysia National Health Accounts (MNHA) Health Expenditure Report 1997–2017 showed that OOP health expenditure to public and private providers of health care increased from RM3,166 million in 1997 to RM21,573 in 2017 (Ministry of Health, 2019). Of that 2017 figure, nearly RM20.4 billion goes

Policy Development on Ageing in Malaysia

to private providers and about RM10 billion (44.9%) is spent on private hospitals, followed by private medical clinics (22.3%) and private pharmacies (14.4%).

Considering that in 2019 there are only 17,325 beds at 250 private hospitals, compared to the 46,988 beds at 154 government hospitals, with the number of government hospital admissions (2.6 million) and outpatient attendances (21.6 million) surpassing that of private hospital admissions (1.2 million) and outpatient attendances (3.5 million), we are looking at a situation where the public healthcare sector shoulders the bulk of work but receiving only half of the financing. Of the RM57.4 billion total expenditure on health in 2017, 51.1% was financed publicly (Ministry of Health, 2019). Public healthcare facilities are overcrowded, understaffed and inadequately funded. With a growing demand due to population ageing, the national healthcare system needs serious reform and resource investment. The COVID-19 pandemic has our public healthcare system bursting at the seams, and we need to seriously contemplate a national health insurance to inject the much-needed capital to upgrade our public health infrastructure. While decentralization of the health system may raise issues of equity and efficiency, these are opportunities for better resource allocation, priority setting and financial management functions to increase organizational capacity and accountability.

The Ministry of Health is the main custodian of elderly healthcare programmes in Malaysia, and there are major similarities to UK's NHS. However, if we do not address the growing gap between the public and private healthcare services, the shortage of facilities and expertise in government hospitals and clinics will only worsen. Without the investment of capital from a national health insurance, it is difficult to imagine or put in place an equitable long-term care financing model for a rapidly ageing population. Less than ten public hospitals have a geriatric unit, and there is only one rehabilitation hospital. Although the Ministry of Health has trained many primary care professionals, nurses, medical attendants and care workers through post-basic geriatric care training, there is a need for more comprehensive accreditation and certification programmes. Without sufficient manpower, the aged care industry will have to continue relying on cheap, foreign labour to break-even as operators could not make the job positions attractive enough when compared to other nursing jobs.

Old age and ageing are multidisciplinary, and there are considerable branches in the medical and allied health fields. The National Oral Health Plan 2011–2020 (Ministry of Health, 2011), the National Plan of Action for Nutrition of Malaysia III, 2016–2025 (Ministry of Health, 2016), the National Strategic Plan for Active Living, 2017–2025 (Ministry of Health, 2018) and the National Palliative Care Strategy and Policy. 2019–2030 (Ministry of Health, 2019) all contain significant references to the elderly and older population. This is not limited to other related and important policy documents such as the National Strategic Plan for Non-Communicable Diseases, 2016–2025 (2016) and others such as the National Dementia Plan that are still in the works. The ambit and purview of the Ministry of Health in Malaysia is broad with multiple roles as service provider, researcher, regulator and funder, and unfortunately too much of a focus on curative care. A properly designed national health insurance can go a long way in promoting healthy lifestyles and good habits, rewarding good behaviour with reduced premiums or other incentives.

Apart from financing and human resource issues, the fragmentation of healthcare services and social care services has resulted in a poor quality of care for the elderly in Malaysia. Assistance with activities of daily living or other daily tasks such as doing groceries, housework or paying bills is not costly, but it can help an older person to continue living in the community. Institutionalization is costly, and the government needs to support and promote home-based and community care as an alternative. Mobile or home-based nursing regulations are needed to ensure uniform minimum standards, and the International Guidelines for Home Health Nursing and other similar initiatives should be adopted (Narayan et al., 2017). Home visits and home help are more social in nature, and we need better home-based long-term care services and products in the market.

This brings us to the most pressing issue of enforcement and regulatory matters. The long-standing issue of registration and licensing of aged care facilities must be resolved with direct input from industry players. It is in the operators' own interest to weed out bad apples and protect the aged care industry from unscrupulous and unfair practices that damage public confidence and consumer trust in their services. Although the Private Aged Healthcare Facilities and Services Act 2018 (Act 802) has been gazetted, it is still not in force pending the passing of its regulations. The COVID-19 testing, infection control training and vaccination drive represent an opportunity for multisectoral stakeholders, especially the Ministry of Health, the Department of Social Welfare and the local authorities, to dialogue and work together in tandem to resolve the many outstanding issues that have been plaguing the aged care sector for decades. While overnight solutions will be hard to come by, significant progress can be made if the authorities, operators and their staff, clients and their family members can standardize some of the operating procedures to ensure minimum standards of care are achieved and minimize risks to all parties involved. We need to put in place best practices as well as proper monitoring and regulatory framework so that the aged care industry can still be within the reach of middle- and lower-income families.

The challenges facing the long-term care industry in Malaysia can be summarized into three, a. funding issues affecting the sustainability and services of aged care operators, especially the ability of NGOs and civil society groups to contain the cost of care and also the unregulated pricing of aged care services by private businesses. We do not have a national long-term care insurance, and out-of-pocket payments are coming out from adult children instead of the elderly clients themselves. Secondly, b. issues related to human resources and the career pathways of care workers. Remuneration is low, and the limited opportunities for advancement have resulted in high staff turnover. Without a national, regional or internationally recognized training and certification programme, care work is a dead-end job with little prospect for career development. Lack of proper training may well contribute to elder abuse in institutions. Finally, c. the regulatory oversight of older persons cut across different government ministries, departments and agencies, as well as different levels of government. The lack of an industry watchdog or independent ombudsman means that consumers and clients are left with little recourse when dispute arises and there is a genuine need for an oversight entity or tribunal to promote the proper growth of the aged care industry. The interests of all stakeholders are better served if there is a platform where grievances could be heard and addressed quickly, transparently and fairly.

Policy Development on Ageing in Malaysia

INCOME SECURITY AND FINANCING OLD AGE

Financing old age and income security in later life are major concerns for both the Government and the individual elderly. The rapid increase in the number of older persons in the society has fiscal implications in terms of social protection and healthcare expenditure, while for the older persons, questions of retirement savings adequacy will persist as longer life expectancy means we need to stretch our dollars to make it last.

The Government's dilemma can be approached from two perspectives, namely the non-contributory and contributory pension systems. As illustrated earlier in Figure 4.4, social assistance schemes such as the BOT and occupational pension for civil servants are paid out from general revenue. As the value for cash transfer programmes increases, as well as the adjusted salary increments, the Government will have to spend a significant portion of its income on pensions and gratuities as well as on subsidies and welfare programmes. The Government expenditure on pension and gratuities was RM25.8 billion in 2018, and the expenditure on emolument was RM81.3 billion (Ministry of Finance, 2019). As a share of total current expenditure, the government is spending about 11% on pensions and 35% on salaries, translating to about 1.8% and 5.6% of our national GDP at current prices. At present, the civil service pension is unfunded and charged using proceeds from the Federal Consolidated Fund, as provided under the Pensions Act 1980 and the Federal Constitution. When the Pensions Trust Fund Act was enacted in 1991, it was aimed to assist the government in funding its future pension liability as an employer. The Federal Government contributes only 5% of the total emolument budget for their employees, while statutory bodies, local authorities and agencies contribute 17.5% of the basic salary of their pensionable staff. Compared to the total EPF contribution rates of 24%, it is evident that the Government is not actualizing the true cost of hiring Federal employees.

On the other hand, the Government is also not spending anything for the EPF – a defined contribution retirement savings plan for private sector workers. The average savings of active members at age 54 were RM227,861 in 2019 (Employees' Provident Fund, 2020). If we use the average life expectancy of 75 to estimate remaining years of life, the average amount to last for 20 years is only slightly less than RM950 a month. Technically, there is zero pension replacement rate for EPF as the retirement savings are disbursed on a lump-sum basis at the withdrawal age of 55. Unfortunately, changes in the population age-sex structure, labour force trends as well as general expectations of retirement living have led to the need for a critical reassessment of our social protection system's adequacy, equitability and sustainability.

One way forward is to reduce differences in benefits by introducing simultaneous reforms to make wages more sustainable for all. Civil servants could start making some contributions to their own pension fund, while private sector workers should receive their retirement income via an annuity plan. Similarly, contributions to EPF should be capped for those earning over RM24,000 a month. Setting a contribution ceiling would improve flow of excess funds to the financial market, including the PRS and other bond or mutual fund products. However, precautions must be taken against property speculation where higher stamp duty charges can be set for high net-worth individuals purchasing low or medium cost properties or enact rent control measures and empty homes tax penalties. Researchers need to analyse both the EPF and Civil Service pension data over time to understand its trends and patterns, as productivity gains benefit the society whether the employer is the government or a private company. Individual accounts, notional or fully funded, are the way forward, with strong built-in elements of risk pooling and redistribution. When individual pension or retirement savings run out, then perhaps the old-age social welfare assistance scheme can then kick in or a new long-term care insurance can be introduced.

It is important to note that any reforms must happen hand in hand with public mindset change. If the Government is to undertake the responsibility of covering for any longevity shortfalls in the annuity scheme, the amount pledged under the annuity scheme no longer belongs to the personal account holder as the Government's risk pooling exercise must come with caveats. Pension schemes, especially defined benefit plans, must be designed to be sustainable as it is highly susceptible to longevity risks. The current thinking on social assistance is also outdated as the fixed amount of aid for specific target welfare recipients provides more administrative convenience than actual relief to beneficiaries. It would have been more family-friendly if financial aid is given based on an assessment of the household as a whole and the quantum is variate according to need. An increase in aid cash value might just result in less aid coverage. The Government needs to seriously consider the use of a Household Registration System to streamline routine population data collection and census tracking, which will make it easier for other reforms such as automatic voter registration and targeted fuel subsidies.

It must be pointed out that old-age poverty is not as straightforward as income poverty due to a few factors. The problem of targeting is not satisfactorily addressed with the adoption of a flat-rate universal pension, considering the many alternative options that are available to us. Solutions to a sustainable pension system must be evaluated as a whole and not from a limited perspective that divides the population into working or non-working groups, nor from a flawed dichotomy of public sector vs. private sector workers. The two key ingredients missing from our social protection system are **redistribution** (reducing inequalities in income, opportunities and access) and **risk pooling** (sharing of risks on the principle of solidarity) elements. There is a gross public misunderstanding of what it takes for Malaysia to put in place an equitable and sustainable pension system for older persons without having to choose between the extremities of a welfare state and laissez-faire capitalism. Without underscoring the importance of intergenerational equity and improving public understanding of lifecycle deficits, it is difficult to effect meaningful reforms for a second demographic dividend.

ASSISTIVE TECHNOLOGY, BUILT AND SOCIAL ENVIRONMENTS

As urbanity rises, more people will grow into old age in towns and cities. Currently, there are numerous challenges concerning the adequacy, suitability and availability of facilities and services for older persons living in the community, especially in rural areas. Our own study has shown that most adults and the elderly (77.6%) do not plan to move from their current house (Universiti Putra Malaysia, 2017). Yet, our housing design, both indoor and outdoor spaces and public transportation system are not age-friendly. We spoke about baby proofing a home in the anticipation of newborns to the family, but modifications to senior proof your dwelling are both uncommon and expensive. Little thought is given to home safety and neighbourhood security for the elderly, something that can be easily addressed with the application of universal design principles.

Our society needs to provide opportunities for older persons to participate in policymaking, environmental or urban planning, civil society movements and legislative engagements. Recently, the Government has announced the intention of drafting a bill for senior citizens, but there is little public outreach on the matter. Cities and town planners need to focus on making their public spaces more conducive for healthy and active ageing, by putting in place enablers for greater mobility and participation in neighbourhood activities. Housing and transportation needs rank high among low-income older persons with poor health (Black and Jester, 2020), as this affects their accessibility to work and health services. This is supported by a local study by Lai and her colleagues (2016) where they found that built environment barriers hindered the social interactions of the aged in the community. Social connectedness is a mediator between active ageing and the age-friendliness of the individual's environment. As indicated by Barton and Grant (2006), a well-designed outdoor space can enhance long-term health, promote physical activity and reduce social isolation (Figure 4.6).

Policymakers in Malaysia are not leveraging on technological innovations and ICT-based solutions in aged care or tackling the challenges of population ageing using new tools. Consider the experience of countries such as Japan and Sweden where there are strong policies to promote the use of ICT and healthcare technologies in the care of older persons (Onaya et al., 2015; Atarodi et al., 2019). The Japanese government not only promoted the use of next-generation ICT through special task force and senior-level committees, but also allocated budgets for the digitization of healthcare, medical care and nursing care fields. Similarly, in Sweden, government departments would test new Internet-based healthcare monitoring systems, telehealth or other assistive devices through pilot projects with residents in selected municipalities. By doing the science to compile evidence and making improvements based on user and expert feedback, we see a surge in gerontechnology innovations being adopted.

Tracing the major policies and programmes since the first National Policy for the Elderly (NPE, 1995) till the current National Policy for Older Persons (Ministry of Women, Family and Community Development, 2011), it is evident that there has been a growing emphasis on old age and ageing issues in national development plans. As more data on ageing and older persons become available, policymakers and key stakeholders must develop the will to invest in novel solutions to new problems. Ageing is multidisciplinary and multisectoral, and there must be greater inter-ministerial coordination and communication. As a country, Malaysia has its own governance and structural legacies that must be overcome. While Malaysia is undergoing transitions to become a high-income nation, we are at the same time confronted with the challenges of new generations, young and old. Malaysia's strong socio-economic development and growth can coexist with a vibrant care economy and silver-haired market.

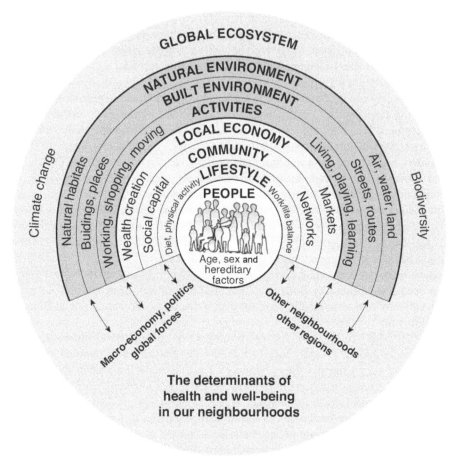

FIGURE 4.6 Health map for local human habitat. Barton and Grant, 2006

CONCLUSION

Malaysia has a short time frame of about 24 years to prepare for the looming "aged nation" status. Hence, there is an urgent need to focus on putting in place policies and programmes that will cater to the needs of the current and future aged. The future aged are already born, and each cohort of older persons differ in their background and experiences. Older persons are also spatially distributed in ways that are aligned with the historical ethnic segregations during her colonial days. Therefore, it has been noted that the Malaysian Chinese in urban areas enjoy longer life expectancy than other communities. With fewer children, however, there is a greater demand for aged care products and services. As such, the ethnic dimension in population ageing cannot be denied. Similarly, gender concerns must be incorporated in policy design and thinking as women remain disadvantaged throughout the life course in Malaysia.

Each successive cohort of older Malaysians are living longer, healthier and wealthier as a successful delay in the onset of diseases added not just years but also life to years. More is needed to encourage the population to adopt a healthy lifestyle for the prevention of non-communicable diseases. Malaysia has not really developed a comprehensive long-term care system, and public financing models are still inadequate. It has to be pointed out that a strong, centralized and Federal-driven response might not be the best way forward as different States and districts are ageing at different rates. As the last mile public service provider would be the local government, we need to think about reforms that can empower communities and municipalities to act in tandem. Federal allocations for growth and development must be more equitable as the richer States will have more resources that can be utilized to address their citizens' needs. A high percentage of older persons want to age in place, but there are very few local services available outside of major cities and towns. There is a dire need to address the missing gap in aged care products and services to ensure the well-being of all older Malaysians. There must be closer collaboration between the actors in the government, business and civil society organizations. Explaining policy choices and their consequences can help the public understand why some hard decisions must be made.

With increased longevity, there must be concomitant changes to our lifespan approach to education, work and leisure. Policies must be in place to encourage older persons to remain active and productive into old age. There is a need to reduce cultural barriers in work and labour force participation to tap into the experiences of older persons for development. We also need to reappraise our social relationships and the importance of social networks in later life. As Malaysia moves along the path of economic growth into the future, longevity issues have to be looked into as a developmental matter and not as a welfare problem. An inclusive society and a society for all ages as advocated by the SDGs call for new ways of addressing Malaysia's vision of Shared Prosperity 2030. With more and more countries in Southeast Asia experiencing similar demographic transitions, Malaysia cannot rely indefinitely on cheap, foreign labour or domestic helpers in the care of older persons. Population ageing is a human success story (United Nations, 2019b), and it is up to us to decide how best we can make Malaysia a better place for everyone to live in.

REFERENCES

Abdul Khalid, M. (2016) *SDD-SSPS Project Working Paper Series: Income Security for Older Persons in Asia and the Pacific: Income security for older persons in Malaysia.* Bangkok: UNESCAP.

Abdullah, R. (1993) Changing population policies and women's lives in Malaysia. *Reproductive Health Matters*, 1(1), 67–77.

Atarodi, S., Berardi, A. M. and Toniolo, A. (2019) Comparing local policy practices to implement ICT-based home care services for aging-in-place in Finland, France, Italy, Spain & Sweden. *Gerontechnology*, 18(2), 108–121.

Barraclough, S. (2000) The politics of privatization in the Malaysian health care system. *Contemporary Southeast Asia*, 22(2), 340–359.

Barton, H. and Grant, M. (2006) A health map for the local human habitat. *The Journal of the Royal Society for the Promotion of Health*, 126(6), 252–253.

Black, K. and Jester, D. J. (2020) Examining older adults' perspectives on the built environment and correlates of healthy aging in an American age-friendly community. *International Journal of Environmental Research and Public Health*, 17(19), 7056.

Chander, R. (Ed.) (1975) *The Population of Malaysia*. Paris: CICRED Series.

Chen, A. J. and Jones, G. (1989) *Ageing in ASEAN: Its Socio-Economic Consequences*. Singapore: Institute of Southeast Asian Studies.

Chen, C. Y. P., Andrews, G. R., Josef, R., Chan, K. E. and Arokiasamy, J. T. (1986) *Health and Ageing in Malaysia. A Study Sponsored by the World Health Organization*. Kuala Lumpur: Faculty of Medicine, University of Malaya.

Coulmas, F. (2007) *Population Decline and Ageing in Japan: The Social Consequences*. London: Routledge.

Cowgill, D. O. and Holmes, L. D. (1972) *Aging and Modernization*. New York: Appleton-Century-Croft.

Department of Statistics Malaysia (1991) *Labour Force Survey Report 1990*. Kuala Lumpur: DOSM.

———— (2001a) *Population Distribution and Basic Demographic Characteristics 2000. Population and Housing Census of Malaysia 2000*. Putrajaya: DOSM.

———— (2001b) *Labour Force Survey Report 2000*. Putrajaya: DOSM.

———— (2007) *Intercensal Population Estimates by Age Group, Ethnic Group and Sex, Malaysia, 1970–2020* [Unpublished tabulated data]. Putrajaya: DOSM.

———— (2011a) Population Distribution and Basic Demographic Characteristic 2010. *Population and Housing Census of Malaysia 2010*. DOSM: Putrajaya.

———— (2011b) *Labour Force Survey Report 2010*. Putrajaya: DOSM.

———— (2012) *30% Sample for Household Expenditure Survey 1998/99, 2004 & 2009* [Unpublished microdata]. Putrajaya: DOSM.

———— (2015) *Vital Statistic Malaysia, 2014*. Putrajaya: DOSM.

———— (2016a) *Population Projections (Revised), Malaysia, 2010–2040*. Putrajaya: DOSM.

———— (2016b) *Population by Age Group, Sex and Ethnic Group, Malaysia, 2010–2040* [Unpublished tabulated data]. Putrajaya: DOSM.

———— (2019) *Abridged Life Tables, Malaysia, 2017–2019*. Putrajaya: DOSM.

———— (2020a) *Household Expenditure Survey Report 2019*. Putrajaya: DOSM.

———— (2020b) *Malaysia Economic Statistics - Time Series 2019*. Putrajaya: DOSM. Accessed from www.dosm.go.my

———— (2020bc). *Social Statistics Bulletin 2020*. Putrajaya: DOSM

———— (2020d) *30% Sample for Household Income and Expenditure Survey 2019* [Unpublished microdata], Putrajaya: DOSM.

———— (2021) *Labour Force Survey Report 2020*. Putrajaya: DOSM.

Department of Social Welfare (2020) *Number of Care Centers Registered with the Department of Social Welfare, MWFCD*. Putrajaya: MAMPU. Malaysia Open Data Portal. Accessed fromwww.data.gov.my

Department of Social Welfare (2021) *Senarai Pusat Aktiviti Warga Emas (PAWE)*. Accessed from www.jkm.gov.my

Dwyer, D. (1987) New population policies in Malaysia and Singapore, *Geography*, 72, 248–250.

Economic Planning Unit (1995) *Seventh Malaysia Plan, 1996–2000*. Kuala Lumpur: Percetakan Nasional Malaysia Berhad.

———— (2000) *Eighth Malaysia Plan, 2001–2005*. Kuala Lumpur: Percetakan Nasional Malaysia Berhad.

———— (2005) *Ninth Malaysia Plan, 2006–2010*. Kuala Lumpur: Percetakan Nasional Malaysia Berhad.

———— (2010) *Tenth Malaysia Plan, 2011–2015*. Kuala Lumpur: Percetakan Nasional Malaysia Berhad.

———— (2015) *Eleventh Malaysia Plan, 2016–2020*. Kuala Lumpur: Percetakan Nasional Malaysia Berhad.

Policy Development on Ageing in Malaysia

———— (2018). *Mid-term Review 11ᵗʰ Malaysian Plan 2016–2020: New Priorities and Emphases*. Putrajaya: Percetakan Nasional Malaysia Berhad.

Employees' Provident Fund (2020). *Annual Report 2019*. Kuala Lumpur: EPF.

Haerpfer, C., Inglehart, R., Moreno, A., Welzel, C., Kizilova, K., Diez-Medrano, J. M., Lagos, P., Norris, E., Ponarin, B. and Puranen, B. et al. (Eds.) (2020). *World Values Survey: Round Seven - Country-Pooled Datafile*. Madrid, Spain & Vienna, Austria: JD Systems Institute & WVSA Secretariat. doi.org/10.14281/18241.1

Hamid, T. A. (2017) *Ageing and Elderly Population in Perak [Unpublished project report]*. Putrajaya: UNDP Malaysia.

Hamid, T. A. and Chai, S. T. (2017) Meeting the needs of older Malaysians: Expansion, diversification and multi-sector collaboration. *Malaysian Journal of Economic Studies*, 50(2), 157–174

Hamid, T. A. and Yahya, N. (2008) National policy for the elderly in Malaysia: Achievements and challenges. In: Lee, H. G. (Ed.) *Ageing in Southeast and East Asia: Family, Social Protection and Policy Challenges*, pp. 108–133. Singapore: Institute of Southeast Asian Studies (ISEAS).

Hamid, T. A., Zakaria, N. S., Abd Rahim, N. A., Chai, S. T. and Nor Akahbar, S. A. (2019). Moving the needle on U3A in Malaysia: Recent developments and prospects. In: Formosa, M. (Ed.) *The University of the Third Age and Active Ageing: International Perspectives on Aging*, vol. 23, pp. 195–206. New York: Springer International.

Hansard (1959) *House of Representatives Official Report, Parliamentary Debates*, First Parliament, First Session, 3 December 1959. Hansard, 1(10). Accessed from www.parlimen.gov.my/hansard-dewan-rakyat.html

———— (1973) *House of Representatives Official Report, Parliamentary Debates*, Third Parliament, Third Session, 18 December 1973. Hansard, 3(42). Accessed from www.parlimen.gov.my/hansard-dewan-rakyat.html

———— (2009) *Senate Official Report*, Twelfth Parliament, Second Session, 6 July 2009. Hansard, 8. Accessed from www.parlimen.gov.my/hansard-dewan-negara.html

Haron, L., Hamid, T.A., Chai, S. T., Othman, A. G. and Ahmad, H. (2019) *Transitional Housing and Long-term Elderly Care Services: Final report*, Volume 1 & 2. Penang: Universiti Sains Malaysia.

Hasmuk, K., Mohammad Sallehuddin, H., Tan, M. P., Cheah, W. K., Ibrahim, R. and Chai, S. T. (2020) *The long-term care COVID-19 situation in Malaysia* (Online Report). London: International Long-Term Care Policy Network, Care Policy and Evaluation Centre (CPEC). Accessed from ltccovid.org/wp-content/uploads/2020/10/Malaysia-LTC-COVID-situation-report-2-October-2020-1.pdf

Hirschman, C. (1980) Demographic trends in Peninsular Malaysia, 1947–75. *Population and Development Review*, 6(1), 103–125.

Ho, B. K., Jasvindar, K., Gurpreet, K., Ambigga, D., Suthahar, A., Cheong, S. M. and Lim, K. H. (2014) Prevalence, awareness, treatment, and control of diabetes mellitus among the elderly: The 2011 National Health and Morbidity Survey, Malaysia. *Malaysian Family Physician*, 9(3), 12–19.

Ho, B. K., Omar, M. A., Sooryanarayana, R., Ghazali, S. S., Zainal Abidin, S. I., Krishnapillai, A., Ariaratnam, S., Tohit, N. M., Abdul Majid, N. L. and Mohd Yusof, M. F. (2020) Trends in population blood pressure and prevalence, awareness, treatment and control of hypertension among older persons: The 2006 & 2015 National Health and Morbidity Survey in Malaysia. *PLOS One*, 15(9), e0238780.

Holzmann, R. (2015). *Old-Age Financial Protection in Malaysia: Challenges and Options*. IZA Policy Paper No. 6. Bonn: Institute for the Study of Labor.

Hurd, M. D. (1990). Research on the elderly: Economic status, retirement, and consumption and saving. *Journal of Economic Literature*, 28(2), 565–637.

Ibrahim, R., Hamid, T. A., Chai, S. T. and Ashari, A. (2018) Malaysia. In: Loichinger, E. and Pothisiri, W. (Eds.) *Research Project on Care for the Elderly in ASEAN+3: The Role of Families and Local and National Support Systems*, pp. 113–140. Bangkok: Department of Older Persons, Ministry of Social Development and Human Security.

ILMIA (2019). *National Employment Returns (NER) 2019.* Selangor: Institute of Labour Market Information and Analysis (ILMIA). Accessed from https://www.ilmia.gov.my/index.php/en/component/zoo/item/national-employment-returns-ner-2019

Institute for Public Health (2019). *National Health and Morbidity Survey (NHMS) 2018: Elderly Health. Volume II: Elderly Health Findings.* Putrajaya: IPH, National Institutes of Health, Ministry of Health Malaysia.

Institute of Labour Market Information and Analysis (2019) *National Strategic Development Plan on Ageing Population: Inclusion and Employment of Malaysia's Ageing Population.* Cyberjaya: Ministry of Human Resources.

Jones, G. W. and Tan, P. C. (1985) Recent and prospective population trends in Malaysia. *Journal of Southeast Asian Studies*, 16, 262–280.

Kinsella, K. and He, W. (2009) An Aging World: 2008. *International Population Reports, P95/09-1.* U.S. Census Bureau: Washington.

Koris, R., Mohamed Nor, N., Haron, S. A., Hamid, T. A., Aljunid, S. M., Muhammad Nur, A., Wana Ismail, N., Shafie, A. A., Yusuff, S. and Maimaiti, N. (2019) The cost of healthcare among Malaysian community-dwelling elderly. *Jurnal Ekonomi Malaysia*, 53(1), 89–103.

Lai, M., Lein, S., Lau, S. and Lai, M. (2016) Modeling age-friendly environment, active ageing and social connectedness in an emerging Asian economy. *Journal of Aging Research*, Article ID: 2052380. doi.org/10.1155/2016/2052380

Lee, C. and Lee, C. (2017) The evolution of development planning in Malaysia. *Journal of Southeast Asian Economies*, 34(3), 436–461.

Leete, R. and Kwok, K. K. (1986) Demographic changes in East Malaysia and their relationship with those in the Peninsula 1960–80. *Population Studies*, 40(1), 83–100.

Mat Zin, R. (2012) Towards a social protection system in an advanced equitable Society. *ASEAN Economic Bulletin*, 29(3), 197–217.

Ministry of Finance (2019). *Economic Outlook 2020.* Putrajaya: MOF.

Ministry of Health (2019). *Health Expenditure Report 1997–2017.* Malaysia National Health Accounts. Putrajaya: Planning Division, MOH.

Ministry of Health (2020) *Annual Report 2019.* Putrajaya: MOH.

Ministry of Women, Family and Community Development (2011) *National Policy for Older Persons 2011–2020.* Putrajaya: MWFCD.

Mohd. Yatim, M. and Ramli, N. (1988). *Malaysia Country Report on Socio-economic Consequences of the Ageing of Population Survey 1986.* Kuala Lumpur: National Population and Family Development Board Malaysia.

Narayan, M., Farris, C., Harris, M. D., & Hiong, F. Y. (2017). Development of the International Guidelines for Home Health Nursing. *Home Healthcare Now*, 35(9), 494–506.

NPFDB (2015). *Fifth Malaysian Population and Family Survey.* Kuala Lumpur: Population and Family Research Sector, National Population and Family Development Board. Accessed from http://www.lppkn.gov.my/index.php?option=com_content&view=article&id=211&Itemid=787(=en

Onaya, T., Taketomi, M., Fujii, H. and Negishi, T. (2015) ICT Trends in Japan's healthcare policy. *Fujitsu Scientific & Technical Journal*, 51(3), 10–17.

Ong, F. S. (2002) Ageing in Malaysia: A review of national policies and programmes. In: Phillips, D. R. and Chan, A. C. M. (Eds.) *Ageing and Long-term Care: National Policies in the Asia-Pacific*, pp. 107–149. Singapore: Institute of Southeast Asian Studies (ISEAS).

Ong, F. S. (2007) Health care and long-term care issues for the elderly. In: Chee, H. L. and Barraclough, S. (Eds.) *Health Care in Malaysia: The Dynamics of Provision, Financing and Access*, pp. 170–186. Oxford: Routledge.

Ong, F.S. and Hamid, T. A. (2010). Social protection in Malaysia: Current state and challenges. In: Asher, M. G., Oum, S. and Parulian, F. (Eds.) *Social Protection in East Asia: Current State and Challenges*, pp. 182–219. Jakarta: Economic Research Institute for ASEAN and East Asia (ERIA).

Pala, J. (1998) *Senior Citizens and Population Ageing in Malaysia*. Population Census Monograph Series. No. 4. Kuala Lumpur: Department of Statistics Malaysia.

Pala, J. (2005) *Population Ageing Trends in Malaysia. Monograph Series, Population Census 2000*. Putrajaya: Department of Statistics Malaysia.

Shrestha, L. (2000) Population aging in developing countries. *Health Affairs*, 19(3), 204–212.

Sushama, P. C. (1985) Malaysia. In: Dixon, J. and Hyung, S. K. (Eds.) *Social Welfare in Asia*. London: Croom Helm.

Tan, M. P., Kamaruzzaman, S. B. and Poi, P. J. H. (2018) An analysis of geriatric medicine in Malaysia: Riding the wave of political change. *Geriatrics*, 3(4), 80.

Tey, N. P. and Lai S. L. (2018) The changing demographic landscape of the Chinese Community in Malaysia since 1970. *Malaysian Journal of Chinese Studies*, 7(1), 19–35.

United Nations (2017). *Living Arrangements of Older Persons: A Report on an Expanded International Dataset* (ST/ESA/SER.A/407). New York: Population Division, Department of Economic and Social Affairs.

United Nations (2019a) *World Population Prospects, 2019 Revision*. New York: Population Division, Department of Economic and Social Affairs. Accessed from population.un.org/wpp/

United Nations (2019b) *World Population Ageing 2019: Highlights* (ST/ESA/SER.A/430). New York: Population Division, Department of Economic and Social Affairs.

Universiti Putra Malaysia (2017a) *Kajian kemudahan dan perkhidmatan bagi memenuhi keperluan warga emas menjelang 2030*. Department of Social Welfare: UPM Consultancy & Services.

Universiti Putra Malaysia (2017b) *Kajian keberkesanan bantuan kewangan Jabatan Kebajikan Masyarakat*. Department of Social Welfare: UPM Consultancy & Services.

Vanoh, D., Shahar, S., Che Din, N., Omar, A., Chin, A. V., Razali, R., Ibrahim, R. and Hamid, T. A. (2016) Predictors of poor cognitive status among older Malaysian adults: baseline findings from the LRGS TUA cohort study. *Aging Clinical and Experimental Research*, 29(2), 173–182.

World Bank (2020) World Development Indicators. Washington: World Bank. Accessed from databank.worldbank.org/

Yaakob, U., Masron, T. and Fujimaki, M. (2011) Ninety years of urbanization in Malaysia: A geographical investigation of its trends and characteristics. *Journal of Ritsumeikan Social Sciences and Humanities*, 4, 79–102.

5 Enriching the Lives of Seniors in Japan (Ikigai Healthy Ageing Policy in Japan)

Tomonori Maruyama
The Japan Mibyou Institute United

CONTENTS

The Problem of the Best Longevity Country in the World 63
Government Policies for Supporting "100-Year Life Society"................................64
Key Values to Live Longer with a Healthy Body and Mind – ikigai......................65
Challenges for Creating Innovation for the Well-Ageing Society 67
    Well-Ageing Society Summit Asia-Japan..67
    Regional Councils on Healthcare Industry of Next Generation and
    Other Organizations 68
    Challenge for Co-Creation of Wellness Tourism 69
Socio-industrial Structural Changes Required: Expectations for the Future 70

THE PROBLEM OF THE BEST LONGEVITY COUNTRY IN THE WORLD

Japan is the world's best longevity country. According to the WHO, in 2018, the average life expectancy in Japan is 84.2 years old. (Men live an average of 81.1 years and women live an average of 87.1 years.)

However, we have problems that Japan's population is rapidly declining and ageing. A report from OECD in April 2018 says that the total population is projected to decline by almost 25% between 2015 and 2050, falling below 100 million. Meantime, the elderly dependency ratio (the elderly population as a share of the working-age population), which was also the highest in the OECD (at 44% in 2015), is projected to remain the highest (at 73% in 2050)[1].

And we have another problem also that there is a gap of about 10 years between "healthy lifespan" and "average lifespan". The healthy lifespan (or healthy life

---

[1] OECD, *JAPAN: PROMOTING INCLUSIVE GROWTH FOR AN AGEING SOCIETY,* 2018 (https://www.oecd.org/about/secretary-general/BPS-Japan-EN-April-2018.pdf)

DOI: 10.1201/9781003043270-5

expectancy: average number of years that a person can expect to live in "full health" by taking into account years lived in less than full health due to disease and/or injury) of Japanese men increased by 0.95 years to 72.14 years from 2013 to 2016, while that of women increased by 0.58 years to 74.79 years during this period, the Ministry of Health reported March 2018. On the other hand, the average life expectancy of Japanese people in 2016 was 80.98 years for men and 87.14 years for women.

As Japan's healthcare system is one of the most accessible in the world because the government pays 70% of the cost of all health procedures and up to 90% for low-income citizens, many Japanese do not feel a big financial pressure to use medical treatments even if they had severe disease. Thus, consequently, the Japanese spend most of the medical expense in those 10 years (the period between "healthy lifespan" and "average lifespan"). And at the same time, the population ageing will increase medical spending pressures and aggravate Japan's fiscal problems also.

Can we say that this unhealthy last 10 years of life, extended by medical technology, is a happy one for us? I believe that the value of "Well-being/Wellness" is essential to make our lives happy and meaningful.

GOVERNMENT POLICIES FOR SUPPORTING "100-YEAR LIFE SOCIETY"

To solve those problems, the government of Japan has been addressing many efforts. In September 2017, ex-Prime Minister Shinzo Abe held the first meeting of the Council for the Design of the "100-Year Life Society" at the Prime Minister's Office. At this meeting, discussions were held on how the Council should proceed in future. Human resource development ("Hito-zukuri") for the era of "100-Year Life Society" is an initiative of the Abe Cabinet to realize a society in which all citizens including the elderly can play an active role. Along with the productivity revolution, it is one of the major themes of the Abe administration.

"In any case, Japan's population will continue to decline. On the other hand, the baby-boom generation will steadily grow older. This may sound gloomy, but we can change the future if we make thorough improvements here. There was an opinion that it is important to enhance the abilities of each individual and to respond to their desire to learn and work. Another comment was "The elderly have a lot of experience, and we can use that experience to create new initiatives". Others stated that people would be able to *contribute to society and live their 100-year lives more fully* by continuing their education and embarking on new lifestyles". Abe stated at the meeting.

Following this, the Ministry of Health, Labour and Welfare (MHLW) reported in December 2017 on "Six Schemes to Support Society in the Era of 100-Year Life Society". Three of these are measures for the elderly, including "improving the treatment of nursing care personnel", "recurrent education (upgrading the skills of the elderly)" and "promoting employment of the elderly". In particular, specific measures for" promoting employment of the elderly" include "subsidies for employing elderly people aged 65 and over" and "support for employers by the Japan Organization for Employment of the Elderly, Persons with Disabilities and Job Seekers". Among the G7 countries, the elderly in Japan work the most, and this is considered to be the key

Enriching the Lives of Seniors in Japan

to realizing the 100-Year Life Society concept. According to the Japan Institute for Labour Policy and Training (JILPT), the employment rate of older men (65–69 years old) in Japan (as of 2018) is 52.9%, and the employment rate of older women in Japan is 33.4%. The rates of both men and women in Japan show the highest in G7 countries. In the employment rates of older people, the USA ranks the second country after Japan (men: 35.5% and women: 27.0%), and the third is the UK (men: 25.7% and women: 16.6%). And nearly 40% of senior Japanese employees say they want to work as long as they can. The Institute of Gerontology of the University of Tokyo conducted a survey on the employment attitudes of 171 seniors living in Kashiwa City who participated in the 2012 Employment Seminar. And the result shows that 83.5% of older people think working is important to keep healthy. (48% of them answered "very important" and 35.5% of them answered "important".) And 54% of them think working is important to contribute to colleagues. (15.3% of them answered "very important" and 38.7% of them answered "important".)

Considering the above-mentioned situations, the motivation for "working" and "contributing to the society (including colleagues)" could be thought of as key factors to realize 100-Year Life Society and enriching the lives of seniors in Japan.

KEY VALUES TO LIVE LONGER WITH A HEALTHY BODY AND MIND – IKIGAI

According to an article in the Nihon Keizai Shimbun dated 9 March 2018, Professor Ichiro Tsuji of Tohoku University, who served as the head of the research team for the Comprehensive Survey of Living Conditions in Japan (a large-scale survey conducted every 3 years by the Ministry of Health, Labour and Welfare), suggests that the following two factors may have contributed to the increase in healthy lifespan between 2006 and 2016.

1. The number of patients with cerebrovascular disease, a major cause of needing nursing care, is decreasing due to improved lifestyles.
2. Social participation opportunities for the elderly are expanding.

We used to exercise naturally through daily life in former times. To keep a healthy lifestyle, it's better to work for traditional production activities like farm work or gardening. Many Japanese seniors want to work with the communities they love as their "ikigai".

In order to conduct an in-depth field study of "ikigai", the secret of healthy longevity, two Western researchers interviewed 100 villagers in Ogimi Village, Okinawa Prefecture, one of the longest-living areas in Japan, and discovered the characteristics and principles that enable Japanese people to live a long and happy life. In their book "Ikigai: The Japanese Secret to a Long and Happy Life", Héctor García and Francesc Miralles define the rules of "ikigai".

The Japanese word "ikigai (生き甲斐)" is written by combining the word "ikiru (生きる)" (to live) and the Chinese characters "kai/gai (甲斐)" (to be worthy of living) and is understood as a word that means "the joy and tension of living" or "the value of living".

A Western Web article I found, published by Water for Health, says that "ikigai" is a Japanese concept meaning "reason for being". "It is the heart of things, the motivation at the centre of our existence: the source of value in a person's life or the things that makes them put one foot in front of the other each day. As described in the book's introduction, a deep connection with, and appreciation for, ikigai is one probable reason for the remarkable longevity of the Japanese, particularly those residing in Okinawa. Here, there are 24.55 people over the age of 100 for every 100,000 inhabitants: far more than the worldwide average. The authors speculate that there are many factors which might collude to explain Okinawa's disproportionate populace of centenarians: their uncommon sense of community; a non-exclusionary sense of oneness wherein even strangers are treated like brothers; access to lush hills and crystalline waters; Moringa tea; a light, nutritious diet and moderate exercise, even after retirement"[2].

In the last part of the book, you will find ten lessons on ikigai. Although it is composed from the perspective of Western researchers, it makes a lot of sense to me as a Japanese. This is because many of them are ordinary life wisdom that I was taught by my grandmother when I was a little boy, and they are rooted in the cultural habits of the Japanese people. Those must be the secret to a long and happy life.

TEN RULES OF IKIGAI

1. **Stay active; don't retire:** "Those who give up on the things they love doing and do well lose their purpose in life. That's why, it's so important to keep doing things of value, making progress, bringing beauty or utility to others, helping out, and shaping the world around you, even after your 'official' professional activity has ended".

2. **Take it slow:** "Being in a hurry is inversely proportional to quality of life. As the old saying goes, 'walk slowly and you'll go far.' When we leave urgency behind, life and time take on new meaning".

3. **Don't fill your stomach:** "Less is more when it comes to eating for long life, too. According to the 80% rule, in order to stay healthier longer, we should eat a little less than our hunger demands instead of stuffing ourselves".

4. **Surround yourself with good friends:** "Friends are the best medicine, there for confiding worries over a good chat, sharing stories that brighten your day, getting advice, having fun, dreaming... in other words, living".

5. **Get in shape for your next birthday:** "Water moves; it is at its best when it flows fresh and doesn't stagnate. The body you move through life in needs a bit of daily maintenance to keep it running for a long time. Plus, exercise releases hormones that make us feel happy".

---

[2] Water for Health, *Ten Rules of Ikigai: A Blueprint for a Fuller, Healthier Life?*, March 2019 (https://www.water-for-health.co.uk/our-blog/2019/03/ten-rules-of-ikigai-a-blueprint-for-a-fuller-healthier-life/)

6. **Smile:** "A cheerful attitude is not only relaxing – it also helps make friends. It's good to recognize that things aren't so great, but we should never forget what a privilege it is to be in the here and now in a world so full of possibilities".
7. **Reconnect with nature:** "Though most people live in cities these days, human beings are made to be part of the natural world. We should return to it often to recharge our batteries".
8. **Give thanks:** "To your ancestors, to nature, which provides you with the air you breathe and the food you eat, to your friends and family, to everything that brightens your days and makes you feel lucky to be alive. Spend a moment every day giving thanks, and you'll watch your stockpile of happiness grow".
9. **Live in the moment:** "Stop regretting the past and fearing the future. Today is all you have. Make the most of it. Make it worth remembering".
10. **Follow your ikigai:** "There is a passion inside you, a unique talent that gives meaning to your days and drives you to share the best of yourself until the very end. If you don't know what your ikigai is yet, as Viktor Frankl says, your mission is to discover it".[3]

Source: Héctor García and Francesc Miralles, Ikigai : the Japanese secret to a long and happy life, PENGUIN BOOKS, 2016.

---

[3] Héctor García and Francesc Miralles, *Ikigai: the Japanese secret to a long and happy life*, PENGUIN BOOKS, 2016.

CHALLENGES FOR CREATING INNOVATION FOR THE WELL-AGEING SOCIETY

So far, I have described the Japanese government's supportive measures to cope with the ageing of society, and the lifestyle of health and longevity that can be learned from the ancient Japanese sense of value (ikigai). However, for these measures to be effective in our social life, it is essential to develop the Mibyou (pre-disease)-, health- and wellness-related industries and to be convinced of the social industrial structure. In the following, I will introduce some examples of domestic efforts to create innovations for the industrialization of these fields.

WELL-AGEING SOCIETY SUMMIT ASIA-JAPAN

The wellness industry is responsible for providing services that support and promote people to lead healthy and meaningful lives. The government of Japan is strongly promoting to realize that the wellness industry would play the role in reducing the medical/nursing care costs by providing innovative services of preventive medicinal care, collaborating with various industries (including IT, agriculture, tourism, sports and health care).

One of the examples would be the 1st Well Ageing Society Summit Asia-Japan. The Ministry of Economy, Trade and Industry held the Japan Healthcare Business Contest on the 9th of October 2018 in Tokyo, in order to identify and support ventures which contribute to solving the healthcare issues including increases in medical expenditures, lifestyle-related diseases and dementia, medical disparities, and demand for elderly care and support because Japan leads the world as a super-ageing society, and thus is experiencing various social challenges before many other industrialized nations, especially in the healthcare sector. Continuous creation and development of new healthcare solutions that can respond to these diverse demands amidst systemic change are necessary in order to *ensure the quality of life in ageing societies.*

Towards these objectives, the Summit was held as an international conference where large corporations, venture companies, investors and government agencies gathered to discuss global initiatives and solutions for the super-ageing society. Through this opportunity, unique and effective business ideas were devised to address various aspects of the super-ageing society. A number of groundbreaking business innovations were proposed, including a "medical imaging diagnosis system", "physical age assessment for behavioural change", "wearable device for discharge prediction", "visualization of biological clock", "smartphone application for self-checking sperm development" and "application for online medical treatment".

Although it is a small step, such innovation projects will support the "100-Year Life Society" in the near future.

REGIONAL COUNCILS ON HEALTHCARE INDUSTRY OF NEXT GENERATION AND OTHER ORGANIZATIONS

On the other hand, the Japanese government has been also trying to create a strategic regional community for supporting the healthy ageing life all over Japan. At the urging of the Ministry of Economy, 46 of the Regional Councils on Healthcare Industry of Next Generation and other organizations have been established to work with universities, farmers, hospitals, nursing homes, tourism-related companies and local governments to create innovative businesses to solve the health problems associated with the ageing of the population in their respective regions. These include the "Hokkaido Health Care Industry Promotion Council Regional Model Consortium", which aims to create a unique healthcare industry in Hokkaido through "medical, agricultural, and commercial cooperation" utilizing food, tourism and other resources; the "OKINAWA Sports and Healthcare Cluster/REGISTA", which is working to expand sports and healthcare tourism and create industries that contribute to extending the health and longevity of the people of Okinawa by taking advantage of the prefecture's potential, such as its warm climate; the "Wellness City Koshi" in Koshi City, Kumamoto Prefecture, which promotes self-medication using services that are not covered by public insurance, and other examples and so on.

Enriching the Lives of Seniors in Japan

CHALLENGE FOR CO-CREATION OF WELLNESS TOURISM

In Japan, there is a traditional wellness culture of warming the body and mind in onsen (hot springs) to maintain good health. It is also said that bathing in onsen increases blood circulation and improves the human immune system.

Here, I would like to introduce some examples of private companies that offer not only healthy lifestyles but also full-fledged wellness tourism in order to enrich the quality of life.

Hoshino Resorts, one of Japan's leading progressive resort companies that has grown rapidly over the past decade with more than 45 lodging facilities in Japan and abroad, mainly high-end onsen ryokans (Japanese style hotels with hot spring facilities) and resorts, offers a variety of wellness stay programmes at its resort facilities. For example, Hoshinoya Karuizawa, their flagship luxurious onsen resort in Nagano Prefecture, has been offering a wellness stay programme called "Forest Wellness Stay (Shinrin-yojo)" for more than 10 years, which includes curing methods using their onsen facility. Forest Wellness Stay, which I experienced in 2009, was designed to learn the original lifestyle of Japanese people living in Nagano Prefecture in ancient times. (According to the Ministry of Health, Labour and Welfare, Nagano Prefecture has the record of the longest average lifespan of women in 2015. And the lifespan of men in Nagano was the second-longest in Japan.)

The guests learned how to breathe clean air, walk in the forest, eat rice with vegetables, drink tea, take bath at onsen, face oneself in mind, meditate and sleep in the ancient ways of Nagano Prefecture, through more than 3 days of practice led by an oriental medicine expert.

In my case, what I learned there and continued to do over the next year is as follows.

a. Whenever we eat the food, we should better chew it more than 50 times.
b. Make rice 50% of the total amount of food in one meal.
c. Having time for meditation before breakfast.

During my stay there (for 3 days), 2kg of my weight was reduced. Furthermore, my weight continued to drop even 3 months after I returned to my daily life in Tokyo. And reached the level of −4.5 kg from the original weight before I joined Forest Wellness Stay.

It is said that more than 90% of Forest Wellness Stay participants have succeeded in losing weight, and more than 70% of the participants have also succeeded in reducing body fat.

Since then, Forest Wellness Stay has continued to evolve. From 2021, under the supervision of the Physical Education and Medicine Research Foundation, they are offering well-being stays through activities in the forest and hot springs, such as the "Forest Power Walk" and "Deep Breathing Bathing", which aim to improve immunity by strengthening lung function, as well as immunity-enhancing foods and acupressure/acupuncture. This kind of wellness programme is to promote the behaviour change of humans in the natural environment. It is not supposed to be able to realize that in ordinary life in the urban area.

In 2013, at the call of the company, experts from medical institutions, onsen-related research institutes, wellness travel journalism, wellness-related international certification committees and IT consultancies came together to hold a joint study group on "The Japanese Way to Stay in a Destination Spa". Through this study, the "Island Time Wellness Stay (Shima-jikan-yojo)" programme was created under the supervision of Doctor Yokokura, to reset the fatigue of the brain and naturally regulate the body and mind by spending time at Taketomi Island in Okinawa, which is said to be the island of longevity, following one's instincts and regulating the five senses. At present, a variety of unique wellness programmes are being offered at several hot spring inns and resort facilities in Japan and abroad.

In recent years, Hoshinoya Tokyo has been offering a wellness stay programme called "Deep Breathing Regimen (Shinkokyu-yojo)", in which guests can learn breathing techniques at the hot springs to strengthen their lung function and enhance their immunity. Hoshinoya Fuji also offers a stay programme, where guests can experience the unique wellness of body and mind through the precious natural experience of climbing Mt. Fuji with the cooperation and generous support of professional experts skilled in climbing.

From June 2020, all onsen ryokans of the "KAI" brand (16 facilities at the beginning) offer "Hot Spring Healing", an early morning exercise programme and hot spring bathing to improve blood flow. Hoshino Resorts offers various other unique wellness programmes that take advantage of the unique culture and natural environment of each region of Japan.

I hope that the voluntary activities of these leading private companies will spread to more organizations and groups, including industry, academia and government, and lead to the improvement of QOL. And eventually, I expect that Japan will be able to provide excellent models for enriching the lives of the elderly.

SOCIO-INDUSTRIAL STRUCTURAL CHANGES REQUIRED: EXPECTATIONS FOR THE FUTURE

In this chapter, I have described the government's support measures to improve the quality of life in the "gap between healthy lifespan and average lifespan" (a scheme to support the "100-Year Life Society"), the lifestyle habits for healthy longevity that can be learned from the ancient Japanese sense of value ("ikigai") and examples of efforts to create innovations for industrialization to realize a healthy ageing society. However, even in Japan, a country that is confronted daily with the concrete challenges of an ageing society that is becoming increasingly serious, and that has a great deal of prior knowledge, experience, and government policies in this field, the reality is that there has yet to be full-scale growth in the Mibyou (pre-disease), health promotion and wellness industries sufficient to dispel the problem of ever-increasing medical expenditure.

One of the possible reasons for this may be the overly convenient and comprehensive medical system and Japan's traditional healthy lifestyle. In addition to the fact that most elderly people tend to rely on medical institutions too casually, they have fewer opportunities than Westerners to consciously implement voluntary health promotion, and they do not feel the need to spend time and money on health maintenance and promotion. As a result, it is difficult to see opportunities for full-fledged growth in this industry as in other industries. It is an ironic dilemma that although everyone in Japan and abroad sees potential growth in this field, the biggest barriers to business are the convenient National Health Insurance System and healthy lifestyles.

However, considering the speed of Japan's ageing population, it is obvious that in the near future, the government will reach the limit of maintaining a well-developed healthcare system for the elderly as before. The government should clearly demonstrate this fact to the public and provide more opportunities for the Mibyou/health/wellness industry to play an active role and contribute as a "leader in realizing sustainable health and longevity".

I am convinced that a change in the socio-industrial structure that can find their/our "ikigai" even at the very end of life will make the lives of all human beings brighter. I sincerely hope that such a future will come.

6 South Korea's Prospect for Aging and Preparation for the Future

Focusing on the Korean Traditional Medicine in the National Health Insurance

Kim Hyung-Ho
Health Insurance Review and Assessment Service (HIRA)

CONTENTS

Introduction 73
Rapid Change in Population Structure 74
Current Status of Korean Traditional Medicine 74
    Korean Medicine 74
    Status of Korean Medical Institutions 75
    Current Status of Korean Medicine Health Insurance 75
Problems of Korean Medicine Health Insurance with Aging 76
    A Rapid Growth in the Usage of Korean Medicine 76
    The Increase in the Duplicate Use of Western Medicine and
    Korean Medicine 76
    Lack of Coverage of Korean Medicine Health Insurance 76
Measures for Korean Medicine Health Insurance with Aging 77
    Expanding Korean Medicine Health Insurance Benefits for the Aged 77
    Expansion of Western Medicine and Korean Medicine Collaborative Care 78
    Other Future Measures for Aging 78
Conclusion 78
References 79

INTRODUCTION

Population aging is a common challenge for many countries around the world. In South Korea, the pace of aging is fast and low fertility is overlapping, so a sense of crisis about aging is prevalent in the national society. For this reason, the South

DOI: 10.1201/9781003043270-6

Korean government is preparing for the future of the country by setting up a special organization under the direct control of the president (Park, 2017). South Korea, which has already realized universal health coverage, recognizes many problems caused by the aging population and is taking active measures against them for the sustainability of national health insurance. This article examined the problems caused by aging in Korea in terms of traditional medicine, especially in the national health insurance. It focuses on changes in the use of traditional medicine due to aging, and pursuit of harmony between Western medicine and traditional medicine. This study is based on the literature review of Korea's related policy data and research results. The development of this article first introduces Korea's aging society in Chapter 2. Chapter 3 researches the current state of traditional Korean medicine (hereinafter referred to as 'Korean medicine') and how it is being applied in the national health insurance. In Chapter 4, the problems of Korean medicine health insurance due to aging are studied. Chapter 5 introduces the countermeasures for Korean medicine health insurance following aging, briefly summarizes this article, and makes suggestions.

RAPID CHANGE IN POPULATION STRUCTURE

The median lifetime expectancy of Koreans has increased by over 20 years in the last 50 years. In contrast, the total fertility rate sharply decreased from 4.53 to 0.98 during the same period. In 2000, Korea became an aging society in which elderly people over 65 of the population make up 7% of the entire population. In 2018, 14% of the population were drawn up of aged people and became an aged society. If this is the trend, in the year 2050, 20% of the population will be made up of old people and get a super-aged society (Lee et al., 2011).

CURRENT STATUS OF KOREAN TRADITIONAL MEDICINE

KOREAN MEDICINE

The involvement and importance of traditional medicine continue to increase worldwide as a means to make do with the aging population, the increase in chronic diseases and rising medical expenses. WHO acknowledges the importance of traditional medical specialty as it commends the role of traditional medicine practitioners in primary health care (Elujoba, Odeleye and Ogunyemi, 2005).

Korean traditional medicine is called 'Korean medicine'. Korean traditional medicine is defined as 'an act of preventing or treating diseases based on traditional oriental medicine from our old ancestors under the social concept, and an act of health and hygiene performed by oriental doctors as a category of wide-ranging medical activities' (Lee and Kwon, 2009).

The usage of Korean medicine, a traditional medicine, has been on the rise in Korea as well. The market share in 2009 was approximately 3.1% of the worldwide market, up 65% from 2004 (The Korean Institute for Oriental Medicine, 2014). The cost of health insurance for Korean medicine is also on the rise. The median growth

South Korea's Prospect for Aging

rate over the past 5 years since 2009 shows that Korean medicine hospitals are 16.0%, far above the intermediate growth rate of 8.2% of all medical institutions (Chae et al., 2015).

STATUS OF KOREAN MEDICAL INSTITUTIONS

The ratio of medical personnel and facilities in Korean medicine in total medical care is very low compared to those in Western medicine. However, the rate of increase is higher in Western medicine. If you look at this in more detail, the number of Korean medicine doctors is about 13% of the total workforce. As of 2013, Western medicine doctors were about 5 times more than Korean medicine doctors. In terms of the number of medical institutions, Western medicine institutions were 2.4 times more than those of Korean medicine institutions. However, Korean medicine doctors increased 3.9% annually between 2009 and 2013, showing a higher rate of increase than Western medicine doctors and dentists. Korean medicine hospitals and Korean medicine clinics account for about 15.6% of all medical institutions. The proportion of Korean medicine clinics is about 15%, and the average annual growth rate in the last 5 years is 2.7%, which is also higher than that of Western medicine (Chae et al., 2015).

CURRENT STATUS OF KOREAN MEDICINE HEALTH INSURANCE

Korea is a country that has achieved universal national health insurance, UHC. National health insurance is applied not only to Western medicine, but also to Korean medicine. However, the coverage of national health insurance for Korean medicine is very low compared to Western medicine (Kim and Kim, 2007).

It is called 'the Cooperative Medical System between Korean Medicine and Western Medicines' (it is hereinafter referred to as 'cooperative health care') to improve the treatment efficiency and the quality of services by establishing a plan for treatment methods, treatment contents, etc., in consultation with a Western medical doctor and a Korean medicine doctor. Korea is making attempts to revitalize it (Lee, 2004). Both the cooperative healthcare institution and the cooperative medical expenses are on the rise. The number of cooperative care institutions increased from 782 in 2009 to 1,355 in 2013, increasing 14.7% annually. The cost of cooperative health care increased by 28.3% annually during the same period.

Collaborative health care was conducted mostly in long-term care hospitals, which are widely used by the elderly for long-term treatment. In 2013, 92% of the medical care costs for collaborative care were incurred at long-term care hospitals. The increased rate of collaborative care in long-term care hospitals rapidly increased to an annual norm of 29.8%. By comparison, only 37,277 cases (4.4%) were taken in 2013 at hospital-level medical institutions other than long-term care hospitals. Of the total patients in the long-term care hospitals, 45.1% were treated with collaborative health care by Western medicine and Korean medicine doctors. The most common Korean medicine treatments in long-term care hospitals is acupuncture 69%, moxibustion 17.2%, and cupping 8.6% (Chae et al., 2015).

PROBLEMS OF KOREAN MEDICINE HEALTH INSURANCE WITH AGING

A RAPID GROWTH IN THE USAGE OF KOREAN MEDICINE

With the aging population, Korean medicine is quickly increasing. It is true that aging leads to an increase in medical use and medical expenses (Lee, 2004; Jeong, 2007). However, the increased rate of Korean medicine is higher than that of Western medicine. In the middle age of 40–64 years, the utilization rate of Korean medicine is the highest, but the average increased rate of users over the age of 65 (7.1%) is more than twice that of the middle age (3.1%). Changes in medical expenses are also presenting the largest growth in the aged population. Korean medicine outpatient treatment used in old age includes unspecified stroke, cerebral infarction, nervous system and circulatory system diseases (Moon, 2017).

The growing preference for Korean traditional medical care valid for chronic and degenerative diseases has contributed to a rising need for Korean medicine in the elderly population. In society to get up for the growth in medical expenses due to aging, it is necessary to seek institutional supplementation (Kim *et al.*, 2018).

THE INCREASE IN THE DUPLICATE USE OF WESTERN MEDICINE AND KOREAN MEDICINE

Korean medicine is often mixed or duplicated with Western medicine in the medical service area in South Korea. In terms of age, middle-aged people in their 40s and 50s and those in their 60s or older have high rates of oriental medicine and overlapping use. With the aging population, the overlapping use of Western medicine and Korean medicine has increased, which has become a problem (Yoon, 2012; Kim et al., 2018).

Duplicate medical treatment of Western medicine and Korean medicine has made troubles such as confusion in medical choices, time and economic losses caused by overlapping medical care, inefficient use of medical resources, and a trend of distrust among medical areas. It can also cause confusion in the selection of medical institutions, worsening the health of individuals and increasing the financial burden by missing the appropriate timing of treatment (Kim, 2004).

By cutting down the utilization of extra medical services in Western medicine and Korean medicine, it is necessary to prevent waste of medical expenses in consumer aspects, to prevent waste of resources in national aspects and to utilize effective resources (Cho, 2001).

LACK OF COVERAGE OF KOREAN MEDICINE HEALTH INSURANCE

Although Korean medicine, which is a traditional Korean medicine, is being used steadily by the masses, it is a reality that most of them are non-insurance areas that are not tracked by national health insurance. Among the total health insurance coverage items, Korean medicine items account for just 5% of the amount in 2012. Most of the applied items are concentrated exclusively on medical behaviour items such as acupuncture, moxibustion and cupping. Health insurance rarely applies to medical devices in the area of diagnosis and treatment, and to herbal medicines (Chae et al., 2015). In 2015, the rate of health insurance coverage for Korean medicine clinics was 47.2%, down 6% from 2014. This was the lowest in the last 9 years. In the same year, the health insurance coverage rate of Korean medicine hospitals was 35.3%, down 1.4% from the previous year's 36.7%. In contrast, the overall health insurance coverage rate rose 0.2% in 2015 from the previous year to 63.4%.

MEASURES FOR KOREAN MEDICINE HEALTH INSURANCE WITH AGING

EXPANDING KOREAN MEDICINE HEALTH INSURANCE BENEFITS FOR THE AGED

The South Korean government has been preparing to expand medical coverage for the elderly in preparation for the aging population by setting up a third basic plan for a low birth rate and aging society. Foremost, the medical insurance was strengthened for the aged, including health care for the elderly, vulnerable, expansion of dental services for the aged, and enhanced dementia screening and prevention (the first plan, 2006–2010). After that, the government expanded the coverage of health insurance based on the characteristics of the disease among the elderly, spread the movement culture of the elderly and expanded the number of professionals, and established an integrated healthcare system centred on the health centre (the second plan, 2011–2015). The plan continues to implement the 3rd round of comprehensive nursing and nursing services (the third plan, 2016–2020) to enhance the prevention and management of diseases in the elderly, reduce the burden of medical expenses for the elderly and strengthen mental health management for the elderly (Byun and Hwang, 2018).

Meanwhile, to amplify the national health policy coverage for Korean medicine, which is comparatively low compared to Western medicine, the government has established and implemented other programmes for the evolution of Korean medicine in the first (2006–2010), the second (2011–2015) and the third (2016–2020) (Lee et al., 2019).

Considering the increasing trend of elderly medical demand for Korean medicine due to the aging population, a policy to strengthen health insurance coverage for Korean medicine reflecting the characteristics of the elderly is needed. The main reason for the low health insurance coverage in Korean medicine is that only acupuncture, moxibustion and other herbal medicines are covered by health insurance and that insurance benefits for herbal medicines are very insufficient (Hong, 2019). Through this analysis, it is considered and implemented step by step to apply the expansion of Korean medicine benefits to (1) herbal medicine (herbal decoction), (2) physical therapy, (3) herbal medicine preparations, (4) Chuna manual therapy, etc. (Chae Jung-mi, et al. 2015). In addition, efforts will be made to secure the safety of Korean medicine such as safety management of medicinal herbs (Kim et al., 2018).

Expansion of Western Medicine and Korean Medicine Collaborative Care

One of the health insurance policies to prepare for the aging population is to reduce the cost of treatment and increase the effectiveness of treatment by cooperative care between Western medicine and Korean medicine. As discussed in Chapter 3, cooperative health care between Korean medicine and Western medicine is being examined, but it is being made out mostly at long-term care hospitals and rarely at other medical establishments. In addition, while the elderly population prefers Korean medicine, it tends to mix or duplicate Western medicine, having various difficulties. It is to expand the collaboration between Western medicine and Korean medicine that can improve the effectiveness of treatment and reduce costs while solving the problems of overlapping treatment. In other words, medical innovation through collaborative health care is a good way to cope with the increasing social demands of aging and accompanying chronic diseases. People with chronic diseases need care relatively more than treatment, compared to people with acute diseases. Elderly people also need more care than younger people. Therefore, it is a desirable form of medical service for the elderly to take advantage of Western medicine while focusing on the treatment of Korean medicine, which aims to continuously care for patients from prevention to treatment and rehabilitation depending on the patient's condition (Kang et al., 2005).

Collective health care is a safe policy to capture two rabbits in the historic period of aging because it can lower the medical expenses of the elderly and provide appropriate medical care for the aged. South Korean government has carried out the first-stage pilot project to confirm the effectiveness of the collaborative health care to prepare for aging and has completed the second-stage pilot project and is conducting the third-stage pilot project (Yoon et al., 2012).

Other Future Measures for Aging

Along with the above measures, Korea is also preparing for a rapid increase in medical resources (Do, 2009) while promoting efficient distribution and provision of medical resources to groom for the aging population (Oh, 2011; 2012).

In improver, the beefing up of the medical delivery system (Kim, 2019) and the expansion of public health care and betterment of medical services are also being pursued continuously (Kang et al., 2009; Jeon and Kan, 2012).

On the other hand, macroscopic discussions are being prepared to reorganize the Korean medical system divided into Western medicine and Korean medicine into a new system suitable for the aging years. It proposes to create institutional changes that include integration of both the relevant academic and licensing systems by integrating the dualized medical supply system (Kim *et al.*, 1998; Cho, 2010; Lee, 2015).

CONCLUSION

In this article, we looked at the current state of traditional medicine in the national health insurance and future measures of traditional Korean medicine in accordance with the aging population. The problems of Korean medicine health insurance due to aging were firstly the rapid increase in the use of Korean medicine, secondly the increase in the expenditure of mixing and duplication with Western medicine, and thirdly the vulnerability of Korean medicine health insurance coverage. When analysing the measures, the initiative is the expansion of health insurance coverage for Korean medicine for the elderly, which should also be accompanied by improved safety and quality of Korean medicine. Second is the expansion of collaborative health care between Western medicine and Korean medicine. Third, other policy considerations include the effective allocation and provision of medical resources, strengthening the medical delivery system, extending public health care and improving medical services. In the end, the discourse on medical integration of Korean medicine and Western medicine is also underway. This study observed the current state of Korean traditional medicine in the national health insurance and the aging population because other Asian countries may have similar difficulties. I trust this will be a slight hint to countries' efforts to achieve medical development in harmony with Western medicine and traditional medicine in the age of aging. The limitation of this article is that it is a rough study, and I hope there will be more in-depth research, such as comparisons with Asian countries.

REFERENCES

Byun, S. J., and Hwang, N. H., (2018) "The major contents and future tasks of the basic plan for low birthrate and aging society". *Health and Welfare Forum* 258: 41–61.

Chae, J. M., Choi, Y. J., and Choi, Y. M. (2015) "A study on the rationalization of insurance benefits for Korean medicine services." HIRA research institution.

Cho, J. K. (2010) "Changes in health care environment and medical integration of Korean medicine and western medicine". *Health and Welfare Issue & Focus* 27: 1–8.

Cho, K. S. (2001) *"Difference in the Behavior of Oriental Medicine."* PhD Thesis. Graduate School of Yonsei University.

Do, S. R. (2009) "Medical use status and policy tasks of the elderly". *Health and Welfare Forum* 2009(11): 66–79.

Jeon, H. S., and Kang, S. K. (2012) "Age differences in the predictors of medical service use between young-old and old-old: implications for medical service in aging society". *Health and Social Studi*es 32(1): 28–57.

Jeong, H. S., Lee, K. S., and Song, Y. M. (2007) "Population aging and medical expenses". *Health Economy and Policy Studies* 13(1): 95–116.

Kang, E. J., Seol, H. H. and Choi, W. J. (2005) "A study for integrated traditional Korean/western medicine to reform public medicine". *Journal of Health and Social Affair*s, 25(1): 3–36.

Kang, S. M., Jeong, H. S., Song, Y. M., and Lee, K. S. (2009) "The future projection of public medical expenses considering population aging". *Health and Policy Studies* (formerly Health and Economic Research) 15(2): 1–20.

Kim, J. S., et al. (1998) "Unification of oriental and western medicine with study on oriental and western medicine". *Korean Journal of Medical History* 7(1): 47–60.

Kim, K. H. (2004) "A Study on the Status of Physicians Collaborating with Oriental Medicine Hospital." Research Report by the Medical Policy Institute of the Korean Medical Association: 1–88.

Kim, Y. M. (2019) "A study on the establishment of patient-oriented medical delivery system-oriented to the European Union's examples of primary health care reinforcement". *Medical Law*, 20(3): 235–262.

Kim, Y. J. (2018) The korea foundation for the promotion of oriental medicine, and the korea institute for health and social affairs, "Oriental Medicine Utilization and Oriental Medicine Consumption Survey." Ministry of Health and Welfare.

'Korea Medicine Doctor' is a doctor or an oriental medical doctor? (2013, June 11.). Retrieved from http://medicaltimes.com/News/1083719.

Lee, H. S. (2004) "A study on factors related to elderly health and medical expenditure". *Korean Elderly Studies* 24(2): 163–179.

Lee, H. J., Kim, S. R., Jang, S. I., and Park, E. C. (2019) "The present state of long-term planning for domestic health and welfare". *Journal of Health and Administration* 29(3): 368–373.

Lee, M. S., and Kwon, Y. K. (2009) "Reviewing the legal basis of oriental medicine through case analysis". *Journal of the Korea Institute of Oriental Medicine* 15(3): 19–28.

Lee, P. S. (2015) "The contents and challenges of medical integration of korean medicine and western medicine". *Medical Policy Forum* 13(4): 39–46.

Lee, S. Y. (2004) "Policy direction for vitalization of the Cooperative Medical System between Korean Medicines and Western Medicines". *Health and Welfare Forum* 97: 66–70.

Moon, K. H. (2017) "The analysis of trends and determinants of korean medical service utilization in outpatients." PhD Thesis. Graduate School of Kyung Hee University.

Oh, Y. H. (2011) "The problems and improvement plans of medical staff supply and demand". *HIRA Policy Tr*end. 5(6): 12–20.

The Korean Institute of Oriental Medicine (2014) "Trends and Environmental Analysis of Korean Medicine Standards at home and abroad." *The Korean Institute of Oriental Medicine.*

Universal health coverage. (4 April 2020). Retrieved from https://www.who.int/health-topics/universal-health-coverage#tab=tab_1.

Yoon, K. J., Lee, A. Y., Kim, H. S., Choi, J. H., Lee, J. A., Kim, N. K. and Lee, S. Y. (2019) "A Study on the Evaluation of the 2nd Phase Pilot Project in Western Medicine and Korean Medicine Collaborative Care". *The Korea Institute for Health and Social Affairs.*

Yoon, K. J. (2012) "The utilization and recognition of oriental medicine by the Korean people". *Health and Welfare Issue & Focus* 140: 1–8.

i. In Korea, there was a dispute between the Doctors Association and the Oriental Medicine Association whether it is appropriate to name the 'Korean Medicine' in the English name of Korean traditional medicine. In this regard, the Supreme Court of Korea finally recognized the use of the name 'Korean Medicine' (Medical Times, 2013, June 11).

ii. The definition of WHO for UHC is as follows: "Universal health coverage means that all people have access to the health services they need, when and where they need them, without financial hardship. It includes the full range of essential health services, from health promotion to prevention, treatment, rehabilitation, and palliative care" (World Health Organization, 2020, April 4).

7 The Triple Response to Population Ageing

Systems, Networks and Culture Change Perspectives from the UK and Europe

Muir Gray
Green Templeton College
University of Oxford

CONTENTS

Introduction 81
The Science of Living Longer 81
The Evidence Base for Living Longer Better 82
The System Century 83
The Aims of the System 83
The Objectives 84
Creating Networks 86
Creating the Right Culture 86
References 88

INTRODUCTION

Every society is faced with the challenge of population ageing, both absolute and relative. One of the reasons why this is seen as a frightening challenge is that it is assumed that the increase in the number of older people will be matched by a proportional increase in the number of people who are very dependent because of frailty, dementia and disability. However, this fear is not supported by scientific evidence.

THE SCIENCE OF LIVING LONGER

When the word 'science' is used, the assumption is that this is laboratory studies connected with senescence and the opportunities for finding drugs that will stop or

DOI: 10.1201/9781003043270-7

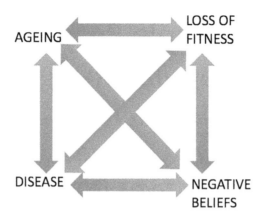

FIGURE 7.1 Problems as people live longer

slow some of the processes that take place as part of normal ageing.. There are three interrelated causes of the problems that occur more frequently as people live longer:

1. Loss of fitness, physical and mental
2. Disease, much of which is preventable, and the disability that results is usually complicated by accelerated loss of fitness which results from
3. Pessimistic and negative beliefs and attitudes (Figure 7.1)

There is now a consensus emerging that the normal process of ageing is not a cause of significant problems until the nineties and that most of the problems seen before that age are caused by the three factors discussed above. Of course, ageing and genetics have some part to play. The effects of ageing are to reduce maximal ability such as maximum heart rate and to reduce resilience, which means there is a need to increase activity with every year that happens. Also, you do need luck to avoid problems like Parkinson's disease or rheumatoid arthritis which do not appear to be caused by environment or lifestyle, but our better understanding now of what happens as we live longer provides the opportunity for intervention and the evidence of the benefits of intervening is getting stronger.

THE EVIDENCE BASE FOR LIVING LONGER BETTER

There is now a strong evidence base that the diseases once thought of as being due to the ageing process, and therefore not preventable, can be delayed or prevented. The United Kingdom, through, for example, the National Institute for Health and Care Excellence, has published guidelines on preventing and delaying frailty, dementia and disability (https://www.nice.org.uk/guidance/ng16), and the Lancet Commission on Dementia (2020), and many other respected agencies, have produced guidance on reducing the risk of dementia even though Alzheimer's disease cannot yet be prevented or treated.

Perhaps one of the most interesting bits of evidence that we have about the changing evidence base and culture is that the first Editorial in JAMA in 2020, often a

The Triple Response to Population Ageing Systems 83

significant indicator of the way in which the Editorial Board's mind is moving, was called a 'Longevity Prescription for the 21st Century' and it was written by a distinguished physician who is a laboratory scientist, but the human genome is not mentioned and the subtitle of the article was 'Renewing Purpose, Building and Sustaining Social Engagement, and Embracing a Positive Lifestyle' (Pizzo 2020).

On the basis of this evidence, it is possible now to develop a response to meet the challenge of population ageing, to help people live longer better and reduce the need for health and social care. To do this requires not a change in the structure of what we do, but

- the development of a system
- the delivery of the system's objectives by population-based networks and
- a new culture focused on enablement, resilience and wellbeing.

THE SYSTEM CENTURY

The 20th century was the century of the bureaucracy in most countries. In the 19th century, traditional rulers and family firms dominated society, but in the 20th century, the large bureaucracies became increasingly important and influential, both in industry and in healthcare, epitomised by the growing power, size and status of the teaching hospital. Not surprisingly, leaders of health and social services became very focused on bureaucracy, studying how it could be improved, merged or reorganised, but in the last decade of the 20th century, the importance of bureaucracies came under serious questioning.

In many countries the word 'bureaucracy' had become a synonym for inefficiency and self-serving individuals and groups starting in Europe with the novels of Franz Kafka, but as the work of Charles Perrow, in his book 'Complex Organizations' (2014), has made clear, bureaucracies are of vital importance but only for linear tasks such as the fair and open employment of staff. For non-linear or complex tasks a different format is necessary. It is also important to bear in mind the statement attributed to Gandhi that there is no bureaucracy that can make bad people behave well but the wrong bureaucracy can make good people behave badly, so it is important to look at ways in which the bureaucratic structure of health and social services is arranged to see if there are obstacles to good practice. It is also important to recognise the importance of bureaucracy for linear tasks like the uncorrupt management of money, but population ageing is a complex challenge and requires a response – the system. The 21st century is the century of the system where the system is a set of activities with a common aim and a common set of objectives.

THE AIMS OF THE SYSTEM

Two aims have been identified in England - the first of which is to increase health span (Figure 7.2) and the second, to compress morbidity at the end of life (Figure 7.3).

The importance of this concept was first described by Fries and Crapo (1981) in their book 'Vitality and Ageing' where they wrote not only about the 'Rectangularization

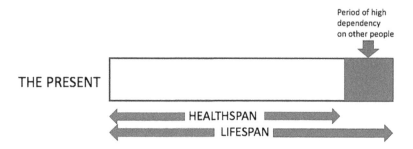

FIGURE 7.2 Increasing the health span

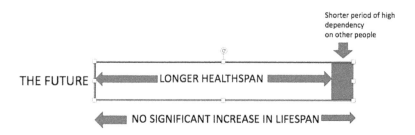

FIGURE 7.3 Compressing morbidity at the end of life

of the Survival Curve', but also the 'Rectangularization of the Morbidity Curve' and the compression of morbidity. Most of the work on longevity by laboratory scientists focuses only on life span but there is little evidence that people are hungry for one or two additional decades above the age of ninety. What is more important in the minds of most people is living longer better, and that is the aim of the system.

There is a second more immediate aim ready to help people 'drop a decade' or to regain the level of ability they had ten years previously, because it is clear that no matter how old people are and no matter how many long-term conditions they have, they can very quickly increase all four aspects of physical fitness – (i) strength, (ii) stamina, (iii) skill and (iv) suppleness. If they reach in the top quartile for their particular age group, they become as physically able as the average person ten years younger.

The benefits of the system is that it will reduce the need for both social care and acute healthcare because frailty reduces resilience, and as a result, minor challenges lead to significant deterioration and the need for emergency admission. The system can shift the last years of life from this (Figure 7.4):

To this (Figure 7.5)

THE OBJECTIVES

Having decided the aims, it is very important to set objectives. Having set the aim, the next step is to set the objectives and the objectives chosen for England are set out below.

The Triple Response to Population Ageing Systems

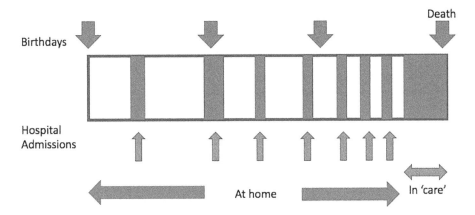

FIGURE 7.4 Ageing in care

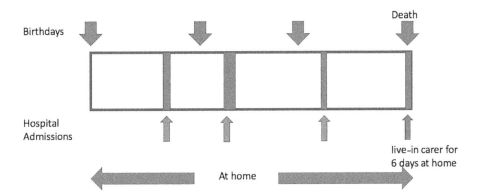

FIGURE 7.5 Ageing at home

- To prevent and mitigate isolation
- To improve physical ability and resilience, prevent and delay frailty and increase healthspan
- To promote knowledge and understanding about living longer better among older people and the wider population to counteract the detrimental effects of ageism
- To create an environment in which people can fulfil their potential
- To activate older people and enable strengthening of purpose
- To support carers better
- To minimise and mitigate the effects of deprivation
- To reduce the risk of and to delay or prevent dementia
- To prevent and minimise the effects of disease and multimorbidity
- To enable both living well and dying well

These include outcome objectives. But because it may take years to achieve these objectives, it is very important also to set process and structure objectives and have measures of progress, or the lack of it, of both:

- The rate of process or activity and
- Measures of the structure that needs to be in place

This concept of structure, process and outcome has been in use in healthcare worldwide for many years being based on the excellent work of Donabedian (2005). It is particularly important to note the objective of involving older people in developing the network that will deliver the systems objectives to a defined population.

CREATING NETWORKS

The 20th century was the century of the hierarchy; the 21st century is the century of the network not only because of the internet but also because we are in the third healthcare revolution. The first revolution was the public health revolution of the 19th century based on empiricism and strong government. The second healthcare revolution of the 20th century was the high-tech revolution epitomised by MRI and hip replacement. But, we are now in the third healthcare revolution driven by citizens, knowledge and the internet and of course the internet, using this as a metaphor for everything that is digital, is of vital importance in changing reality.

A network is a set of individuals and organisations committed to delivering the systems objectives.

The same system specification should do for one or even more than one country; but to achieve the objective, the network needs to take into account local history and geography, to use the military distinction between strategic and operational command. The network needs individuals identified by the main organisations as being part of the group that provides leadership for the network, given responsibility by their employing organisations are involved in joint decision making that may not always be of benefit to their particular organisation but of benefit to the population as a whole. This means what is needed is a collaborative culture, and this is one aspect of the new culture that the network must create as part of its leadership responsibility.

CREATING THE RIGHT CULTURE

The management and leadership literature has identified culture as the feature that distinguishes leadership from management using the definition of culture prepared by Edgar Schein, generally regarded as the leading author in this field.

> When we examine culture and leadership closely, we see that they are two sides of the same coin; neither can really be understood by itself. If one wishes to distinguish leadership from management or administration, one can argue that leadership creates and changes cultures, while management and administration act within a culture.

Schein E.H. (2010, pp. 10–11)

The culture of an organisation may be understood through what is called their spoken values, for example its mission statement and website; but to really understand, it is important to speak to people within the network, or who are being supported in the network because what is written and what is actually done maybe dramatically different. The collaborative culture is one feature of the optimal response to the challenge of population ageing, but the other is the very culture of what we are trying to achieve.

In Europe, the word 'care' is used and the mission has been to develop a culture of 'caring', but there is increasing reservation about this because in many countries caring means doing things for older people on the mistaken assumption that they cannot do things for themselves. This is inadvertently accelerating the rate of decline as shown in the figure below, widening the fitness gap and accelerating the loss of ability, and it this loss of ability, from the negative thinking, that creates frailty and precipitates the drop below the line at which independent living is possible. (Figure 7.6).

Negative societal beliefs and attitudes that assume that all problems are due to ageing and that older people cannot recover lost ability, lead to a 'culture of care'. This is in contrast to taking action to help the individual recover the lost ability – physical, cognitive and emotional.

New language is emerging in different countries. In England, there has been discussion about 'enablement' as the appropriate word or even 'coaching', a term derived from sport science, with a coach being someone who aims to help a person reduce the gap between potential and performance. For this reason, physical trainers and the fitness industry are playing a central role in the *Living Longer Better* system in England not just in providing services but also in changing the culture, and what

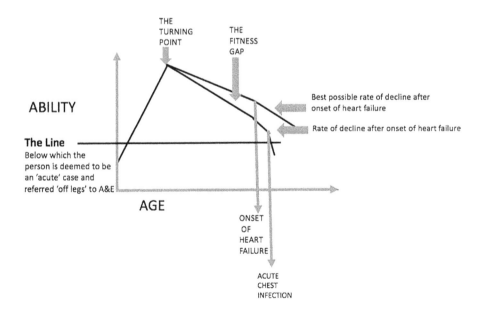

FIGURE 7.6 Accelerating the rate of decline

is needed is not structural reorganisation of health and social services but a cultural revolution.

International models of healthy ageing can serve as points of reference for Asia in framing the region's own local and national agendas based on culturally relevant approaches to:

- the development of a system for healthy ageing
- the delivery of the system's objectives by population-based networks
- a new culture focused on enablement, resilience and wellbeing.

REFERENCES

Donabedian, A. 2005. Evaluating the quality of medical care, *The Milbank Quarterly*, 83(4): 691–729.

Fries, J. F. and Crapo, L. M. 1981. *Vitality and Aging*. San Francisco: W.H. Freeman

Livingston, G. et al. 2020. Dementia prevention, intervention, and care: 2020 report of the Lancet Commission, *The Lancet*, 396, No. 10248 Published: July 30, 2020.

Perrow, C. 2014. *Complex Organizations: A Critical Essay*. Brattleboro VT: Echo Point Books & Media.

Pizzo, P. A. 2020. A prescription for longevity in the 21st century: renewing purpose, building and sustaining social engagement, and embracing a positive lifestyle, *JAMA*, 323(5): 415–416. doi:10.1001/jama.2019.21087

Schein, E. H. 2010. *Organizational Culture and Leadership*. 2, pp. 10–11. San Francisco, CA: John Wiley & Sons.

8 The Health and Well-Being of the Left-Behind Elderly in Rural China

Paul Kadetz
Queen Margaret University

CONTENTS

Introduction 89
    Factors Impacting the Left-Behind Elderly Phenomenon in China 90
        Wealth Inequality 90
        Rapid Urbanization 91
        The Hukou System 91
        Rural Pension System 92
        The One-Child Policy 92
    The Impact of Rural Migration on the Health and Well-Being of
    Left-Behind Elderly 92
    Understanding the Complex Impact of Adult-Child Migration on the
    Well-Being of Their Parents 94
        The Number of Children Who Have Migrated 94
        Who Has Migrated and for How Long 94
        Change in Workload and Responsibilities 95
        Differences in Vulnerability 95
        The Role of Rural HealthCare: Access and Quality 96
        The Capacity of Rural Healthcare for Multi-Morbidities among
        Elderly Patients 97
        The Influence of Neoliberalism 97
    The Role of Agency, Recuperation, Social Cohesion, and Social Capital
    in the Health of Left-Behind Elderly 98
Conclusions 100
References 101

INTRODUCTION

Demographic changes of a growing population of elderly, coupled with increased urbanization, and an increased requirement of mobility for work have presented

DOI: 10.1201/9781003043270-8

challenges for the health and well-being of the elderly throughout the world, particularly for those living in rural areas. But, nowhere have these factors been tested on a larger scale than in China. According to the 2019 Chinese census, 17.9% of China's total population (249 million) were at least 60 years of age and 11% (158 million) at least 65 years of age (Li et al. 2020). According to Ma et al. (2020), the population over 60 years of age in China increased from 10.3% in 2000 to 17.6% in 2018, while there was an increase from 15.4% to 23.6% in those aged between 45 and 60 over the same 8-year period. Nor is this trend predicted to abate; by 2050, nearly one-third (31%) of the population of China, nearly 450 million people, is projected to comprise one-quarter of the world's population aged 60 or older (Tse, 2013; Huang and Li, 2019). Part of this demographic shift is an outcome of the change in life expectancy, which increased from 50 years in 1950 to 73 years in 2010 and is expected to rise to 80 years in 2050 (Huang and Li, 2019). The rural Chinese account for 40.4% of the total population in China, and those aged 60 or older comprise 20.5% of the rural Chinese and 16.1% of the urban Chinese (Ma, He and Xu, 2020).

The elderly in rural areas of China whose children have migrated to urban areas for employment have been labelled the "left-behind" elderly. The idea of elderly parents being left behind by their children is a concept that is foreign to Chinese culture and is quite contrary to the historical role of a central pillar of Chinese societies: filial piety (*Xiao*, 孝). Dating to the 4th century BCE, Confucian thought emphasized the importance of filial piety as not merely a virtue, but rather a law of nature for an ordered society. Traditionally, welfare support for the elderly in rural China has been the responsibility of the family, partly due to these cultural traditions and partly due to a lack of a social safety network (Xiang, Jiang and Zhao, 2016). Given inadequate support from rural governments, elderly parents are supposed to turn to their families for physical, financial, and psychological assistance (Tse, 2013). However, rural adult-child migration has eroded this foundation of traditional family support and has led to the presence of millions of left-behind parents in rural areas. The creation of the overwhelming number of left-behind elderly in rural China, some of whom are incapable of fully caring for themselves, has been the outcome of a confluence of social and demographic changes instituted by the Chinese Communist Party (CCP).

This chapter will examine the factors that have resulted in left-behind elderly, the impact of adult-child migration on the well-being of those elders left behind, and what the state and communities could do to improve the health and well-being of the left-behind elderly in rural China.

FACTORS IMPACTING THE LEFT-BEHIND ELDERLY PHENOMENON IN CHINA

Wealth Inequality

The remarkable economic growth of China over the past two decades has not been achieved without consequence. Rapid economic growth that ignores impacts has resulted in some of the worst air and water pollution in the world; marked inequality in the distribution of this wealth (as reflected in a Gini coefficient of 0.465)—ranked 31 in the world for wealth inequality (CIA, 2020); unbridled urbanization; and a permanent underclass of rural migrant workers. Wealth inequality in China is

The Health and Well-Being

particularly evident in the ratio of the urban to rural per capita income that was 2.6 in 1978 and increased to approximately 3.3 in 2010.

Rapid Urbanization

China's unprecedented speed of urbanization over the past thirty years has predominantly been an outcome of internal migration, with rural migrants currently comprising an estimated 40% of urban populations and a further 200 million rural residents predicted to settle permanently in cities by 2025 (National Bureau of Statistics, 2018). These dramatic population movements have been fostered by China's rigid belief in the need for rapid economic growth, fuelled by the development of a domestic market of a growing urban middle-class of consumers in tandem with the perpetuation of a low-paid domestic rural migrant underclass. China's ability to serve as the "workshop for the world" and continue to produce goods at globally competitive low cost is, at least in part, possible because of the so-called household registration or *hukou* system.

The Hukou System

The boundaries between rural and urban in China are complex and have been constructed beyond geography or administrative designations, extending to socioeconomic and historically embedded cultural distinctions. The official legal determination of rural or urban status is designated through a household registration system known as *hukou* (户口). According to Zhang (2012: 244), family registers were in existence as early as the Xia Dynasty (BCE 2100–1600). The modern household registration system of hukou, constructed by the Chinese Communist Party in 1958, turned distinctions of residence into legally designated boundaries (*Ibid.*). The hukou was partly intended to control the movement of China's vast population, particularly following the decentralization of state welfare to provincial, city, and town levels after the Cultural Revolution, in addition to fiscal decentralization that began in the 1980s.[1]

The establishment of residence designates where one has access to state welfare benefits including education, housing, pension, and medical care. Medical care and social health insurance are also tied to permanent employment. Hence, residing in an area outside of one's legal *hukou* can restrict access to permanent jobs issued with a formal contract, public schooling, and medical insurance, as well as healthcare services and facilities (Ma and Zhou, 2009).

However, the hukou system is changing in some urban areas, particularly in eastern cities such as Beijing, Shanghai, and Guangzhou, where city governments can grant local permanent hukou often to those who are either very rich, highly educated, and/or are employed in good jobs in the public sector or in large private companies (Fields and Song 2020). Beginning in March 2014, China's Plan for New Urbanization (2014–2020) proposed that 100 million migrants should have

---

[1] There is disagreement in the literature concerning the starting point of fiscal decentralization in China. For example, Su and Zhao (2004) place the start of fiscal decentralization at 1980, whereas Lin and Liu (2000:10) identify that the changes in fiscal relationships "between the central and provincial governments were, to a large extent, experimental and temporary" from 1980 to 1984, and recognize 1985 as the actual starting point of fiscal decentralization.

their hukou registered in the place they work (Zhang et al. 2020). However, for a majority of rural migrants the contingencies to receive an urban hukou render it difficult, if not prohibitive.

Although the hukou system is changing and dynamic, rural benefits are usually markedly inferior to those in urban areas (particularly in terms of healthcare), due to the lack of access to urban social health insurance. Rural migrant access to urban healthcare is usually contingent on the ability to pay out of pocket, which can be prohibitive for most rural migrants. Thus, when rural migrants require hospitalization, they often need to return to their rural hometowns, or counties where hospitals are located. Hence, though the hukou system may not act as a deterrent for the migration of young, healthy, rural workers, it may serve to keep their less healthy, elderly parents in their rural villages, where they are more likely to be the recipient of welfare services that are inferior to those available in urban areas.

Rural Pension System

The current pension system for rural elderly is considered woefully inadequate, forcing the rural elderly to depend on their working children as the main source of their income. Given how unreliable migrant children's own income may be, the rural elderly are placed at a greater risk of falling into poverty (Scheffel and Zhang, 2019). While nearly half of urban elderly over the age of 60 rely on retirement pension funds, a mere 4.6% of rural elderly receive pension incomes (*Ibid.*).

The One-Child Policy

Possibly more than any other factor, the one-child policy introduced in 1979, which restricted the number of children a couple could have to one without being subject to financial penalties, has resulted in long-term demographic changes that have reduced the number of children who can care for one's parents. Household size in rural China has decreased from 3.61 in 2004 to 3.19 in 2013 (Xiang, Jiang and Zhao, 2016). Furthermore, in a society where males are strongly favoured, some parents have resorted to sex-selective abortion and female infanticide to secure male heirs (Hu and Shi, 2020). The resulting imbalanced sex ratio (116 males per 100 females in 2010) further problematizes elder care that normatively is the domain of daughters, who are now solely responsible for the care of their own parents as well as those of her husband's (*Ibid.*).

Thus, urbanization, the restrictions of the hukou system, shifts in rural healthcare insurance, inadequate rural pension coverage, and the marked shift in demographics resulting from the one-child policy have all resulted in a perfect storm through which rural elderly must navigate in the absence of their adult children.

THE IMPACT OF RURAL MIGRATION ON THE HEALTH AND WELL-BEING OF LEFT-BEHIND ELDERLY

The literature concerning the impacts of adult-child migration on the health of elderly parents spans a spectrum from overwhelmingly negative to its polar opposite. Analysing data from the China Health and Nutrition Survey (CHNS) and from the China Health and Retirement Longitudinal Study (CHARLS), Huang et al. (2016)

The Health and Well-Being 93

and Li et al. (2020) respectively conclude that migration of adult children significantly impairs the health of their parents. Specifically, both studies identify lower self-reported health and activities of daily living, and higher depression scores in the elderly studied. Furthermore, with every additional migrant child, left-behind parents are diagnosed with 0.30% more illnesses, a 7.2% increased likelihood of reporting worst self-rated health (Tse, 2013, p. 14), and have an 8% increased probability of poor health (Xiang et al. 2016; Xiang, 2015).

Mental health has also been found to be impacted by child migration. For example, Scheffel and Zhang (2019) found that child migration is associated with lower levels of happiness, as well as significantly higher levels of loneliness and depressive symptoms in left-behind parents. Such feelings of loneliness and abandonment may impact mental health (Tse, 2013), which may also be exacerbated in Chinese culture where there is an expectation that one's children will be present and caring for the parent. Where Xiang et al. (2016) identify that child migration adversely affects the mental health of the parents, but not their physical health, Tse (2013) identified that both physical and mental health, as well as memory, deteriorated in those left-behind elderly who present with poor memory and are reportedly more likely to suffer a serious fall. Scheffel and Zhang (2018) found adult-child migration reduces left-behind parent-reported happiness by 6.6% and increases the probability of loneliness by 3.3%, in addition to feelings of powerlessness. The impacts of child migration on mental health should be understood to potentially impact physical health as well, and vice versa (*Ibid.*). Ma et al. (2020) found that chronic physical illnesses have been associated with an increased risk of depressive symptoms and that patients with one, two, and three or more chronic physical conditions were 21%, 66%, and 111% more likely to experience depressive symptoms than those without any chronic physical conditions.

However, not all impacts of adult-child migration on the health of left-behind elderly were found to be negative. In rural China, off-farm migrant labour earns much higher wages than farmwork. The greater the earnings, the more migrant children can potentially provide for their parents. Chang et al. (2016) studied 2,000 households in five provinces over a 4-year period and identified that the improved finances from urban employment contributed to improved health outcomes for left-behind elderly. Specifically, they identified an increase in the proportion of elderly for whom at least one of their children migrated from 48.8% to 54.3% between 2007 and 2011, and though 19% of their elderly sample's health declined according to self-report, 27% reported an improvement in health over this same period and were more likely to have a decrease, rather than an increase, in incidents of annual illness. Increased income could improve elderly daily life in multiple ways including the ability to afford a healthier diet, less stress, and more financial access to quality medical care (*Ibid.*). Ma and Zhou (2009), who found that migrant labour income remittances accounted for about one-quarter of the total rural household income, identify that the positive health impacts of child remittances may balance the deleterious impacts of being left behind for the elderly, as migration improved the self-perceived economic sufficiency of nearly 70% of the left-behind elderly.

However, some studies do not identify any significant associations between adult-child urban migration in China and the health of left-behind elders (Song 2014), or identify mixed or "compensated" associations, particularly regarding the impact of remittances. For example, Tse (2013, p. 14) identified that remittances only increased the likelihood of left-behind parents suffering depression and poor mental health, whereas the impacts on other health outcomes were minimal. Tse argues that the fact that remittances have insignificant impact on physical health suggests that financial contributions from migrant children may merely have a modest compensating effect on the overall health of the left-behind elderly. Similarly, Ma and Zhou (2009) found that the distribution of life satisfaction or dissatisfaction, which they used as a proxy to measure well-being, was not very different between migrant and non-migrant households, indicating that the negative and positive effects of long-distance migration may be more or less balanced. They hypothesize that for elderly living in a household with a migrant child, the loss of care or increase in familial burden over time and distance will be compensated by enhanced income transfer to the elderly, to the extent that the overall well-being and life satisfaction of the elderly would not be severely affected.

Ambiguous and/or contradictory findings of the ultimate impacts of internal migration on elder health are also demonstrated across the international literature (Kuhn, Everett and Silvey, 2011; Antman, 2012; Böhme, Persian and Stöhr, 2015; Chang et al. 2016), where internal migration of children can result either in elder parent health deterioration or in an increased income that benefits elder health. Hence, the impact of adult-child migration on the health of elders may be far less straightforward and far more nuanced than expected.

UNDERSTANDING THE COMPLEX IMPACT OF ADULT-CHILD MIGRATION ON THE WELL-BEING OF THEIR PARENTS

Several factors may interact in myriad complex ways to impact the health and well-being of left-behind elders including: the number of children who have migrated; who in the family is migrating; changes to the workload or responsibilities in those left behind; the quality and capacity of rural healthcare; and the influence of neoliberalism.

The Number of Children Who Have Migrated

According to Tse (2013), the greater the number of adult-child migrants, the poorer the self-rated health and depression of their elderly parents; although, other health outcomes, including poor physical health, memory, and occurrence of serious fall, were not reported to demonstrate significant correlation with one's adult-child migration status. In general, Tse concludes that left-behind elderly with more children demonstrate better health outcomes and are less likely to suffer depression and poor memory.

Who Has Migrated and for How Long

Tse (2013) identifies that migration of one's daughter has a greater impact on parental health than migration of the son. Although migration of sons and daughters both cause parents to report lower self-rated health and poor memory status, the effects are significantly greater with the migration of the daughter. Furthermore, migration

The Health and Well-Being 95

of only daughters has resulted in parents suffering more physical illnesses, depression, and increased occurrences of serious falls (*Ibid.*).

Although Xiang et al. (2016) conclude that having someone at home to take care of the elderly is more important than sending home money, especially for poor households, other studies contradict what seems to be an obvious finding. For example, Ma and Zhou (2009) found the life satisfaction of left-behind elderly was greater over longer-term migration (50.4%) than where there was either no migration (45.7%) or short-term migration (37.9%). Similarly counter-intuitive, Chang et al. (2016) identified that those elderly whose adult children either returned home over the duration of the study or never migrated from home during this period were more likely to experience a decrease in health status and more likely to demonstrate an increase in the number of incidents of annual illness than children who migrated for a longer term.

Change in Workload and Responsibilities

Li et al. (2020) find that the impact of the migration of adult children on their parents is linked to the specific change in parental workload, economic support, and emotional support. In general, they identified the negative influence of the burden of a greater workload on parental health to be more significant than the influence of economic and emotional support on parental health.

Differences in Vulnerability

Although all of the above-mentioned factors can interact in complex ways to render the left-behind elderly more vulnerable, some inherent factors in the elderly were also identified in the literature. Clearly, part of the issue with many of the debates in the literature is an issue of aggregated data and generalizability. Although recognition of trends may be valuable, highly aggregated data may hide the individual differences between elderly and result in depicting a hegemonic group of "the elderly". This issue is particularly apparent when attempting to differentiate between the variations in vulnerability among the elderly.

Much of the literature identified left-behind elderly females to be more vulnerable than males. For example, Xiang et al. (2015) note that a left-behind mother is 4% more likely to report poor health than a father. And Tse (2013, p. 14) identifies that left-behind female parents report significantly worse status in every health measure in comparison with male parents. Other studies identified that being female compounds vulnerability with factors such as being widowed (Sheffel and Zhang 2019), poorly educated (Li et al. 2020a), and being more likely to have multiple chronic illnesses (Ma et al. 2020). Lei et al. (2014) also distinguish that the prevalence of depressive symptoms in an aged and older sample was highest among rural women (49%), followed by urban women (35%), rural men (35%), and urban men (23%).

Other factors leading to vulnerability in left-behind elderly include having only one child, low-income households, and being older than 60 years of age (Xiang et al. 2016). Being over 60 with only one child was considered the most important factor in vulnerability of left-behind parents (Xiang et al. 2015). Scheffel and Zhang (2019) find that widowhood, coupled with difficulties in performing activities of daily living (ADLs) and instrumental activities of daily living (IADLs), as well as lower self-rated health are the most important determinants associated with considerably reduced emotional health of left-behind elderly.

Both the likelihood and amount of migrant child remittances follow a pattern that may also distinguish vulnerability. For example, Ma and Zhou (2009) found the propensity of income transfer to favour females, who are older, widowed or divorced, and serve as caretakers of their grandchildren, while the amount of income transferred favoured elderly females from more developed regions who maintained close family and social ties.

The Role of Rural HealthCare: Access and Quality

It is questionable if some of the impacts of the health of left-behind elderly in rural China are not primarily a function of rural healthcare itself. As a result of the dramatic shift from economic communism to state-controlled capitalism, with the death of Mao and the economic reforms and "opening-up" of Deng Xiaoping, health insurance coverage rates dropped dramatically from 90% in 1980 to 5% in 1985 (Liu & Cao, 1992). Many rural residents remained uninsured until 2003, when the Chinese government implemented a nationwide project known as the New Cooperative Medical Scheme (NCMS) in rural China. By 2010, the NCMS covered 835.6 million rural residents, nearly two-thirds of the Chinese population. Though health insurance coverage has markedly increased in rural areas, the objective of the NCMS is primarily to provide low-cost basic health care services, though the benefit level for rural recipients is considerably lower than for their urban counterpart (Xiang et al. 2016). Although the NCMS has substantially improved rural residents' use of healthcare services, it has not reduced out-of-pocket expenses for patients. Due to limited coverage and insufficient benefits provided by public pension and health insurance systems, adult children remain the primary source of financial and instrumental support for their left-behind parents (Li et al. 2020a).

Regardless of the many policies that have attempted to improve access to rural healthcare, the quality of healthcare in rural China remains inferior to urban healthcare (Li et al. 2020b). The substandard quality of rural healthcare may be an outcome of the struggle to recruit and maintain healthcare human resources in rural areas, as well as the prevalence of poorly trained village doctors, many of whom are a layover of the Maoist barefoot doctors (Ma et al., 2020). Chen et al. (2020) illustrate that rural clinicians are well aware of the substandard care and a lack of needed medical resources in rural village clinics and township hospitals.

Even though China served as a global model for primary and integrative healthcare in the World Health Organization's 1978 Declaration of Alma Ata, Li et al. (2020b) argue that the quality of care, particularly in rural areas, may be deleteriously impacted by the lack of primary healthcare's integration into the general healthcare system; particularly exemplified by the lack of integration of mental health services at the primary care level, as well as throughout the Chinese healthcare system. This issue has resulted in a lack of accurate estimation of mental health needs, a lack of financing and funding and development of affordable and sustainable care for mental health, a lack of mental health human resources and training, and a lack of integration of mental healthcare with physical healthcare.

Furthermore, there is a lack of capacity to deliver care to specific subpopulations in order to meet the needs of China's diverse population (*Ibid.*). The shortcomings of the rural healthcare system are compounded by the elderly who are presenting with multi-morbidities.

The Capacity of Rural Healthcare for Multi-Morbidities among Elderly Patients

Globally, the impact of populations living longer presents the potential for elderly to simultaneously experience more than one chronic condition, i.e. multi-morbidities. Rural healthcare systems in China are not prepared to handle patients with one chronic condition, much less those with multi-morbidities. Ma et al. (2020) identified that 70.4% of patients in China with a chronic illness were multi-morbid and that multi-morbidity is more prevalent among rural (58.3%) than among urban populations (50.4%). They attribute this difference to a higher prevalence of mental depression in rural areas. For example, Ma et al. (2020) identified that 36.8% of rural residents above the age of 45 had depressive symptoms compared to 24.7% of urban residents.

The Influence of Neoliberalism

Few, if any, studies have considered the impact of economic neoliberalism on elder well-being. Neoliberalism describes both an economic system and an accompanying philosophy. The economic system of neoliberalism is mostly concerned with an unfettered market in which trade is free from the regulations of the state, including tariffs and taxes. The philosophy of neoliberalism not only results in the marked withdrawal of the role of the state, particularly concerning the welfare of its citizens, but also reinforces the importance of the autonomous individual who bears the responsibility for their own well-being. Although post-Maoist China, since the economic changes of the 1980s, may be considered to practise state-controlled capitalism, the neoliberal autonomous individual has been reinforced and superimposed on the historical Confucian central responsibilities of the family in the welfare of citizens. This placing of responsibility on the family for the welfare of its members was made a legal mandate in 1996 (Article 10 of the law on the Protection of the Rights of the Elderly) and 2001 (Article 21 of the Marriage Law) in which elderly parents are entitled to the support provided by their children, as well as in a July 2013 law which "requires migrant members to 'often' visit relatives over 60 years old, in addition to caring for their psychological needs. Migrants who fail to do so can face possible fines and detentions" (Tse 2013, p. 3). However, migrant children may be limited in the amount that can be sent back to parents, which is an outcome of the unequal distribution of wealth throughout China. Tse (2013) identified a correlation between the inequitable distribution of community wealth and elder health outcomes, finding that higher village GDP per capita increases the overall health quality of elders, in terms of self-rated health, mental status, and memory.

Thus, there are myriad and varied factors that can interact in complex ways to impact the health of rural left-behind elderly. However, there are also several ways to mitigate these deleterious factors and improve the health and well-being of left-behind elderly.

The Role of Agency, Recuperation, Social Cohesion, and Social Capital in the Health of Left-Behind Elderly

Much of the literature on the left-behind elderly depicts them as being acted upon and agentless, rather than capable of acting. This brief examination identifies how agency, recuperation, social cohesion, and social capital can benefit the health and well-being of the left-behind elderly.

Recuperation is commonly classified in terms of recovery of one's health and well-being through rest or activities that foster recovery. However, to understand recuperation, we need to understand from what one is recuperating. Hence, recuperation is relative to one's state of being. For example, if one has been too solitary, recuperation would be fostered through social activities. This concept of recuperation and revitalization is central to traditional and ancient Chinese medical thought, where treatment aims to harmonize imbalances caused by excesses or deficiencies in one's life, and preventative health measures, including moderation and regularity in lifestyle and diet, living in harmony with the seasons, and avoiding physical overexertion and emotional excess, are emphasized.

The Essential Prescriptions for Every Emergency Worth a Thousand in Gold (*Beiji qian jin yaofang*, 備急千金要方), c. 652 CE, is illustrative for Physician-Scholar Sun Simiao's (孫思邈) seventh-century philosophy of *Yangsheng* (养生). "The ancients, in their knowledge of the Dao, followed the pattern of yin and yang, harmonised [their actions] with skills and calculations, were moderate in their food and drink and regular in their living habits, and did not recklessly overexert themselves. Therefore, they were able to keep their body and spirit complete and live out their heavenly years to the fullest, only leaving after a hundred years had passed" (quoted in Wilms, 2010). Yangsheng may be understood as a system of beliefs and practices designed for self-health cultivation, or what Lo (2001) calls "Techniques of nurturing life", which are aimed at physical cultivation and longevity, dating to the Western Han period, and which in the present may broadly include such popular activities as *taijiquan* (太極拳) and *qigong* (氣功). These cultivation-of-longevity practices were originally performed in hopes of attaining one's proper life expectancy, with the possession of their full vital forces (Engelhardt, 2000).

According to Yang (2006, p. iv), yangsheng practice "enables the elderly to maintain a positive attitude towards ageing [and] allows for more control over the social, economic and cultural implications of ageing in today's China". Although commonly practised individually, yangsheng practices are also often practised in groups, thereby serving as a bridge from physical well-being to social well-being, which is particularly valuable for left-behind elders. Yang (2006, p. 208) argues: "Yangsheng, as an effective means through which the aging body can be transformed into an active, independent, and useful social body". In other words, yangsheng practices may not only provide a means for physical and psychical recuperation, but may also serve as a means to exercise sociality through social cohesion and social capital.

Social cohesion can be defined as the interactions among members of a group that are characterized by "attitudes and norms that includes trust, a sense of belonging, and the willingness to participate and help" (Chan, To and Chan, 2006, p. 298). Hence, social cohesion allows one to feel that they "belong" to a group and helps

The Health and Well-Being

to give their life meaning through their interactions with others. Roca and Helbing (2011, p. 11370) assert that well-being in modern societies relies on social cohesion. While Coburn (2000, p. 135) identifies "a particular affinity between neoliberal (market-oriented) political doctrines, income inequality, and lowered social cohesion". Neoliberalism, it is argued, produces both higher income inequality and lowered social cohesion. Considering that neoliberalism champions competition and full responsibility of the individual for their own life, it is apparent why neoliberalism would not inherently foster social cohesion and why, in turn, social cohesion would be needed to counter the negative social impacts of neoliberalism. Furthermore, fostering social cohesion could serve as a means of recuperation to redress the solitude experienced by the left-behind elderly.

If social cohesion inspires a sense of belonging, social capital can be thought of as the extra benefits of this belonging. Social capital can be understood as both the resources and social status acquired via one's social relationships. According to Bhandari and Yasunobu (2009, p. 480), social capital refers to "a collective asset in the form of shared norms, values, beliefs, trust, networks, social relations, and institutions that facilitate cooperation and collective action for mutual benefits". This definition captures much of the multidimensional aspects of social capital. Social capital, with its elements of social trust, norms of reciprocity, and particularly social cohesion, is foundational for a community's capacity to effectively respond to social change (Kadetz 2018). Social capital is particularly central to Chinese social relations, where success and status are portrayed as a direct outcome of the strength of one's social connections or guanxi (關係) (Chen et al. 2020). The concept of guanxi, which dates to Confucian doctrine, is enacted through one's mutual commitments and reciprocity in social relations and is similar to the transcultural role of gift giving—as the crossing of a threshold marking entry into social relationships—as described by Mauss (2002).

Social capital has been identified as an important determinant of health outcomes (Kawachi et al. 2004). Many studies have demonstrated the relationship between social capital and health, particularly in terms of trust (Subramanian et al. 2002) and reciprocity, perceived social support (Wen et al. 2003), and civic participation (Yip et al. 2007; Yamaoka 2008; Wang et al. 2009). In general, high levels of social capital are believed to enable elderly to maintain independent, productive, and satisfactory lives (Huang and Li, 2019), whereas having low social capital and being left behind were significantly associated with a lower health-related quality of life (i.e. having lower outcomes in physical, psychological, social, and cognitive functioning, as well as poorer general well-being), resulting in significant vulnerabilities (Zhong et al. 2017).

Some have distinguished between cognitive social capital (which mainly concerns trust) and structural social capital (also known as community capital, which mainly concerns the development of social networks and linkages). Cognitive social capital, and trust, in particular, has been positively correlated with self-reported general health, psychological health, and subjective well-being, which were identified as positively associated with both general health and mental health (Wang et al. 2009), whereas mistrust is powerfully associated with worsening mental health (*Ibid.*). Yip et al. (2007, p. 46) also distinguish the health benefits of cognitive social capital, identifying that trust "exhibits stronger and more consistently positive associations with health and well-being in rural China than organizational membership".

According to Putnam et al. (1993), social capital and social cohesion can be understood to overlap: particularly in terms of trust, norms, and networks, all of which can facilitate coordinated actions. Being an important link between both social cohesion and social capital, fostering trust would be an important means to improve the health and well-being of left-behind elderly. In sum, social cohesion and social capital can act as buffers and serve to build community capacity and resilience in both communities and individuals (Kadetz, 2018). Clearly, many of the deleterious health outcomes of being left behind and elderly may be balanced by community activities that foster social cohesion, social capital, and trust. However, this is not to imply that community and individual agency should bear the responsibility for either instituting, developing, or sustaining these activities, which would need to be the responsibility of local governments. Navarro's (2004; 2002) critique of the use of the concept of social capital in the literature is that, similar to the discourse of neoliberalism, social capital can be understood to circumvent and relieve the state of its responsibilities for the welfare of its citizens, placing this burden squarely on the shoulders of individuals and families. However, what may be overlooked in this critique is the sense of meaning and purpose that may be lost when one is left behind and that may be renewed with increased sociality.

CONCLUSIONS

The needed input of the Chinese government in protecting the health of the left-behind elderly across several dimensions has been established by the literature. (i) Although the current demographic crisis resulting from the one-child policy will take years to reverse, if even possible, [2] the hukou system could be overhauled to allow the urban relocation of the entire family of migrant workers, including their elderly parents. (ii) More importantly is having access to rural health care that is of equal quality to urban care. (iii) According to Scheffel and Zhang (2019), the concept of elderly care is not commonly considered acceptable or appropriate in China, and local governments will rarely provide financial support for elder care, and no specific funding is allocated for longer-term elderly care. Hence, the provision of elderly care facilities, such as assisted living or nursing homes, is highly underdeveloped and underfunded in China, and the quality of such services, if they exist at all, is considered very low, particularly in rural areas. (iv) An equitable rural pension system would be necessary to overcome many of the inequalities of the rural elderly. (v) Fostering agency, recuperation, social cohesion, and social capital in communities of left-behind elderly are imperative. (vi) Trust is central to building communities. Wang et al. (2009) call for effective policies that target building a trusting environment in order to improve general health and reduce interpersonal mistrust to improve mental well-being. And (vii) technical innovation could also benefit the health and well-being of left-behind elderly in rural China. For example, digital health can be leveraged to improve rural

---

[2] And actually may not substantially reverse in the near future, given the tepid response to the Universal Two-Child Policy instituted in 2016, for which young couples rationalizse that they cannot afford a second child.

The Health and Well-Being 101

healthcare in China, particularly in facilitating support for patients and front-line providers (Li et al. 2020a).

There is much work that the Chinese government can, and needs to, enact in order to redress the deleterious outcomes of many of its former policies and programs that have compromised the health of the left-behind elderly. Central to the above-mentioned recommendations, local governments need to prioritize the development or improvement of the current social support system for the elderly who are left behind by their migrant working children (Ma and Zhou 2009). The prioritization of social infrastructure that protects the health and well-being of the rural left-behind elderly in China is essential to ameliorate the impacts of years of policies that have exacerbated the vulnerability of the rural elderly. Yip et al. (2007, p. 48) suggest that "policies aimed at producing and enhancing an environment that strengthens existing social networks and facilitates the exchange of social support, at both the individual and village levels, hold promise in improving the health and well-being of the Chinese rural population". In addition, low-cost institutions in source communities of migration, such as day care for the left-behind elderly, would provide needed relief (Ma and Zhou 2009).

In sum, there is no rationale for the People's Republic of China to ignore one of its most vulnerable populations, the left-behind elderly, and exclude them from enjoying the benefits of the nation's dramatic economic growth, for which the work of their children is, in large part, responsible.

REFERENCES

Adulyadej, B. (1999a) 'The practice of the arts of healing act B.E. 2542', *The Royal Thai Gazette*, 116 Article(39a).

Adulyadej, B. (1999b) The protection and promotion of thai traditional medicine wisdom act B.E. 2542, *Thai Royal Gazette*, Available at: https://thailawonline.com/fr/thai-laws/laws-of-thailand/301-protection-and-promotion-of-traditional-thai-medicine-wisdom-act-be-2542-1999-.html (Accessed: 10 September 2020).

Afshar, S. et al. (2015) 'Multi-morbidity and the inequalities of global ageing: A cross-sectional study of 28 countries using the World Health Surveys', *BMC Public Health*, 15(776). doi: 10.1186/s12889-015–2008-7.

Aizenstein, H. J. et al. (2016) 'Vascular depression consensus report - a critical update', *BMC Medicine*, 14(1), pp. 1–16. doi: 10.1186/s12916-016-0720–5.

Al-Hashel, J. Y. et al. (2018) 'Use of traditional medicine for primary headache disorders in Kuwait', *Journal of Headache and Pain*, 19(1), pp. 3–9. doi: 10.1186/s10194-018-0950–3.

Al-Kindi, R. et al. (2011) 'Complementary and alternative medicine use among adults with diabetes in muscat region, Oman', *Sultan Qaboos University Medical Journal*, 11(1), p. 62.

Al-Rowais, N. et al. (2010) 'Traditional healers in riyadh region: Reasons and health problems for seeking their advice. A household survey', *Journal of Alternative and Complementary Medicine*, 16(2), pp. 199–204. doi: 10.1089/acm.2009.0283.

Ang, J. Y. et al. (2021) 'A Malaysian retrospective study of acupuncture-assisted anesthesia in breast lump excision', *Acupuncture in Medicine*, 39(1), pp. 64–68. doi: 10.1177/0964528420920307.

Antman, F. (2012) 'How does adult child migration affect the health of elderly parents left behind? Evidence from Mexico', *SSRN Electronic Journal*. doi: 10.2139/ssrn.1578465.

Ao, X., Jiang, D. and Zhao, Z. (2016) 'The impact of rural-urban migration on the health of the left-behind parents', *China Economic Review*, 37, pp. 126–139. doi: 10.1016/j. chieco.2015.09.007.

Awad, A. I., Al-Ajmi, S. and Waheedi, M. A. (2012) 'Knowledge, perceptions and attitudes toward complementary and alternative therapies among Kuwaiti medical and pharmacy students', *Medical Principles and Practice*, 21(4), pp. 350–354. doi: 10.1159/000336216.

Barcella, C. A. et al. (2021) 'Severe mental illness is associated with increased mortality and severe course of COVID-19', *Acta Psychiatrica Scandinavica*, (March), pp. 1–10. doi: 10.1111/acps.13309.

Bernama (2020) *Malaysia's Population Estimates at 32.7 million in 2020, Astro Awani.* Available at: http://english.astroawani.com/malaysia-news/malaysias-population-estimates-32-7-million-2020-251323 (Accessed: 15 July 2020).

Bhandari, H. and Yasunobu, K. (2009) 'What is social capital? A comprehensive review of the concept', *Asian Journal of Social Science*, 37(3). doi: 10.1163/156853109X436847.

Bodeker, G. et al. (2018) *Mental Wellness: Pathways, Evidence, Horizons.* Edited by G. Bodeker. Miammi.

Bodeker, G. and Kronenberg, F. (2015) 'Tackling obesity: Challenges ahead', *The Lancet*, 386(9995), pp. 740–741. doi: 10.1016/S0140–6736(15)61539-2.

Böhme, M. H., Persian, R. and Stöhr, T. (2015) 'Alone but better off? Adult child migration and health of elderly parents in Moldova', *Journal of Health Economics*, 39, pp. 211–227. doi: 10.1016/j.jhealeco.2014.09.001.

Bowman, G. L. et al. (2012) 'Nutrient biomarker patterns, cognitive function, and MRI measures of brain aging', *Neurology*, 78(4), pp. 241–249. doi: 10.1212/WNL.0b013e3182436598.

Brooks, S. J. et al. (2020) 'The psychologial impact of quarantine and how to reduce it: Rapid review of the evidence', *The Lancet*, 295(10227), pp. 912–920.

Byrow, Y. et al. (2020) 'Perceptions of mental health and perceived barriers to mental health help-seeking amongst refugees: A systematic review', *Clinical Psychology Review*, 75(July 2018), p. 101812. doi: 10.1016/j.cpr.2019.101812.

Chan, J., To, H. P. and Chan, E. (2006) 'Reconsidering social cohesion: Developing a definition and analytical framework for empirical research', *Social Indicators Research*, 75(2), pp. 273–302. doi: 10.1007/s11205-005-2118-1.

Chang, F. et al. (2016) 'Adult child migration and elderly parental health in rural China', *China Agricultural Economic Review*, 8(4), pp. 677–697. doi: 10.1108/CAER-11–2015–0169.

Chen, M. et al. (2020) 'Prescribing Antibiotics in Rural China: The Influence of Capital on Clinical Realities', *Frontiers in Sociology*, 5(October), pp. 0–10. doi: 10.3389/fsoc.2020.00066.

China, N. S. B. o. t. P. s. R. o. (2018) *National Statistical Bureau of the People's Republic of China.* Available at: http://www.stats.gov.cn/english/Statisticaldata/AnnualData.

Chokevivat, V. and Chuthaputti, A. (2005). 'The Role of Thai Traditional Medicine in Health Promotion', in *Department for the Development of Thai Traditional and Alternative Medicine*, pp. 1–25. Available at: http://citeseerx.ist.psu.edu/viewdoc/download?doi=10 .1.1.496.5656&rep=rep1&type=pdf.

Chong, S. A. et al. (2016) 'Recognition of mental disorders among a multiracial population in Southeast Asia', *BMC Psychiatry*, 16(1). doi: 10.1186/s12888-016-0837-2.

CIA (2020) *The World Factbook.* Available at: https://www.cia.gov/library/publications/the-world-factbook/fields/223rank.html.

Coburn D (2000) 'Income inequality, social cohesion, and the health status of populations', *Social Science and Medicine*, 51, pp. 135–146.

Crawford Shearer, N. B., Fleury, J. D. and Belyea, M. (2010) 'An innovative approach to recruiting homebound older adults', *Research in Gerontological Nursing*, 3(1), pp. 11–17. doi: 10.3928/19404921–20091029-01.

The Health and Well-Being 103

Crosette, B. (1986) Vietnamese Revive Ancient Medical Arts, The New York Times. Available at: https://www.nytimes.com/1986/08/12/science/vietnamese-revive-ancient-medical-arts.html (Accessed: 16 October 2020).

Crunfli, F. et al. (2021) 'SARS-CoV-2 infects brain astrocytes of COVID-19 patients and impairs neuronal viability', *medRxiv*, p. 2020. doi: 10.1101/2020.10.09.20207464.

Dai, Y. et al. (2016) 'Social Support and self-rated health of older people: A comparative study in Tainan Taiwan and Fuzhou Fujian Province', *Medicine*, 95(24), p. 3881. doi: 10.1097/MD.0000000000003881.

De La Rubia Ortí, J. E. et al. (2018) 'Does music therapy improve anxiety and depression in alzheimer's patients?', *Journal of Alternative and Complementary Medicine*, 24(1), pp. 33–36. doi: 10.1089/acm.2016.0346.

Department of AYUSH (2012) *Ayurveda: The Science of Life*. Department of AYUSH.

Department of Statistics (2020) *Current Population Estimates, Malaysia, Online*. Available at: https://www.dosm.gov.my/v1/index.php?r=column/cthemeByCat&cat=155&bul_id=OVByWjg5YkQ3MWFZRTN5bDJiaEVhZz09&menu_id=L0pheU43NWJwRWVSZklWdzQ4TlhUUT09 (Accessed: 22 February 2021).

Douaud, G. et al. (2013). 'Preventing Alzheimer's disease-related gray matter atrophy by B-vitamin treatment', *Proceedings of the National Academy of Sciences of the United States of America*, 110(23), pp. 9523–9528. doi: 10.1073/pnas.1301816110.

Engelhardt, U. (2000) 'Longevity techniques and Chinese medicine', in *Daoism handbook*. Brill, pp. 74–108.

Fasullo, L., Hernandez, A. and Bodeker, G. (2020) 'The innate human potential of elevated and ecstatic states of consciousness: Examining freeform dance as a means of access', *Dance, Movement & Spiritualities*, 6(1–2), pp. 87–117. doi: 10.1386/dmas_00005_1.

Fields, G. and Song, Y. (2020) 'Modeling migration barriers in a two-sector framework: A welfare analysis of the hukou reform in China', *Economic Modelling*, 84(59), pp. 293–301. doi: 10.1016/j.econmod.2019.04.019.

Fotoukian, Z. et al. (2014) 'Concept analysis of empowerment in old people with chronic diseases using a hybrid model', *Asian Nursing Research*, 8(2), pp. 118–127. doi: 10.1016/j.anr.2014.04.002.

Fu, S., Huang, N. and Chou, Y.-J. (2014) 'Trends in the prevalence of multiple chronic conditions in Taiwan From 2000 to 2010: a population-based study'. doi: 10.5888/pcd11.140205.

Fujikawa, Y. (1904) *Nihon igakushi (History of Japanese Medicine)*. Shokabo.

Galderisi, S. et al. (2015) 'Toward a new defition of mental health', *World Psychiatry*, 14(2), p. 231.

García, H. and Miralles, F. (2016) *IKIGAI. The Japanese Secret to a Long and Happy Life*.

Google (2020) *Singapore Ethnic Composition in 2019, Online*. Available at: https://www.google.com.my/search?q=singapore+ethnic+composition+in+2019&tbm=isch&ved=2ahUKEwiy6OHQs5DsAhVJB3IKHWjwCukQ2-cCegQIABAA&oq=singapore+ethnic+composition+in+2019&gs_lcp=CgNpbWcQAzoECAAQGFDp2gFYg8kCYPzNAmgAcAB4AIABXIgBrgqSAQIyOJgBAKABAaoBC2d3cy13a (Accessed: 30 September 2020).

Hansa Jayadeva, S. (2010) *Yoga Teacher's Manual for School Teachers*. Morarji Desai National Institute of Yoga.

Hu, Y. and Shi, X. (2020) 'The impact of China's one-child policy on intergenerational and gender relations', *Contemporary Social Science*, 15(3), pp. 360–377. doi: 10.1080/21582041.2018.1448941.

Huang, B., Lian, Y. and Li, W. (2016) 'How far is Chinese left-behind parents' health left behind?', *China Economic Review*, 37(71002056), pp. 15–26. doi: 10.1016/j.chieco.2015.07.002.

Huang, C. and Li, Y. (2019) 'Understanding leisure satisfaction of Chinese seniors: human capital, family capital, and community capital', *Journal of Chinese Sociology*, 6(1). doi: 10.1186/s40711-019-0094-0.

Huang, Y. and Liu, X. (2015) 'Improvement of balance control ability and flexibility in the elderly Tai Chi Chuan (TCC) practitioners: A systematic review and meta-analysis', *Archives of Gerontology and Geriatrics*, 60(2), pp. 233–238. doi: 10.1016/j.archger.2014.10.016.

Ibrahim, I. et al. (2016) 'A qualitative insight on complementary and alternative medicines used by hypertensive patients', *Journal of Pharmacology and Bioallied Science*, 8(4), pp. 284–288.

Institute for Public Health (2015) *National Health and Morbidity Survey 2015: Traditional and Complementary Medicine, Ministry of Health Malaysia*. Putrajaya.

Institute for Public Health (2020) *National Health and Morbidity Survey 2019: Non-Communicable Diseases, Health Demand, and Health Literacy - Key Findings*. Available at: http://iku.gov.my/images/IKU/Document/REPORT/NHMS2019/Fact_Sheet_NHMS_2019-English.pdf.

Institute of Medicine (US) Committe on the Use of Complementary and Alternative Medicine by the American Public (2005) *Complementary Alternative Medicine in the United States*. Washington, D.C. Available at: https://www.ncbi.nlm.nih.gov/books/NBK83804/.

Jaiswal, Y. and Williams, L. (2017) 'A glimpse of Ayurveda – The forgotten history and principles of Indian traditional medicine', *Journal of Traditional and Complementary Medicine*, 7(1), pp. 50–53. doi: 10.1016/j.jtcme.2016.02.002.

John W Brick Foundation (2021) *Move you mental wellness*. Available at: www.johnwbrickfoundation.org/move-your-mental-health-report/ (Accessed: 24 June 2021).

Kadetz, P. (2018) 'Collective efficacy, social capital and resilience: An inquiry into the relationship between social infrastructure and resilience after Hurricane Katrina', in *Creating Katrina, Rebuilding Resilience*. Butterworth-Heinemann, pp. 283–304.

Kalil, A. (2020) 'Treating COVID-19 Off-label drug use, compassionate use, and randomized clinical trials during pandemics', *Journal of the American Medical Association*, 323(19), pp. 1897–1898.

Kavadar, G. et al. (2019) 'Use of traditional and complementary medicine for musculoskeletal diseases', *Turkish Journal of Medical Sciences*, 49(3), pp. 809–814. doi: 10.3906/sag-1509-71.

Kawachi, I. et al. (2004) 'Commentary: Reconciling the three accounts of social capital', *International Journal of Epidemiology*, 33(4), pp. 682–690. doi: 10.1093/ije/dyh177.

Keshet, Y. and Popper-Giveon, A. (2013) 'Integrative health care in israel and traditional arab herbal medicine: when health care interfaces with culture and politics', *Medical Anthropology Quarterly*, 27(3), pp. 368–384. doi: 10.1111/maq.12049.

Khalaf, A. J. and Whitford, D. L. (2008) 'The use of complementary and alternative medicine by patients with osteoporosis', *Nature Clinical Practice Endocrinology and Metabolism*, 4(3), p. 120. doi: 10.1038/ncpendmet0732.

Kuhn, R., Everett, B. and Silvey, R. (2011) 'The effects of children's migration on Elderly Kin's health: A counterfactual approach', *Demography*, 48(1), pp. 183–209. doi: 10.1007/s13524-010-0002-3.

Lauber, C. and Rössler, W. (2007) 'Stigma towards people with mental illness in developing countries in Asia', *International Review of Psychiatry*, 19(2), pp. 157–178. doi: 10.1080/09540260701278903.

Lee, D. Y. W. et al. (2021) 'Traditional Chinese herbal medicine at the forefront battle against COVID-19: Clinical experience and scientific basis', *Phytomedicine*, 80(September 2020), p. 153337. doi: 10.1016/j.phymed.2020.153337.

Lei, X. et al. (2014) 'Depressive symptoms and SES among the mid-aged and elderly in China: Evidence from the China Health and Retirement Longitudinal Study national baseline', *Social Science and Medicine*, 120, pp. 224–232. doi: 10.1016/j.socscimed.2014.09.028.

The Health and Well-Being

Lei, Y. et al. (2021) 'SARS-CoV-2 spike protein impairs endothelial function via downregulation of ACE 2', *Circulation Research*, 128, pp. 1323–1326.

Lhamo, N. and Nebel, S. (2011) 'Perceptions and attitudes of Bhutanese people on Sowa Rigpa, traditional bhutanese medicine: A preliminary study from Thimphu', *Journal of Ethnobiology and Ethnomedicine*, 7(January), pp. 1–9. doi: 10.1186/1746-4269-7-3.

Li, C. et al. (2020) 'Discussion on TCM theory and modern pharmacological mechanism of Qinfei Paidu decoction in the treatment of COVID-19', *Journal of Traditional Chinese Medicine*, pp. 1–4.

Li, T. et al. (2020) 'What happens to the health of elderly parents when adult child migration splits households? Evidence from rural China', *International Journal of Environmental Research and Public Health*, 17(5). doi: 10.3390/ijerph17051609.

Li, X. et al. (2020) 'Quality of primary health care in China: challenges and recommendations', *The Lancet*, 395(10239), pp. 1802–1812. doi: 10.1016/S0140-6736(20)30122-7.

Lo, V. (2001) 'The influence of nurturing life culture on early Chinese medical theory', *In* Hsu, E. (ed.) *Innovation in Chinese medicine*. Cambridge University Press, pp. 19–50.

Logue, J. K. et al. (2021) 'Sequelae in adults at 6 months after COVID-19 infection', *JAMA Network Open*, 4(2), pp. 8–11. doi: 10.1001/jamanetworkopen.2021.0830.

Luo, H. et al. (2020) 'Reflections on treatment of COVID-19 with traditional Chinese medicine', *Chinese Medicine (United Kingdom)*, 15(1), pp. 1–14. doi: 10.1186/s13020-020-00375-1.

Ma, X., He, Y. and Xu, J. (2020) 'Urban-rural disparity in prevalence of multimorbidity in China: A cross-sectional nationally representative study', *BMJ Open*, 10(11), pp. 1–9. doi: 10.1136/bmjopen-2020-038404.

Ma, Z. and Zhou, G. (2009) 'Isolated or compensated: the impact of temporary migration of adult children on the wellbeing of the elderly in rural China', *Geographical review of Japan series B*, 81(1), pp. 47–59. doi: 10.4157/geogrevjapanb.81.47.

Malaysian Government (2016) *The Traditional and Complementary Medicine Act 2016*.

Mauss, M. (2002) *The Gift: The Form and Reason for Exchange in Archaic Societies*. London: Routledge.

Miller, V. et al. (2017) 'Prospective Urban Rural Epidemiology (PURE) study investigators. Fruit, vegetable, and legume intake, and cardiovascular disease and deaths in 18 countries: A prospective cohort study', *The Lancet*, 390(10107), pp. 2037–2049.

Ministry of AYUSH (2015) *Homeopathy: Science of Gentle Healing. Ministry of AYUSH*.

Ministry of AYUSH (2016) *Unani System of Medicine: The Science of Health and Healing*.

Ministry of AYUSH (2019) *Introduction to Sowa-Rigpa, About the Systems*.

Ministry of Health and National Institute of Health Research and Development (2018) *National report on basic health research, Riskesdas, 2018. Jakarta, Indonesia*.

Ministry of Health Turkey (2016) *Traditioal and Complementary Medicine Practices and Related Legislation*.

Ministry of Health Turkey (2020) *What is Traditiona and Complementary Medicine, Traditional, Complementary and Functional Medicine Practices, Department*.

Minton, S. and Faber, R. (2016) *Thinking with the Dancing Brain: Embodying Neuroscience*. Lanham, Maryland: Rowman and Littlefield.

Mofredj, A. et al. (2016) 'Music therapy, a review of the potential therapeutic benefits for the critically ill', *Journal of Critical Care*, 35, pp. 195–199. doi: 10.1016/j.jcrc.2016.05.021.

Mohanty, S., Sharma, P. and Sharma, G. (2020) 'Yoga for infirmity in geriatric population amidst COVID-19 pandemic: Comment on "Age and Ageism in COVID-19: Elderly mental health-care vulnerabilities and needs", *Asian Journal of Psychiatry*, 53, p. 102199.

Moreno, C. et al. (2020) 'How mental health care should change as a consequence of the COVID-19 pandemic', *Lancet Psychiatry*, 7(9), pp. 813–824. doi: 10.1016/S2215-0366(20)30307-2.

Nadareishvili, I. et al. (2019) 'Georgia's healthcare system and integration of complementary medicine', *Complementary Therapies in Medicine*, 45(January), pp. 205–210. doi: 10.1016/j.ctim.2019.06.016.

Nagasu, M., Muto, K. and Yamamoto, I. (2021) 'Impacts of anxiety and socioeconomic factors on mental health in the early phases of the COVID-19 pandemic in the general population in Japan: A web-based survey', *PLoS ONE*, 16(3 March), pp. 1–19. doi: 10.1371/journal.pone.0247705.

National Health Services (2018) *A Guide to Tai Chi, NHS UK*. UK. Available at: http://www.nhs.uk/Livewell/fitness/Pages/taichi.aspx (Accessed: 24 June 2021).

National Institute on Aging (2011) *Global Health and Aging*.

Nutbeam, D. and Kickbusch, I. (1998) 'Health promotion glossary', *Health Promotion International*, 13(4), pp. 349–364. doi: 10.1093/heapro/13.4.349.

Ogbo, F. A. et al. (2018) 'The burden of depressive disorders in South Asia, 1990–2016: Findings from the global burden of disease study', *BMC Psychiatry*, 18(1), pp. 1–11. doi: 10.1186/s12888-018-1918-1.

Ozer, O., Santaş, F. and Yildirim, H. H. (2012) 'An evaluation on levels of knowledge, attitude and behavior of people at 65 years and above about alternative medicine living in Ankara', *African Journal of Traditional, Complementary, and Alternative Medicines : AJTCAM / African Networks on Ethnomedicines*, 10(1), pp. 134–141. doi: 10.4314/ajtcam.v10i1.18.

Pang, W. et al. (2020) 'Chinese herbal medicine for coronavirus disease 2019: A systematic review and meta-analysis', Integrative Medicine Research, 9(160) (March), p. 100477. doi: 10.1016/j.phrs.2020.105056.

Park, B. J. et al. (2010) 'The physiological effects of Shinrin-yoku (taking in the forest atmosphere or forest bathing): Evidence from field experiments in 24 forests across Japan', *Environmental Health and Preventive Medicine*, 15(1), pp. 18–26. doi: 10.1007/s12199-009-0086-9.

Park, H. (2003) *North Korea Handbook*. Yonhap News Agency. Available at: https://books.google.com.my/books?id=JIlh9nNeadMC&pg=PA439&lpg=PA439&dq=KORYO+MEDICINE&source=bl&ots=gy-.

Patel, V. et al. (2018) 'The Lancet Commission on global mental health and sustainable development', *The Lancet*, 392(10157), pp. 1553–1598. doi: 10.1016/S0140–6736(18)31612-X.

Pusan National University School of Korean Medicine (2015) *Korean Medicine: Current Status and Future Prospects*.

Putnam, R., Leonardi, R. and Nanetti, R. (1993) 'What makes democracy work: civic traditions in modern Italy', *International Affairs*.

Ravishankar, B. and Shukla, V. J. (2007) 'Indian systems of medicine: A brief review', *Arfrican Journal of Traditional, Complementary and Alternative Medicine*, 4(3), pp. 319–337.

Republic of Phillipines (1997) *Traditional and Alternative Medicine Act of 1997*.

Reyburn, S. (2019) *Rosa Parks: In her own Words*. Atlanta: University of Georgia Press.

Roca, C. P. and Helbing, D. (2011) 'Emergence of social cohesion in a model society of greedy, mobile individuals', *Proceedings of the National Academy of Sciences of the United States of America*, 108(28), pp. 11370–11374. doi: 10.1073/pnas.1101044108.

Sarris, J. et al. (2015) 'Nutritional medicine as mainstream in psychiatry', *The Lancet Psychiatry*, 2(3), pp. 271–274. doi: 10.1016/S2215–0366(14)00051-0.

Scheffel, J. and Zhang, Y. (2019) 'How does internal migration affect the emotional health of elderly parents left-behind?', *Journal of Population Economics*, 32(3), pp. 953–980. doi: 10.1007/s00148-018-0715-y.

Shengelia, R. (1999) 'Study of the history of medicine in Georgia', *Croatian Medical Journal*, 40(1), pp. 38–41.

Shi, N. et al. (2021) 'Efficacy and safety of Chinese herbal medicine versus Lopinavir-Ritonavir in adult patients with coronavirus disease 2019: A non-randomized controlled trial', *Phytomedicine*, 81(January). doi: 10.1016/j.phymed.2020.153367.

Shih, C. C. et al. (2015) 'Use of Folk Therapy in Taiwan: A Nationwide Cross-Sectional Survey of Prevalence and Associated Factors', *Evidence-based Complementary and Alternative Medicine*, 2015. doi: 10.1155/2015/649265.

Shuval, J. T. and Averbuch, E. (2012) 'Complementary and alternative health care in Israel', *Israel Journal of Health Policy Research*, 1(1), pp. 1–12. doi: 10.1186/2045-4015-1-7.

Song, L. et al. (2007) 'Effects of a sun style Tai Chi exercise on arthritic symptoms, motivation and performance of health behaviours in women with osteoarthritis', *Taehan Kanho Hakhoe chi*, 37(2), pp. 249–256.

Song, Y. (2014) 'Mental support or economic giving: migrating children's elderly care behaviour and health conditions of left-behind elderly in rural China', *Population and Developemtn*, 20(4), pp. 37–44.

Stickley, A. et al. (2013) 'Prevalence and factors associated with the use of alternative (folk) medicine practitioners in 8 countries of the former Soviet Union', *BMC Complementary and Alternative Medicine*, 13(83). doi: 10.1186/1472-6882-13-83.

Subramanian, S. V., Kim, D. J. and Kawachi, I. (2002) 'Social trust and self-rated health in US communities: A multilevel analysis', *Journal of Urban Health*, 79(1), pp. 21–34. doi: 10.1093/jurban/79.suppl_1.s21.

Thas, J. J. (2008) 'Siddha Medicine-background and principles and the application for skin diseases', *Clinics in Dermatology*, 26(1), pp. 62–78. doi: 10.1016/j.clindermatol.2007.11.010.

The Law Commission Revisions (2015) *The Statutes of the Republic of Singapore - COPYRIGHT ACT*.

The State Council Information Office (2016) *Traditioanal Chinese Medicine in China*. Available at: http://english.www.gov.cn/archive/white_paper/2016/12/06/content_281475509333700.htm.

Al Thiab Al Kendi, A. (2014) *Health and Medicall Care in the First Hijri Century (1–101 AH/ 622–719 AD)*. National Center for Complementary and Alternative Medicine.

Thompson, N. and Thompson, S. (2001) 'Empowering Older People', *Journal of Social Work*, 1(1), pp. 61–76.

Tiemeier, H. (2003) 'Biological risk factors for late life depression', *European Journal of Epidemiology*, 18(8), pp. 745–750. Available at: http://ovidsp.ovid.com/ovidweb.cgi?T=JS&PAGE=reference&D=emed6&NEWS=N&AN=2003347329.

Traditional and Complementary Medicine (2020) *Guidelines for Registration of Traditional and Complementary Medicine Practitioners in Brunei Darussalam, Ministry of Health Brunei*.

Traditional and Complementary Medicine Division (2007) *National Policy on Traditional/ Complementary Medicine, Malaysia*. 2nd edn.

Tse, C. (2013) 'Migration and health outcomes of left-behind elderly in rural China', *Available at SSRN 2440403*.

United Nations (2016) *ESCAP population data sheet Population and Development Indicators for Asia and the Pacific, 2012*. Available at: https://www.unescap.org/sites/default/d8files/knowledge-products/SPPS PS data sheet 2016 v15-2.pdf.

United Nations (2020) *Policy Brief: The Impact of COVID-19 on Older Person, Online2*. Available at: https://www.un.org/development/desa/ageing/wp-content/uploads/sites/24/2020/05/COVID-Older-persons.pdf (Accessed: 5 June 2021).

Uttley, L. et al. (2015) 'Systematic review and economic modelling of the clinical effectiveness and cost-effectiveness of art therapy among people with non-psychotic mental health disorders', *Health Technology Assessment*, 19(18). doi: 10.3310/hta19180.

Verghese, J. et al. (2003) 'Leisure Activities and the Risk of Dementia in the Elderly', *The New England Journal of Medicine*, 348, pp. 2508–2516.

Wang, Hongmei et al. (2009) 'The flip-side of social capital: The distinctive influences of trust and mistrust on health in rural China', *Social Science and Medicine*, 68(1), pp. 133–142. doi: 10.1016/j.socscimed.2008.09.038.

Watanabe, K. et al. (2011) 'Traditional Japanese Kampo medicine: Clinical research between modernity and traditional medicine - The state of research and methodological suggestions for the future', *Evidence-based Complementary and Alternative Medicine*. doi: 10.1093/ecam/neq067.

Water for Health (2019) *Ten Rules of Ikigai: A Blueprint for a Fuller, Healthier Life?*, *Online*. Available at: Water for Health (Accessed: 24 June 2021).

Wen, M., Browning, C. R. and Cagney, K. A. (2003) 'Poverty, affluence, and income inequality: Neighborhood economic structure and its implications for health', *Social Science and Medicine*, 57(5), pp. 843–860. doi: 10.1016/S0277–9536(02)00457–4.

WHO (2002) *WHO Traditional Medicine Strategy 2002–2005*. Geneva, Switzerland.

WHO (2013) *WHO Traditional Medicine Strategy*. Geneva, Switzerland.

WHO (2018) *Traditional, Complementary and Integrative Medicine*, *WHO TM Strategy*. Available at: https://www.who.int/health-topics/traditional-complementary-and-integrative-medicine#tab=tab_1 (Accessed: 30 August 2020).

WHO (2019) *WHO Global Report on Traditional and Complementary Medicine 2019*.

Wilms, S. (2010) 'Nurturing Life in Classical Chinese Medicine: Sun Simiao on Healing without Drugs, Transforming Bodies and Cultivating Life', *Journal of Chinese Medicine*, 93.

World Health Organization (2002) *Active Ageing: A Policy Framework*.

World Health Organization (2009) *WHO Guidelines on Hand Hygiene in Health Care*. Available at: https://www.ncbi.nlm.nih.gov/books/NBK144013/pdf/Bookshelf_NBK144013.pdf.

World Health Organization (2017) *Depression and Other Common Mental Disorders: Global Health Estimates*. Geneva, Switzerland. Available at: https://apps.who.int/iris/bitstream/handle/10665/254610/WHO-MSD-MER-2017.2-eng.pdf.

World Health Organization (2018) *Mental Health Atlas 2017*. Geneva.

World Health Organization (2020a) *COVID-19 Strategy Update*, *Online*.

World Health Organization (2020b) *Nutrition for Older Persons*, *Online*. Available at: https://www.who.int/nutrition/topics/ageing/en/index1.html.

World Health Organization (2020c) *WHO Timeline COVID-19*, *Online*. Available at: https://www.who.int/news/item/27-04-2020-who-timeline—covid-19 (Accessed: 24 June 2021).

Xiang, A., Jiang, D. and Zhao, Z. (2016) 'The impact of rural-urban migration on the health of the left-behind parents', *China Economic Review*, 37, pp. 126–139. doi: 10.1016/j.chieco.2015.09.007.

Yamaoka, K. (2008) 'Social capital and health and well-being in East Asia: A population-based study', *Social Science and Medicine*, 66(4), pp. 885–899. doi: 10.1016/j.socscimed.2007.10.024.

Yang, D. (2006) *Dusk Without Sunset: Actively Aging in Traditional Chinese Medicine*. University of Pittsburgh.

Yip, W. et al. (2007) 'Does social capital enhance health and well-being? Evidence from rural China', *Social Science and Medicine*, 64(1), pp. 35–49. doi: 10.1016/j.socscimed.2006.08.027.

Zhang, Y. (2020) 'A case of severe COVID19 cured by Qinfei Paide decoction combined with Western Medicine', *Tianjin Journal of Traditional Chinese Medicine*, pp. 1–4.

Zhao, K. et al. (2016) 'A systematic review and meta-analysis of music therapy for the older adults with depression', *International Journal of Geriatric Psychiatry*, 31(11), pp. 1188–1198. doi: 10.1002/gps.4494.

Zhong, Y. et al. (2017) 'Association between social capital and health-related quality of life among left behind and not left behind older people in rural China', *BMC Geriatrics*, 17(1), pp. 1–11. doi: 10.1186/s12877-017-0679-x.

9 The Definition of TM
Perspectives from WHO and Countries across Asia

Goh Cheng Soon
T&CM Division, MOH Malaysia

CONTENTS

Introduction 109
    Definition of Traditional Medicine 110
    Perspective from WHO 111
    Perspective from the Asian Countries Located in the WPR 111
    Perspective from the Asian Countries Located in the SEAR 115
    Perspective from the Asian Countries Located in the EMR 118
    Perspective from the Asian Countries Located in the EUR 120
    Perspective from Taiwan 123
    Discussion 123
Conclusion 125
References 125

INTRODUCTION

The World Health Organization (WHO) seeks to bring traditional medicine (TM) "into mainstream of healthcare, appropriately, effectively, and above all, safely" since it contributes to people's health and wellness (WHO 2013). TM is meeting the healthcare needs of ageing population since it plays a key role in primary healthcare through empowering people and communities by creating an more readily accessible medical assistance which also provides comfort and familiarity to elderly.

Ageing and its health challenges are one of the priorities that have emerged as the issues in many countries in this fast-changing world. In particular, traditional and complementary medicine (T&CM) could play an essential role in serving the elderly category of population who believe T&CM and require a greater health care need such as ageing with chronic illnesses (Fu, Huang and Chou, 2014). As reported in *the National Health and Morbidity Survey 2015*, an estimated 29.25% of the Malaysian population had ever used any T&CM practices with consultation and health problems related to musculoskeletal system (Institute for Public Health, 2015). Myalgia, joint and muscle ache and back pain contribute to the highest usage of T&CM practices in Malaysia. 8.7% of Malaysia's population aged 13 years and over experienced chronic bodily pain, and among them, 29.3% were elderly affected by chronic pain as pain

DOI: 10.1201/9781003043270-9

prevalence increases with age (Institute for Public Health, 2020). As indicated by the Chief Statistician of Malaysia, Datuk Seri Dr Mohd Uzir Mahidin, the percentage of the population aged 65 years and over had increased from 6.7% to 7% over a one-year period, and Malaysia was expected to have ageing population with the age of 60 years and over at 15.3% by 2030 (Bernama, 2020)

As there is an increasing role for TM in the health maintenance and disease prevention, the internationally acceptable definition for TM may be relevant in facilitating international standardisation and harmonisation of TM practices and products within Asia. The use of common terms in the definition may enable collections of uniform data concerning TM practice and its utilisation in Asian countries. It aims to obtain recognition from the medical fraternity and inclusion into the national healthcare system by allowing exchange of health records and inclusion of TM data in health information systems in a manner compatible with data collected in the practice of modern medicine. Modern medicine is a dominant practice in the majority of the countries in Asia. In order to move towards better health outcomes and enter into the Universal Health Coverage (UHC) era, greater communication and respect is needed between the respective systems. In a recent global report, the WHO has again indicated that T&CM can contribute significantly to the goal of UHC (WHO, 2019).

Furthermore, a definition of TM may allow an easy reference, providing summaries of the traditional medical practices within the country, especially practice that is originated within that particular country. Through country-specific traditional medical knowledge and practices, information sharing on history, culture, religion, policy, legislation, education and training between nations can be beneficial. Hence, the purpose of this write-up is to find out whether a standard definition of TM among countries across Asia is a necessity. However, my range of interest is rather narrow, focusing on the definition of "traditional medicine" which could be merely the "tip of the iceberg" as compared to the wide range of practice of "complementary and alternative medicine" (CAM) (Institute of Medicine (US) Committee on the Use of Complementary and Alternative Medicine by the American Public, 2005). CAM could be used in certain countries to denote TM especially in developed countries. Moreover, the term "folk medicine" has been used as interchangeable with the TM in certain countries such as Israel, Kazakhstan and Russia.

DEFINITION OF TRADITIONAL MEDICINE

The practice of TM can vary from country to country and from region to region. Similarly, the definition of the TM could be varied in 50 countries across Asia based on their TM practices. It may involve a complex process in defining TM that includes stakeholder's engagement, identifying the country TM practices, having policy debates and getting recognition officially. However, they do understand that a working definition of TM is useful to them.

In order to look into the perspectives from WHO and countries across Asia pertaining to the definition of TM, the 50 Asian countries will be categorised into 4 groups in accordance with WHO regions. One-quarter of the 194 WHO Member States are in Asia. Eleven of the Asian countries locate in the Western Pacific Region (WPR),

The Definition of TM

South-East Asia Region (SEAR) and European Region (EUR) of WHO, respectively. Sixteen out of the 50 Asian countries situate in the Eastern Mediterranean Region (EMR). Taiwan is the only one Asian country that has yet to be accepted by the WHO.

PERSPECTIVE FROM WHO

In accordance with WHO, TM is "the sum total of the knowledge, skill, and practices based on the theories, beliefs, and experiences indigenous to different cultures, whether explicable or not, used in the maintenance of health as well as in the prevention, diagnosis, improvement or treatment of physical and mental illness" (WHO, 2018). WHO uses the term "traditional medicine" to refer to both TM systems such as traditional Chinese medicine (TCM) and Indian traditional systems of medicine, and a variety of indigenous medicine that benefit from thousands of years of experience. TM can be categorised into medication therapies including the usage of herbal medicines, animal parts and/or minerals and non-medication therapies including acupuncture and manual therapies and exercises (tai ji, qigong and yoga). Their fundamental theory and application are different from modern medicine. TM and indigenous medicine have been developed under the influence of history, culture, personal attitudes and philosophy (WHO, 2002). Traditional medical knowledge may be passed on verbally from one generation to another and may also be officially taught in recognised universities.

On the other hand, complementary medicine (CM) refers to "a broad set of health care practices that are not part of that country's own tradition or conventional medicine and are not fully integrated into the dominant healthcare system (WHO, 2018)." The merging of both the terms is known to be T&CM, encompassing products, practices and practitioners (WHO, 2019). The terms CM and alternative medicine are used interchangeably with TM in some countries. For example, while acupuncture is regarded as a TCM therapy in China, it has been known as a CAM therapy in many European countries because acupuncture was not established as part of their own health care traditions. A particular practice is not constraint to the term TM only, and it could be of CM or alternative medicine and T&CM, depending on its geographical location. The usage of TM is more common in developing countries, whereas the usage of CM is more popular in developed countries.

PERSPECTIVE FROM THE ASIAN COUNTRIES LOCATED IN THE WPR

Within the WHO WPR, the definition of TM in Malaysia, the Philippines and Singapore has been clearly spelled out in the respective country's relevant act, whereas for several countries its interpretation could be extracted from official governmental websites and published articles. Table 9.1 indicates that the definition of T&CM in Brunei, Malaysia and the Philippines mainly focuses on practices that take care of both physical and mental health, but exclude modern medical and dental practices. Similar to the definition of TM by WHO, the element of "culture" is being one of the significant components in the definition of T&CM in Malaysia and the Philippines.

TABLE 9.1
Definition of TM of Those Asian Countries in the WPR

No.	Country	T&CM Definition	Website Link
1	Brunei	A form of health-related practice used in the maintenance of health as well as in the prevention, diagnosis, improvement or treatment of physical and mental illnesses, and excludes medical or dental practices utilised by registered medical and dental practitioners.	http://www.moh.gov.bn/Shared Documents/Brunei MEDICAL BOARD/team Guidelines for Registration of Traditional and Complementary Medicine Practitioners in Brunei Darussalam.pdf
2	Cambodia	N/A	N/A
3	China	Traditional Chinese medicine (TCM) is a medical science that was formed and developed in the daily life of the people and in the process of their fight against diseases over thousands of years.	http://english.www.gov.cn/archive/white paper/2016/12/06/content 281475509333700.htm (China's State Council Information Office issued a white paper on the development of TCM in China on 6 June 2016)
4	Japan	N/A	N/A
5	Laos	N/A	N/A
6	Malaysia	A form of health-related practice designed to prevent, treat or manage ailment or illness or preserve the mental and physical well-being of an individual, and includes practices such as traditional Malay medicine, traditional Chinese medicine, traditional Indian medicine, homoeopathy and complementary therapies, but excludes medical and dental practices used by a medical and dental practitioner, respectively.	http://tcm.moh.gov.my/en/upload/aktaBI2016.pdf Traditional and Complementary Medicine Act 2016)
7	Mongolia	N/A	N/A
8	Philippines	The sum total of knowledge, skills and practice on health care, not necessarily explicable in the context of modern, scientific philosophical framework, but recognised by the people to help maintain and improve their health towards the wholeness of their being, the community and society, and their interrelations based on culture, history, heritage and consciousness.	https://pitahc.gov.ph/about/republic-act-no-8423/ (Traditional and Alternative Medicine Act 1997)

(Continued)

The Definition of TM

TABLE 9.1 (*Continued*)
Definition of TM of Those Asian Countries in the WPR

No.	Country	T&CM Definition	Website Link
9	Singapore	"Practice of Traditional Chinese Medicine" means any of the following acts or activities: a. acupuncture; b. the diagnosis, treatment, prevention or alleviation of any disease or any symptoms of a disease or the prescription of any herbal medicine; c. the regulation of the functional states of the human body; d. the preparation or supply of any herbal medicine on or in accordance with a prescription given by the person preparing or supplying the herbal medicine or by another registered person; e. the preparation or supply of any of the substance specified in the Schedule; f. the processing of any herbal medicine; g. retailing of any herbal medicine; on the basis of traditional Chinese medicine.	https://sso.agc.gov.sg/Act/TCMPA2000 (Traditional Chinese Medicine Practitioners Act (Chapter 333A) 2001)
10	South Korea	N/A	N/A
11	Vietnam	Traditional medicine in the Socialist Republic of Vietnam comprises two components: a plant remedy-based form of medicine referred to as thuôc nam (southern medicine) and a Sino-Vietnamese theory and system of healing referred to as thuôc nam (northern medicine), which includes herbal medicine, acupuncture, massage and exercise techniques.	https://www.kingsfund.org.uk/sites/files/kf/All%20Case%20Studies1.pdf

In Malaysia, the definition of "Practice of traditional and complementary medicine" reflects the uniqueness of Malaysia as a multi-ethnic and multicultural country with a confluence of three traditional systems of medicine – Malay, Chinese and Indian – and other medical systems from the indigenous ethnic groups (60,000 years) (Traditional and Complementary Medicine Act, 2016). It is also acknowledged that the practice of T&CM is supported by Malaysia's rich tropical biodiversity as a reliable source for natural health products. The definition is further strengthened by the statement from the *National Policy of Traditional and Complementary Medicine*: "T&CM system shall be an important component of the healthcare system. It will co-exist with modern medicine and contribute towards enhancing the health and quality of life of all Malaysians" (Traditional and Complementary Medicine Division, 2007). The Ministry of Health (MOH) Malaysia is currently embarking on the integration of T&CM into the national healthcare system with a focus on anaesthesiology and pain-free clinic (Ang et al., 2021). Malaysia moves in line with the strategic direction of WHO aiming to include T&CM into the mainstream health system, by promoting safe, quality and effective use of T&CM, and to increase its accessibility to everyone.

Similarly, the definition of TM in the Philippines which has been inked in the **Traditional and Alternative Medicine Act 1997** is under the influence of the policy of the State with the main concerns on the development of safe and quality TM and healthcare integration, and indigenous societies and intellectual property right pertaining to their traditional medical knowledge (Republic of Philippines, 1997).

Brunei is located on the northern coast of the island of Borneo and has bordered with Malaysia and the South China Sea. The *Guideline for Registration of Traditional and Complementary Medicine Practitioners in Brunei Darussalam* has a list of priority T&CM practice areas to facilitate registration of practitioners, namely traditional Malay medicine, TCM, traditional Indian medicine, acupuncture, osteopathy, chiropractic, homoeopathy, manipulative therapies, cupping and herbalists (Traditional and Complementary Medicine, 2020). These practice areas are almost similar to the practice areas in Malaysia which have been mentioned in the definition of T&CM. T&CM practices in both Malaysia and Brunei have a close relationship with ethnicity and culture.

On the contrary, the definition of TCM in China, Singapore and the Socialist Republic of Vietnam is based on the accumulated clinical experiences and activities being conducted as well as its rich history. TCM has been identified as the TM in China and Singapore mainly because of the majority Chinese community there. More than 70% of Singapore's population are Chinese (Google, 2020). As denoted by the **Traditional Chinese Medicine Practitioners Act (Chapter 333A) 2001**, the definition of TM in Singapore mainly focuses on TCM (The Law Commission Revisions, 2015). Moreover, TCM in China represents the Chinese civilisation, embracing the philosophical ideas of the Chinese nation with five thousands of years of continuous history of absorption and innovation in disease management (The State Council Information Office, 2016). Their philosophy of TCM emphasises on the Yin–Yang balance inside human body and thus enhances the body's resistance to diseases.

The Socialist Republic of Vietnam had experienced a significant "revival" in the medical practice due to shortage of medicines, medical equipment and budget and resulted in the usage of affordable and easily accessible TM for thousands of years (Crosette, 1986). It is situated in the tropical region with a high diversity of fauna and flora as well as wildlife species with medicinal value. After years of use of TM, Vietnam has formulated its own theory and principle on TM. Hence, its TM comprises two components: "a plant remedy-based form of medicine referred to as *thuôc nam* (southern medicine) and a Sino-Vietnamese theory and system of healing referred to as *thuôc bâc* (northern medicine), which includes herbal medicine, acupuncture, massage and exercise techniques (Watanabe et al., 2011)."

Shifting our focus to Japan, its TM is known as "*Kampo medicine,*" which has a long historical development, mainly rooted from the Chinese tradition which was clearly indicated by the term "*Kampo,*" meaning "method from the Han period (206 BC to 220 AD) of ancient China (Watanabe et al., 2011)." Under the influence of modern medicine, abdomen palpation technique *(fukuship)* had been introduced into Kampo diagnosis (sho) (Fujikawa, 1904). Today, Kampo medicine is based on diagnostic methods that directly relate the symptoms to the therapy, but not on the principle of Yin–Yang and five-element theory. Interestingly, a total of 148 Kampo herbal prescriptions can be prescribed under the national health insurance system in Japan.

The Definition of TM 115

Korea has a strong tie with China, Japan and Vietnam because they share the Chinese characters. Under this mutually influential relationship, the traditional medical knowledge from China, Japan and Vietnam has greatly influenced and contributed to the development of Korean TM known as Korean medicine. "Korean medicine" is a combination of medicine from local Korean Peninsula and Liaodong China, and the medical technologies that are shared in East Asian countries (Pusan National University School of Korean Medicine, 2015). Korean medicine is based on the theory of essence, qi and spirit for herbal therapy as well as meridian theory for acupuncture and moxibustion. It also values the importance of diet and lifestyle and introduces them into the Korean medicine practice. To date, with the element of localisation, Korean medicine has coexisted with modern medicine in the Korean National Healthcare System.

Perspective from the Asian Countries Located in the SEAR

In the SEAR, only Thai TM has been spelled out clearly in the act, namely Protection and Promotion of Thai Traditional Medicine Wisdom Act B.E. 2542 in 1999. The definition of the TM in the majority of the other countries in the SEAR comprises phases such as "indigenous or generation knowledge" and "principles of the ancient wisdom" (refer to Table 9.2). In short, the definitions of TM in the majority of the countries in the SEAR have lots of similarities with WHO's definition on TM. They agree that TM is composed of knowledge that passed down from generation to generation. However, the geographical factor does influence the practice of medicine in Bhutan, which shares a border with Tibet, China to the north and India to the south. The Bhutan traditional medical system is known as *Sowa-Rigpa* (Tibetan medicine), meaning "the science of healing" **(Lhamo and Nebel, 2011),** which was rigorously transmitted through canonical text and verbal teachings.

The Indian Systems of Medicine (Traditional System of Medicine) are rather unique with a confluence of systems of medicine within India and outside India which have been assimilated into Indian culture **(Ravishankar and Shukla, 2007)**. However, the present form of Traditional System of Medicine is the outcome of continued scientific inputs. The Indian TM is known as AYUSH embracing Ayurveda, yoga and naturopathy, Unani, Siddha, Sowa-Rigpa and homoeopathy **(Jaiswal and Williams, 2017)**. Ayurveda is the "science of life" considering that the human body is constituted from five elements (air, water, space, earth and fire) **(Department of AYUSH, 2012)**. Siddha means "truth" establishment and is based upon the principle similar to Ayurveda, along with one of its characteristics of using plant and mineral preparation to treat psychosomatic system (perception) (Thas, 2008), and Unani is the "science of health and healing" that describes the wet and dry characteristic of each humour that constitutes the human body (Ministry of AYUSH, 2016). Naturopathy uses the curative power of nature in combination with the traditional techniques such as yoga to help restore good health. Yoga means "union" establishment with the Supreme Universal Spirit contributing to pain relief and suffering and health improvement (Hansa Jayadeva, 2010).

Homoeopathy is also recognised as the "Science of Gentle Healing" as it is a specialised system of rational therapy based on fixed and definite laws of nature that has

TABLE 9.2
Definition of TM of Those Asian Countries in the SEAR

No.	Country	T&CM Definition	Website Link
1	Bangladesh	The sum total of the knowledge, skills and practices based on the theories, beliefs and experiences indigenous to different cultures, whether explicable or not, used in the maintenance of health as well as in the prevention, diagnosis, improvement or treatment of physical and mental illness.	https://www.ncbi.nlm.nih.gov/pmc/articles/PMC3974044/pdf/1471-2458-14-202.pdf
2	Bhutan	In Bhutan, traditional medical practice is one of the country's tangible heritages. The country hosts two forms of traditional medicines: local healing practices and the official traditional medical system known as Sowa-Rigpa, meaning "the science of healing." Sowa-Rigpa (Wylie transliteration of Tibetan, gso-ba rig-pa, or "knowledge field of healing"), also known as Tibetan medicine, is a scholarly Asian traditional medical system rigorously transmitted through canonical text and oral teachings.	https://pubmed.ncbi.nlm.nih.gov/21457504/ https://www.sciencedirect.com/science/article/abs/pii/S1876382019305165
3	India	India has a rich history of traditional system of medicine based upon six systems of medicine – Ayurveda, Siddha, Unani, homoeopathy, yoga and naturopathy. Sowa-Rigpa is formally recognised and promoted as traditional medical system by the Government of India.	https://www.ncbi.nlm.nih.gov/pmc/articles/PMC5198827/ https://www.sciencedirect.com/science/article/abs/pii/S1876382019305165
4	Indonesia	Drugs and treatments utilized in Traditional health services refer to experiences and skills passed down from generation to generation empirically that can be accounted for and applied in accordance with the norms prevailing in society.	http://ditjenpp.kemenkumham.go.id/arsip/bn/2018/bn940-2018.pdf
5	Maldives	Knowledge, skills and practices based on theories and experiences indigenous to a local community or region. Traditional medicines are often used synonymously with the terms alternative and complementary medicines. Hence, for the Maldivian context, traditional medicines are the herbal medicines produced by local practitioners and have been passed on generations.	http://health.gov.mv/Uploads/Downloads/Informations/Informations(310).pdf
6	Myanmar	N/A	N/A

(Continued)

TABLE 9.2 (*Continued*)
Definition of TM of Those Asian Countries in the SEAR

No.	Country	T&CM Definition	Website Link
7	Nepal	N/A	N/A
8	North Korea	The Korean people's medicine, created in the course of history and a treasure medical heritage of Korean people that has contributed to treating patients and improving people's health.	https://books.google.com.my/books?id=JIlh9nNeadMC&pg=PA439&lpg=PA439&dq=KORYO+MEDICINE&source=bl&ots=gy-
9	Sri Lanka	N/A	N/A
10	Thailand	The medical processes dealing with the examination, diagnosis, therapy, treatment or prevention of diseases, or promotion and rehabilitation of the health of humans or animals, midwifery, Thai massage, and the preparation and production of Thai traditional drugs and the making of devices and instruments for medical purposes. All of these are based on the knowledge or textbooks that were passed on and developed from generation to generation.	https://thailawonline.com/fr/thai-laws/laws-of-thailand/301-protection-and-promotion-of-traditional-thai-medicine-wisdom-act-be-2542-1999-.html
11	Timor-Leste	N/A	N/A

a similarity to the pharmacological aspects of the drug and the disease (Ministry of AYUSH, 2015). Last but not least, Sowa-Rigpa which can be defined as "Knowledge of Healing" is a combination of Tibetan traditions and Ayurvedic principles which is officially recognised and promoted as traditional medical system by the Government of India (Ministry of AYUSH, 2019). Indian TM emphasises on preservation and promotion of health and prevention of diseases through diet and healthy lifestyle. Diet and physical and mental activities are one of the causative factors considered to affect the harmony equilibrium of human beings. In short, the Indian Systems of Medicine focus on restoring and harmonising the metabolic equilibrium of human beings through a holistic approach by looking into their physical, mental, mind and spiritual planes of living. Their ultimate goal is to take care of the physical and mental health of man, which is similar to the objective of WHO on promoting TM.

The TM in the North Korea is known as "Koryo medicine," which is interpreted as "the Korean people's medicine, created in the course of history and a treasured medical heritage of Korean people that has contributed to treating patients and improving people's health (Park, 2003)." North Korea culture including traditional medical knowledge is inseparably related to that of South Korea since they had been united during the Goryeo Dynasty. During this dynasty, a medical policy hub called the "Taeuigam" was introduced in the Korean Peninsula (Pusan National University School of Korean Medicine, 2015). With its long frame for ginseng (Goryeo Ginseng), Koryo medicine was promoted to improve and strengthen the public health in North Korea.

The Thai TM knowledge and massage skill have been passed down from Thai ancestors since the Sukhothai period (1238–1377) that are congruent with local Thai culture, religion and lifestyle (Chokevivat and Chuthaputti, 2005). The legal definition of Thai TM in the Protection and Promotion of Thai Traditional Medicine Wisdom Act B.E. 2542 is "the medical processes dealing with the examination, diagnosis, therapy, treatment, or prevention of diseases, or promotion and rehabilitation of the health of humans or animals, midwifery, Thai massage, as well as the preparation and production of Thai traditional drugs and the making of devices and instruments for medical purposes. All of these are based on the knowledge or textbooks that were passed on and developed from generation to generation (Adulyadej, 1999b)." Prior to this, the Practice of the Arts of Healing Act B.E. 2542 interprets Thai TM as "the practice of the art of healing that is based on Thai traditional knowledge or textbooks that have been passed on and developed from generation to generation, or based on the education from academic institutes that the Professional Committee approved (Adulyadej, 1999a)." In other words, Thai TM as the country's heritage of wisdom of health care has been legally accepted and officially recognised as part of the Thai national healthcare system.

PERSPECTIVE FROM THE ASIAN COUNTRIES LOCATED IN THE EMR

Two-thirds of the Asian countries in the EMR do not have a proper definition for TM. As illustrated in Table 9.3, the *Afghanistan National Medicines Policy 2019* has a definition for TM in Afghanistan, which stems mainly from the pharmaceutical perspective, no much difference from the interpretation by the WHO. Kuwait has totally agreed to the version of WHO in defining TM. The TM practices in Oman include Arab-Greek medicine, ancient Chinese medicine, Indian Ayurveda medicine and other forms of TM. That is to say, the recognised TM practices in a particular country may not be the country's own tradition. Moreover, the Arab-Greek medicine finds a widespread use in Islamic countries in the EMR. Countries such as Bahrain, the Kingdom of Saudi Arabia and Iraq use the term CAM rather than TM, but their CAM carries the same interpretation as TM by WHO.

CAM, especially religious and Quranic healing practices, has been widely used in the Kingdom of Saudi Arabia by women and illiterate population. The practice of CAM in Arab (Arabic medicine or prophetic medicine) has a connection to the Persians, Ethiopians and Romans through trade (Al Thiab Al Kendi, 2014). Prophet Muhammad used to perform Hijama (wet cupping) for disease prevention and health maintenance, as per verses in the Quran that "Prevention is better than cure (Al Thiab Al Kendi, 2014)." Reciting based on the Quran and Sunnah of the Prophet has been used by 25% of CAM practitioners in the Kingdom of Saudi Arabia, and 45% of them use herbal remedies (Al-Rowais et al., 2010). Moreover, people are advised to avoid excessive eating or drinking for mental clarity and encourage fasting for the health benefits (Al Thiab Al Kendi, 2014) (Table 9.4).

Similarly, CAM is growing in popularity among the general population in the other Gulf countries, such as Bahrain (63%) (Khalaf and Whitford, 2008), Oman (42%) (Reyburn, 2019) (Al-Kindi et al., 2011), the United Arab Emirates (67%) and Kuwait (69.5%) (Al-Hashel et al., 2018). This is most likely due to the religious beliefs

The Definition of TM

TABLE 9.3
Definition of TM of Those Asian Countries in the EMR

No.	Country	T&CM Definition	Website Link
1	Afghanistan	A material or product of plant, animal or mineral origin that is used in traditional practices to protect the health and to treat disease, whose effectiveness is proven by reliable traditional medicine sources.	https://pdf.usaid.gov/pdf_docs/pa00kcmr.pdf (Afghanistan National Medicine Policy 2014–2019)
2	Bahrain	The diagnostic, therapeutic, preventive and rehabilitative healthcare systems and practice, with a view to health maintenance, care and protection through different methods and means and the use of diverse products; plant, animal, metal or otherwise, which does not fall under modern medicine and is without prejudice to the provisions of Decree Law No. 18 for the year 1997 on regulating the profession of pharmacy and pharmaceutical centres.	https://www.nhra.bh/Departments/HCP/MediaHandler/GenericHandler/documents/departments/LAU/HCP/HCP110_Resolution_Resolution%20No.%20(33)%20for%20the%20year%202016%20Issuing%20the%20Regulations%20on%20Organizing%20the%20Practice%20of%20Alternative%20and%20Complementary%20Medicine_English.pdf (Decision No. (33) of 2016 Issuing Regulation on the Practice of Alternative and Complementary Medicine)
3	Cyprus	N/A	N/A
4	Iran	N/A	N/A
5	Iraq	CAM is defined by the World Health Organization as the sum total of the knowledge, skills and practices based on the theories, beliefs and experiences indigenous to different cultures, whether explicable or not, used in the maintenance of health as well as in the prevention, diagnosis, improvement or treatment of physical and mental illness.	https://www.ncbi.nlm.nih.gov/pmc/articles/PMC5314826/
6	Jordan	N/A	N/A
7	Kuwait	The World Health Organization (WHO) defined traditional medicine (TM) as the sum total of knowledge, skills and practices based on the theories, beliefs and experiences indigenous to different cultures that are used to maintain health, as well as to prevent, diagnose, improve or treat physical and mental illnesses.	https://www.ncbi.nlm.nih.gov/pmc/articles/PMC6755714/pdf/10194_2018_Article_950.pdf
8	Lebanon	N/A	N/A

(*Continued*)

TABLE 9.3 (*Continued*)
Definition of TM of Those Asian Countries in the EMR

No.	Country	T&CM Definition	Website Link
9	Oman	The term traditional medicine (TM) has an inclusive meaning; it includes all of the Arab-Greek medicine, ancient Chinese medicine, Indian Ayurveda medicine and other forms of TM. Complementary or alternative medicine (CAM) is the TM that is used outside the indigenous community by the other populations.	https://www.ncbi.nlm.nih.gov/pmc/articles/PMC4322628/pdf/IJHPM-4-65.pdf
10	Pakistan	N/A	N/A
11	Palestine	N/A	N/A
12	Qatar	N/A	N/A
13	Saudi Arabia	N/A	N/A
14	Syria	N/A	N/A
15	United Arab Emirates	N/A	N/A
16	Yemen	N/A	N/A

and cultural backgrounds and family factors in the Gulf countries within the EMR. However, the knowledge of the CAM among the public and medical fraternity is generally poor (Awad, Al-Ajmi and Waheedi, 2012).

It is clear that cultural effects, social relations, religious belief and safety of the practices have influenced the decision-making of using CAM by the people in the EMR. They believe that CAM therapy is effective and safe based on its "naturalness," in spite of lacking robust data on the safety and efficacy of CAM (Ibrahim et al., 2016). The majority of the people know the practice of CAM through cultural and social support.

PERSPECTIVE FROM THE ASIAN COUNTRIES LOCATED IN THE EUR

Generally, the TM practice of those Asian countries in the EUR means folk and traditional form of healthcare practice originating from local indigenous population. "Indigenous experiences" have been indicated in the definition of TM by the WHO. In some countries, TM has yet to be officially recognised and incorporated into the mainstream healthcare system, for example TM in Israel. Being surrounded by Arab Muslim Eastern states, local indigenous medicine or TM in Israel has been influenced by the Arabians' culture (Keshet and Popper-Giveon, 2013). Even though the Arabian population is only a minority in Israel, with the Jewish population as its

The Definition of TM

TABLE 9.4

Definition of TM of Those Asian Countries in the EUR

No.	Country	T&CM Definition	Website Link
1	Armenia	N/A	N/A
2	Azerbaijan	N/A	N/A
3	Georgia	Georgian traditional medicine comprises the methods of diagnosis and treatment which exist in Sumerian, Chinese, Indian and Tibetan as well as in Greek and Roman medicine. It has a solid philosophical foundation in the mentality and culture of Georgian people. Georgian traditional medicine comprises ancient written classical documents and folk medicine. The treatments and procedures that are not officially accepted by modern medicine are called "alternative," "complementary," "unconventional" and even "untraditional."	http://neuron.mefst.hr/docs/CMJ/issues/1999/40/1/9933895.pdf
4	Israel	The term traditional medicine is used to denote folk medicines and healing knowledge originating from a local indigenous population. The term complementary medicine is used for medicines and healing practices that often draw on indigenous TM, but are practised in non-indigenous, generally Western healthcare settings. Arabic TM includes local Mediterranean and Arab traditional herbal medicine. This is practised mainly by traditional healers and is not formally integrated into Israeli healthcare organisations.	https://anthrosource.onlinelibrary.wiley.com/doi/abs/10.1111/maq.12049
5	Kazakhstan	Folk medicine (healing) – aggregate of empirical information accumulated by a people in regard to healing remedies, as well as medicinal and hygienic procedures and practices, and practical application thereof, used with the purpose of preservation of health and prevention and treatment of illnesses.	https://www.wto.org/english/thewto_e/acc_e/kaz_e/WTACCKAZ62_LEG_1.pdf (The Law of the Republic of Kazakhstan N 111-1)
6	Kyrgyzstan	N/A	N/A

(Continued)

TABLE 9.4 (*Continued*)
Definition of TM of Those Asian Countries in the EUR

No.	Country	T&CM Definition	Website Link
7	Russia	Traditional medicine – the methods of health improvement, established in folk experience, based on the use of knowledge, skills and practical skills to assess and restore health. Traditional medicine does not include the provision of services of an occult-magical nature, as well as the performance of religious rites. (Google translated from Russian)	http://www.consultant.ru/document/ cons_doc_LAW_121895/1498a4ebc56 ba8cb777c0e0c416523b6b84e7719/ (The Federal Law on the Basis of Protecting the Health of Citizens in the Russian Federation)
8	Tajikistan	N/A	N/A
9	Turkey	Traditional and complementary medicine – the whole of knowledge, skills and practices based on theories, beliefs and experiences that are specific to different cultures, beliefs and experiences that can be used for protection from physical and mental illnesses, diagnosis, improvement or treatment, and can be explained or not. They are supportive and complementary methods of Western medicine. (Google translated)	https://getatportal.saglik.gov.tr/ TR,24683/geleneksel-ve-tamamlayici- tip-nedir.html
10	Turkmenistan	N/A	N/A
11	Uzbekistan	N/A	N/A

majority, TM remains popular among the Arab minority in Israel because of their low socioeconomic levels and lack of accessibility to the national healthcare services. TM treatments may include the process of reciting Quran, prescribing treatments under the guidance of books with astrological and destiny calendars along with medicinal plants (Keshet and Popper-Giveon, 2013). TM in Israel is different from the CAM that includes practices such as homoeopathy, acupuncture, Chinese medicine, naturopathy and osteopathy (Shuval and Averbuch, 2012).

On the other hand, TM in Kazakhstan and Russia was recognised officially with the legal interpretation printed in The Law of the Republic of Kazakhstan N 111-1 and Federal Law on the Basis of Protecting the Health of Citizens in the Russian Federation, respectively. As interpreted from the above two laws of the two neighbouring countries, TM is medicine of an accumulation of the practitioners' experiences during the process of health preservation and disease prevention and treatment. However, a study reported that more rural people in Kazakhstan will consult TM practitioners for an unusual lump under the skin as compared to those in Russia (Stickley et al., 2013).

The Definition of TM

Similar to Kazakhstan and Russia, as one of the countries of the former Soviet Union, Georgia has used the folk medicine, known as Georgian TM. Georgian TM is a combination of local culture with "the methods of diagnosis and treatment which exist in Sumerian, Chinese, Indian, Tibetan, as well as in Greek and Roman medicine," documented in the ancient written classical documents (Shengelia, 1999). It has been officially accepted by their medical healthcare system and principally in rural locations. Surprisingly, 77% of the people in Georgia obtain their knowledge on TM from family and friends, less than half (44%) from books or media, and 11% from medical doctors (Nadareishvili et al., 2019).

The Department of Traditional and Complementary Medicine, Ministry of Health Turkey, has indicated that T&CM is the practice in Turkey and carries almost the same definition of TM by the WHO to protect the physical and mental health (Ministry of Health Turkey, 2020). In accordance with the Regulation on Traditional and Complementary Medicine Practices, the officially listed 15 T&CM practices include acupuncture, apitherapy, phytotherapy, hypnosis, leech therapy (hirudo-therapy), homoeopathy, chiropractic, cupping therapy, maggot therapy, mesotherapy, prolotherapy, osteopathy, ozone therapy, reflexology and music therapy (Ministry of Health Turkey, 2016). The usage of T&CM has been under the influence by social, cultural, religion and economic factors as well as traditional structures of societies (Kavadar et al., 2019). 83.5% of the population believed in T&CM, and herbal therapy is the main preference (Ozer, Santaş and Yildirim, 2012).

Perspective from Taiwan

Taiwan has yet to be accepted as one of the members of the WHO since the People's Republic of China claims that Taiwan is a province of China and not an independent state. Hence, it will not be recruited into any of the WHO regions at this stage.

TCM has been practised in Taiwan since the 16th century. The trends in TCM utilisation through consulting registered TCM practitioners have increased gradually since TCM has been recognised as an important part of its medical system (Shih et al., 2015). TCM includes herbal medicine, acupuncture, moxibustion, bone reduction, traditional trauma treatment, traditional dislocation treatment, traditional fracture treatment, tuina, baguan and other therapies. However, 1.3% of Taiwanese use folk therapies that mean "various types of TCM delivered by non-licensed practitioners and non-board-certified specialists who are not reimbursed by Taiwan's National Health Insurance Program" in non-clinical settings or facilities. These non-licensed TCM practitioners gained their knowledge through apprenticeship. The usage of folk therapies is under the influence of sociodemographic, lifestyle and health behaviours. From the above interpretation, many TCM-related treatments are associated with folk therapies due to their similarities. They are interrelated because they are part of the Taiwanese's culture and daily life that had undergone more than 2000 years of development.

Discussion

It is understood that, where and as appropriate, the definition of TM will be depending on national needs, capacity, priorities, existing health policies, strategies, legislation, resources, culture and history. Most commonly, TM more closely corresponds to the patient's ideology and is practised within the country of origin. Hence, the framing of a definition for TM requires a collaboration with interested stakeholders, nationally and internationally. This write-up has revealed a diversity of approaches pertaining to the interpretation of TM in Asian countries.

The definition of TM by WHO has been listed precisely and comprehensively. It includes all the information about traditional approach, practices, methods and remedies after engaging with experts from all the six regions.

The rich and voluminous information of TM in countries from the WPR allows a better picture on the interpretation of TM and its perspective with respect to WHO's interpretation. There is a rather wide spectrum of interpretation of TM within the Asian countries in the WPR remain linked closely with culture and religion. Particularly, TCM has a rich history and culture and is widely practised around East Asia. Moreover, based on TCM philosophy, every remedy from natural raw materials has its clear-cut role at a definite period of disease and a place in a definite treatment regime.

Furthermore, the Indian TM, which originated from India, is another TM with a rich history and culture. The peculiar feature of Indian TM is of "multiple systems" embracing Ayurveda, yoga, naturopathy, Unani, Siddha, Sowa-Rigpa and homoeopathy. Each system has its philosophy to achieve a common goal on human mental and physical health.

On the other hand, for those Asian countries that do not have a specific interpretation for their TM, namely "Khmer traditional medicine" in Cambodia, traditional Mongolian medicine and traditional Timorese medicine, they have similar salient features as those countries with a definition for their TM, for example a close linkage with their historical and cultural heritage, and under the influence of religions. TM utilisation is officially supported for disease prevention and health promotion in rural areas of these countries.

I have observed that TM in certain countries comprises ancient medical traditions and folk medicine for healing. At times TM could be the only source of healthcare in certain communities that can be easily accessed and perhaps culturally acceptable by that community. A close person's advice or experience was the most common rationale given for frequent self-taking decisions made by patients to receive TM treatment. Healthcare professionals of both the systems should not remain in a black box and should be aware of the existing differences in culture and medicinal history of TM, and must be careful in interpreting the definition of the respective TM system.

Rural residents were more likely to consult TM practitioners than urban residents due to the social and cultural factors and accessibility to traditional medical system. The prevalence of use of TM among developing and developed countries is high. Therefore, there is an apparent need to establish effective health education programmes and implement an appropriate policy and regulation on TM. The health education should be simultaneously provided to patients and medical fraternity including patients' families and friends since they relied heavily on them for advice on the usage of TM.

Furthermore, for those countries with the legal definition on TM, I presume they have explicit policies on the training and licensing of TM practitioners. On the other hand, for those countries without a proper policy and regulation, the TM was applied by non-instituted trained practitioners who may cause harm to patients. Hence,

The Definition of TM

capacity building in practice, education and other aspects are needed to establish evidence-based regulation and standards for TM that ensure informed decision-making and patient safety.

Before concluding, it is wise to mention several possible limitations in this write-up. Firstly, it is not a comprehensive study of the definition of TM in every country in Asia, and it focuses only on limited aspects of TM interpretation in several Asian countries of which information could be gathered through literature search. There is little or no information about the TM interpretation in those countries. In-depth interview or qualitative survey through questionnaires could be considered in the near future in an attempt to fill up the information gap. Next, limited Asian countries have a legal definition on their TM, whereas the majority of the other Asian countries have attempted to explain their TM based on the historical materials, cultural factors and geographical demarcation.

CONCLUSION

The definition of TM has a relationship with the history of medicine which could reflect different epochs, cultures, national specificities and mode of life. As the history, culture, forms, practices, role and development of TM in Asia vary widely, it is not possible to have one model or one set of definitions to deal with the different needs and available resources of all countries. Therefore, the challenges faced and the actions required will vary according to their individual situations. It is recommended that, where appropriate, countries might consider to use the definition of TM by the WHO as a framework or guide for framing a working definition on TM in their countries. This is because WHO has taken consideration of a diversity of medical practices, approaches, knowledge and beliefs incorporating the usage of plant-, animal- and/ or mineral-based medicines, spiritual therapies, manual techniques and exercises for health maintenance and disease treatment, diagnosis or prevention in the definition of TM. Countries that are without a proper interpretation of TM and wish to develop it could consider fostering collaboration among WHO and the neighbouring countries to look into the definition of TM and ultimately may gain a substantial interpretation.

Even though many Asian countries do not plan to have a definition on TM, they would like to move in line with WHO's strategic plan for UHC. Definition is important but is not a must since a demand from the population is there even without a definition. As long as every country understands its traditional medicinal knowledge and recognises the practices, the mandatory matter for each country is to have a directive and strategic plan for TM development and strengthen its healthcare system for "Health for All."

REFERENCES

Adulyadej, B. (1999a) 'The practice of the arts of healing act B.E. 2542', *The Royal Thai Gazette*, 116 Article(39a).

Adulyadej, B. (1999b) The protection and promotion of thai traditional medicine wisdom act B.E. 2542, *Thai Royal Gazette*, Available at: https://thailawonline.com/fr/thai-laws/laws-of-thailand/301-protection-and-promotion-of-traditional-thai-medicine-wisdom-act-be-2542-1999-.html (Accessed: 10 September 2020).

Afshar, S. et al. (2015) 'Multi-morbidity and the inequalities of global ageing: A cross-sectional study of 28 countries using the World Health Surveys', *BMC Public Health*, 15(776). doi: 10.1186/s12889– 015–2008–7.

Aizenstein, H. J. et al. (2016) 'Vascular depression consensus report - a critical update', *BMC Medicine*, 14(1), pp. 1–16. doi: 10.1186/s12916-016-0720–5.

Al-Hashel, J. Y. et al. (2018) 'Use of traditional medicine for primary headache disorders in Kuwait', *Journal of Headache and Pain*, 19(1), pp. 3–9. doi: 10.1186/s10194-018-0950–3.

Al-Kindi, R. et al. (2011) 'Complementary and alternative medicine use among adults with diabetes in muscat region, Oman', *Sultan Qaboos University Medical Journal*, 11(1), p. 62.

Al-Rowais, N. et al. (2010) 'Traditional healers in riyadh region: Reasons and health problems for seeking their advice. A household survey', *Journal of Alternative and Complementary Medicine*, 16(2), pp. 199–204. doi: 10.1089/acm.2009.0283.

Ang, J. Y. et al. (2021) 'A Malaysian retrospective study of acupuncture-assisted anesthesia in breast lump excision', *Acupuncture in Medicine*, 39(1), pp. 64–68. doi: 10.1177/0964528420920307.

Antman, F. (2012) 'How does adult child migration affect the health of elderly parents left behind? Evidence from Mexico', *SSRN Electronic Journal*. doi: 10.2139/ssrn.1578465.

Ao, X., Jiang, D. and Zhao, Z. (2016) 'The impact of rural-urban migration on the health of the left-behind parents', *China Economic Review*, 37, pp. 126–139. doi: 10.1016/j.chieco.2015.09.007.

Awad, A. I., Al-Ajmi, S. and Waheedi, M. A. (2012) 'Knowledge, perceptions and attitudes toward complementary and alternative therapies among Kuwaiti medical and pharmacy students', *Medical Principles and Practice*, 21(4), pp. 350–354. doi: 10.1159/000336216.

Barcella, C. A. et al. (2021) 'Severe mental illness is associated with increased mortality and severe course of COVID-19', *Acta Psychiatrica Scandinavica*, (March), pp. 1–10. doi: 10.1111/acps.13309.

Bernama (2020) *Malaysia's Population Estimates at 32.7 million in 2020, Astro Awani*. Available at: http://english.astroawani.com/malaysia-news/malaysias-population-estimates-32-7-million-2020-251323 (Accessed: 15 July 2020).

Bhandari, H. and Yasunobu, K. (2009) 'What is social capital? A comprehensive review of the concept', *Asian Journal of Social Science*, 37(3). doi: 10.1163/156853109X436847.

Bodeker, G. et al. (2018) *Mental Wellness: Pathways, Evidence, Horizons*. Edited by G. Bodeker. Miammi.

Bodeker, G. and Kronenberg, F. (2015) 'Tackling obesity: Challenges ahead', *The Lancet*, 386(9995), pp. 740–741. doi: 10.1016/S0140–6736(15)61539-2.

Böhme, M. H., Persian, R. and Stöhr, T. (2015) 'Alone but better off? Adult child migration and health of elderly parents in Moldova', *Journal of Health Economics*, 39, pp. 211–227. doi: 10.1016/j.jhealeco.2014.09.001.

Bowman, G. L. et al. (2012) 'Nutrient biomarker patterns, cognitive function, and MRI measures of brain aging', *Neurology*, 78(4), pp. 241–249. doi: 10.1212/WNL.0b013e3182436598.

Brooks, S. J. et al. (2020) 'The psychologial impact of quarantine and how to reduce it: Rapid review of the evidence', *The Lancet*, 295(10227), pp. 912–920.

Byrow, Y. et al. (2020) 'Perceptions of mental health and perceived barriers to mental health help-seeking amongst refugees: A systematic review', *Clinical Psychology Review*, 75(July 2018), p. 101812. doi: 10.1016/j.cpr.2019.101812.

Chan, J., To, H. P. and Chan, E. (2006) 'Reconsidering social cohesion: Developing a definition and analytical framework for empirical research', *Social Indicators Research*, 75(2), pp. 273–302. doi: 10.1007/s11205-005-2118-1.

Chang, F. et al. (2016) 'Adult child migration and elderly parental health in rural China', *China Agricultural Economic Review*, 8(4), pp. 677–697. doi: 10.1108/CAER-11–2015–0169.

The Definition of TM

Chen, M. et al. (2020) 'Prescribing Antibiotics in Rural China: The Influence of Capital on Clinical Realities', *Frontiers in Sociology*, 5(October), pp. 0–10. doi: 10.3389/fsoc.2020.00066.

China, N. S. B. o. t. P. s. R. o. (2018) *National Statistical Bureau of the People's Republic of China*. Available at: http://www.stats.gov.cn/english/Statisticaldata/AnnualData.

Chokevivat, V. and Chuthaputti, A. (2005). 'The Role of Thai Traditional Medicine in Health Promotion', in *Department for the Development of Thai Traditional and Alternative Medicine*, pp. 1–25. Available at: http://citeseerx.ist.psu.edu/viewdoc/download?doi=10.1.1.496.5656&rep=rep1&type=pdf.

Chong, S. A. et al. (2016) 'Recognition of mental disorders among a multiracial population in Southeast Asia', *BMC Psychiatry*, 16(1). doi: 10.1186/s12888-016-0837-2.

CIA (2020) *The World Factbook*. Available at: https://www.cia.gov/library/publications/the-world-factbook/fields/223rank.html.

Coburn D (2000) 'Income inequality, social cohesion, and the health status of populations', *Social Science and Medicine*, 51, pp. 135–146.

Crawford Shearer, N. B., Fleury, J. D. and Belyea, M. (2010) 'An innovative approach to recruiting homebound older adults', *Research in Gerontological Nursing*, 3(1), pp. 11–17. doi: 10.3928/19404921–20091029-01.

Crosette, B. (1986) Vietnamese Revive Ancient Medical Arts, The New York Times. Available at: https://www.nytimes.com/1986/08/12/science/vietnamese-revive-ancient-medical-arts.html (Accessed: 16 October 2020).

Crunfli, F. et al. (2021) 'SARS-CoV-2 infects brain astrocytes of COVID-19 patients and impairs neuronal viability', *medRxiv*, p. 2020. doi: 10.1101/2020.10.09.20207464.

Dai, Y. et al. (2016) 'Social Support and self-rated health of older people: A comparative study in Tainan Taiwan and Fuzhou Fujian Province', *Medicine*, 95(24), p. 3881. doi: 10.1097/MD.0000000000003881.

Department of AYUSH (2012) *Ayurveda: The Science of Life*. Department of AYUSH.

Department of Statistics (2020) *Current Population Estimates, Malaysia, Online*. Available at: https://www.dosm.gov.my/v1/index.php?r=column/cthemeByCat&cat=155&bul_id=OVByWjg5YkQ3MWFZRTN5bDJiaEVhZz09&menu_id=L0pheU43NWJwRWVSZklWdzQ4TlhUUT09 (Accessed: 22 February 2021).

Douaud, G. et al. (2013). 'Preventing Alzheimer's disease-related gray matter atrophy by B-vitamin treatment', *Proceedings of the National Academy of Sciences of the United States of America*, 110(23), pp. 9523–9528. doi: 10.1073/pnas.1301816110.

Engelhardt, U. (2000) 'Longevity techniques and Chinese medicine', in *Daoism handbook*. Brill, pp. 74–108.

Fasullo, L., Hernandez, A. and Bodeker, G. (2020) 'The innate human potential of elevated and ecstatic states of consciousness: Examining freeform dance as a means of access', *Dance, Movement & Spiritualities*, 6(1–2), pp. 87–117. doi: 10.1386/dmas_00005_1.

Fields, G. and Song, Y. (2020) 'Modeling migration barriers in a two-sector framework: A welfare analysis of the hukou reform in China', *Economic Modelling*, 84(59), pp. 293–301. doi: 10.1016/j.econmod.2019.04.019.

Fotoukian, Z. et al. (2014) 'Concept analysis of empowerment in old people with chronic diseases using a hybrid model', *Asian Nursing Research*, 8(2), pp. 118–127. doi: 10.1016/j.anr.2014.04.002.

Fu, S., Huang, N. and Chou, Y.-J. (2014) 'Trends in the prevalence of multiple chronic conditions in Taiwan From 2000 to 2010: a population-based study'. doi: 10.5888/pcd11.140205.

Fujikawa, Y. (1904) *Nihon igakushi (History of Japanese Medicine)*. Shokabo.

Galderisi, S. et al. (2015) 'Toward a new defition of mental health', *World Psychiatry*, 14(2), p. 231.

García, H. and Miralles, F. (2016) *IKIGAI. The Japanese Secret to a Long and Happy Life.*

Google (2020) *Singapore Ethnic Composition in 2019, Online.* Available at: https://www.google.com.my/search?q=singapore+ethnic+composition+in+2019&tbm=isch&ved=2ahUKEwiy6OHQs5DsAhVJB3IKHWjwCukQ2-cCegQIABAA&oq=singapore+ethnic+composition+in+2019&gs_lcp=CgNpbWcQAzoECAAQGFDp2gFYg8kCYPzNAmgAcAB4AIABXIgBrgqSAQIyOJgBAKABAaoBC2d3cy13a (Accessed: 30 September 2020).

Hansa Jayadeva, S. (2010) *Yoga Teacher's Manual for School Teachers.* Morarji Desai National Institute of Yoga.

Hu, Y. and Shi, X. (2020) 'The impact of China's one-child policy on intergenerational and gender relations', *Contemporary Social Science*, 15(3), pp. 360–377. doi: 10.1080/21582041. 2018.1448941.

Huang, B., Lian, Y. and Li, W. (2016) 'How far is Chinese left-behind parents' health left behind?', *China Economic Review*, 37(71002056), pp. 15–26. doi: 10.1016/j.chieco.2015.07.002.

Huang, C. and Li, Y. (2019) 'Understanding leisure satisfaction of Chinese seniors: human capital, family capital, and community capital', *Journal of Chinese Sociology*, 6(1). doi: 10.1186/s40711-019-0094-0.

Huang, Y. and Liu, X. (2015) 'Improvement of balance control ability and flexibility in the elderly Tai Chi Chuan (TCC) practitioners: A systematic review and meta-analysis', *Archives of Gerontology and Geriatrics*, 60(2), pp. 233–238. doi: 10.1016/j.archger.2014.10.016.

Ibrahim, I. et al. (2016) 'A qualitative insight on complementary and alternative medicines used by hypertensive patients', *Journal of Pharmacology and Bioallied Science*, 8(4), pp. 284–288.

Institute for Public Health (2015) *National Health and Morbidity Survey 2015: Traditional and Complementary Medicine, Ministry of Health Malaysia.* Putrajaya.

Institute for Public Health (2020) *National Health and Morbidity Survey 2019: Non-Communicable Diseases, Health Demand, and Health Literacy - Key Findings.* Available at: http://iku.gov.my/images/IKU/Document/REPORT/NHMS2019/Fact_Sheet_NHMS_2019-English.pdf.

Institute of Medicine (US) Committe on the Use of Complementary and Alternative Medicine by the American Public (2005) *Complementary Alternative Medicine in the United States.* Washington, D.C. Available at: https://www.ncbi.nlm.nih.gov/books/NBK83804/.

Jaiswal, Y. and Williams, L. (2017) 'A glimpse of Ayurveda – The forgotten history and principles of Indian traditional medicine', *Journal of Traditional and Complementary Medicine*, 7(1), pp. 50–53. doi: 10.1016/j.jtcme.2016.02.002.

John W Brick Foundation (2021) *Move you mental wellness.* Available at: www.johnwbrickfoundation.org/move-your-mental-health-report/ (Accessed: 24 June 2021).

Kadetz, P. (2018) 'Collective efficacy, social capital and resilience: An inquiry into the relationship between social infrastructure and resilience after Hurricane Katrina', in *Creating Katrina, Rebuilding Resilience.* Butterworth-Heinemann, pp. 283–304.

Kalil, A. (2020) 'Treating COVID-19 Off-label drug use, compassionate use, and randomized clinical trials during pandemics', *Journal of the American Medical Association*, 323(19), pp. 1897–1898.

Kavadar, G. et al. (2019) 'Use of traditional and complementary medicine for musculoskeletal diseases', *Turkish Journal of Medical Sciences*, 49(3), pp. 809–814. doi: 10.3906/sag-1509-71.

Kawachi, I. et al. (2004) 'Commentary: Reconciling the three accounts of social capital', *International Journal of Epidemiology*, 33(4), pp. 682–690. doi: 10.1093/ije/dyh177.

Keshet, Y. and Popper-Giveon, A. (2013) 'Integrative health care in israel and traditional arab herbal medicine: when health care interfaces with culture and politics', *Medical Anthropology Quarterly*, 27(3), pp. 368–384. doi: 10.1111/maq.12049.

Khalaf, A. J. and Whitford, D. L. (2008) 'The use of complementary and alternative medicine by patients with osteoporosis', *Nature Clinical Practice Endocrinology and Metabolism*, 4(3), p. 120. doi: 10.1038/ncpendmet0732.

Kuhn, R., Everett, B. and Silvey, R. (2011) 'The effects of children's migration on Elderly Kin's health: A counterfactual approach', *Demography*, 48(1), pp. 183–209. doi: 10.1007/s13524-010-0002-3.

De La Rubia Ortí, J. E. et al. (2018) 'Does music therapy improve anxiety and depression in alzheimer's patients?', *Journal of Alternative and Complementary Medicine*, 24(1), pp. 33–36. doi: 10.1089/acm.2016.0346.

Lauber, C. and Rössler, W. (2007) 'Stigma towards people with mental illness in developing countries in Asia', *International Review of Psychiatry*, 19(2), pp. 157–178. doi: 10.1080/09540260701278903.

Lee, D. Y. W. et al. (2021) 'Traditional Chinese herbal medicine at the forefront battle against COVID-19: Clinical experience and scientific basis', *Phytomedicine*, 80(September 2020), p. 153337. doi: 10.1016/j.phymed.2020.153337.

Lei, X. et al. (2014) 'Depressive symptoms and SES among the mid-aged and elderly in China: Evidence from the China Health and Retirement Longitudinal Study national baseline', *Social Science and Medicine*, 120, pp. 224–232. doi: 10.1016/j.socscimed.2014.09.028.

Lei, Y. et al. (2021) 'SARS-CoV-2 spike protein impairs endothelial function via downregulation of ACE 2', *Circulation Research*, 128, pp. 1323–1326.

Lhamo, N. and Nebel, S. (2011) 'Perceptions and attitudes of Bhutanese people on Sowa Rigpa, traditional bhutanese medicine: A preliminary study from Thimphu', *Journal of Ethnobiology and Ethnomedicine*, 7(January), pp. 1–9. doi: 10.1186/1746-4269-7-3.

Li, C. et al. (2020) 'Discussion on TCM theory and modern pharmacological mechanism of Qinfei Paidu decoction in the treatment of COVID-19', *Journal of Traditional Chinese Medicine*, pp. 1–4.

Li, T. et al. (2020) 'What happens to the health of elderly parents when adult child migration splits households? Evidence from rural China', *International Journal of Environmental Research and Public Health*, 17(5). doi: 10.3390/ijerph17051609.

Li, X. et al. (2020) 'Quality of primary health care in China: challenges and recommendations', *The Lancet*, 395(10239), pp. 1802–1812. doi: 10.1016/S0140-6736(20)30122-7.

Lo, V. (2001) 'The influence of nurturing life culture on early Chinese medical theory', *In* Hsu, E. (ed.) *Innovation in Chinese medicine*. Cambridge University Press, pp. 19–50.

Logue, J. K. et al. (2021) 'Sequelae in adults at 6 months after COVID-19 infection', *JAMA Network Open*, 4(2), pp. 8–11. doi: 10.1001/jamanetworkopen.2021.0830.

Luo, H. et al. (2020) 'Reflections on treatment of COVID-19 with traditional Chinese medicine', *Chinese Medicine (United Kingdom)*, 15(1), pp. 1–14. doi: 10.1186/s13020-020-00375-1.

Ma, X., He, Y. and Xu, J. (2020) 'Urban-rural disparity in prevalence of multimorbidity in China: A cross-sectional nationally representative study', *BMJ Open*, 10(11), pp. 1–9. doi: 10.1136/bmjopen-2020-038404.

Ma, Z. and Zhou, G. (2009) 'Isolated or compensated: the impact of temporary migration of adult children on the wellbeing of the elderly in rural China', *Geographical review of Japan series B*, 81(1), pp. 47–59. doi: 10.4157/geogrevjapanb.81.47.

Malaysian Government (2016) *The Traditional and Complementary Medicine Act 2016*.

Mauss, M. (2002) *The Gift: The Form and Reason for Exchange in Archaic Societies*. London: Routledge.

Miller, V. et al. (2017) 'Prospective Urban Rural Epidemiology (PURE) study investigators. Fruit, vegetable, and legume intake, and cardiovascular disease and deaths in 18 countries: A prospective cohort study', *The Lancet*, 390(10107), pp. 2037–2049.

Ministry of AYUSH (2015) *Homeopathy: Science of Gentle Healing. Ministry of AYUSH*.

Ministry of AYUSH (2016) *Unani System of Medicine: The Science of Health and Healing*.

Ministry of AYUSH (2019) *Introduction to Sowa-Rigpa, About the Systems.*

Ministry of Health and National Institute of Health Research and Development (2018) *National report on basic health research, Riskesdas, 2018. Jakarta, Indonesia.*

Ministry of Health Turkey (2016) *Traditioal and Complementary Medicine Practices and Related Legislation.*

Ministry of Health Turkey (2020) *What is Traditiona and Complementary Medicine, Traditional, Complementary and Functional Medicine Practices, Department.*

Minton, S. and Faber, R. (2016) *Thinking with the Dancing Brain: Embodying Neuroscience.* Lanham, Maryland: Rowman and Littlefield.

Mofredj, A. et al. (2016) 'Music therapy, a review of the potential therapeutic benefits for the critically ill', *Journal of Critical Care*, 35, pp. 195–199. doi: 10.1016/j.jcrc.2016.05.021.

Mohanty, S., Sharma, P. and Sharma, G. (2020) 'Yoga for infirmity in geriatric population amidst COVID-19 pandemic: Comment on "Age and Ageism in COVID-19: Elderly mental health-care vulnerabilities and needs"', *Asian Journal of Psychiatry*, 53, p. 102199.

Moreno, C. et al. (2020) 'How mental health care should change as a consequence of the COVID-19 pandemic', *Lancet Psychiatry*, 7(9), pp. 813–824. doi: 10.1016/S2215–0366 (20)30307–2.

Nadareishvili, I. et al. (2019) 'Georgia's healthcare system and integration of complementary medicine', *Complementary Therapies in Medicine*, 45(January), pp. 205–210. doi: 10.1016/j.ctim.2019.06.016.

Nagasu, M., Muto, K. and Yamamoto, I. (2021) 'Impacts of anxiety and socioeconomic factors on mental health in the early phases of the COVID-19 pandemic in the general population in Japan: A web-based survey', *PLoS ONE*, 16(3 March), pp. 1–19. doi: 10.1371/journal.pone.0247705.

National Health Services (2018) *A Guide to Tai Chi, NHS UK*. UK. Available at: http://www.nhs.uk/Livewell/fitness/Pages/taichi.aspx (Accessed: 24 June 2021).

National Institute on Aging (2011) *Global Health and Aging.*

Nutbeam, D. and Kickbusch, I. (1998) 'Health promotion glossary', *Health Promotion International*, 13(4), pp. 349–364. doi: 10.1093/heapro/13.4.349.

Ogbo, F. A. et al. (2018) 'The burden of depressive disorders in South Asia, 1990–2016: Findings from the global burden of disease study', *BMC Psychiatry*, 18(1), pp. 1–11. doi: 10.1186/s12888-018-1918–1.

Ozer, O., Santaş, F. and Yildirim, H. H. (2012) 'An evaluation on levels of knowledge, attitude and behavior of people at 65 years and above about alternative medicine living in Ankara', *African Journal of Traditional, Complementary, and Alternative Medicines : AJTCAM / African Networks on Ethnomedicines*, 10(1), pp. 134–141. doi: 10.4314/ajtcam. v10i1.18.

Pang, W. et al. (2020) 'Chinese herbal medicine for coronavirus disease 2019: A systematic review and meta-analysis', Integrative Medicine Research, 9(160) (March), p. 100477. doi: 10.1016/j.phrs.2020.105056.

Park, B. J. et al. (2010) 'The physiological effects of Shinrin-yoku (taking in the forest atmosphere or forest bathing): Evidence from field experiments in 24 forests across Japan', *Environmental Health and Preventive Medicine*, 15(1), pp. 18–26. doi: 10.1007/s12199-009-0086–9.

Park, H. (2003) *North Korea Handbook*. Yonhap News Agency. Available at: https://books.google.com.my/books?id=JIlh9nNeadMC&pg=PA439&lpg=PA439&dq=KORYO+M EDICINE&source=bl&ots=gy-.

Patel, V. et al. (2018) 'The Lancet Commission on global mental health and sustainable development', *The Lancet*, 392(10157), pp. 1553–1598. doi: 10.1016/S0140–6736(18)31612-X.

Pusan National University School of Korean Medicine (2015) *Korean Medicine: Current Status and Future Prospects.*

Putnam, R., Leonardi, R. and Nanetti, R. (1993) 'What makes democracy work: civic traditions in modern Italy', *International Affairs.*

Ravishankar, B. and Shukla, V. J. (2007) 'Indian systems of medicine: A brief review', *Arfrican Journal of Traditional, Complementary and Alternative Medicine*, 4(3), pp. 319–337.

Republic of Phillipines (1997) *Traditional and Alternative Medicine Act of 1997*.

Reyburn, S. (2019) *Rosa Parks: In her own Words*. Atlanta: University of Georgia Press.

Roca, C. P. and Helbing, D. (2011) 'Emergence of social cohesion in a model society of greedy, mobile individuals', *Proceedings of the National Academy of Sciences of the United States of America*, 108(28), pp. 11370–11374. doi: 10.1073/pnas.1101044108.

Sarris, J. et al. (2015) 'Nutritional medicine as mainstream in psychiatry', *The Lancet Psychiatry*, 2(3), pp. 271–274. doi: 10.1016/S2215–0366(14)00051-0.

Scheffel, J. and Zhang, Y. (2019) 'How does internal migration affect the emotional health of elderly parents left-behind?', *Journal of Population Economics*, 32(3), pp. 953–980. doi: 10.1007/s00148-018-0715-y.

Shengelia, R. (1999) 'Study of the history of medicine in Georgia', *Croatian Medical Journal*, 40(1), pp. 38–41.

Shi, N. et al. (2021) 'Efficacy and safety of Chinese herbal medicine versus Lopinavir-Ritonavir in adult patients with coronavirus disease 2019: A non-randomized controlled trial', *Phytomedicine*, 81(January). doi: 10.1016/j.phymed.2020.153367.

Shih, C. C. et al. (2015) 'Use of Folk Therapy in Taiwan: A Nationwide Cross-Sectional Survey of Prevalence and Associated Factors', *Evidence-based Complementary and Alternative Medicine*, 2015. doi: 10.1155/2015/649265.

Shuval, J. T. and Averbuch, E. (2012) 'Complementary and alternative health care in Israel', *Israel Journal of Health Policy Research*, 1(1), pp. 1–12. doi: 10.1186/2045–4015-1–7.

Song, L. et al. (2007) 'Effects of a sun style Tai Chi exercise on arthritic symptoms, motivation and performance of health behaviours in women with osteoarthritis', *Taehan Kanho Hakhoe chi*, 37(2), pp. 249–256.

Song, Y. (2014) 'Mental support or economic giving: migrating children's elderly care behaviour and health conditions of left-behind elderly in rural China', *Population and Developemtn*, 20(4), pp. 37–44.

Stickley, A. et al. (2013) 'Prevalence and factors associated with the use of alternative (folk) medicine practitioners in 8 countries of the former Soviet Union', *BMC Complementary and Alternative Medicine*, 13(83). doi: 10.1186/1472–6882-13–83.

Subramanian, S. V., Kim, D. J. and Kawachi, I. (2002) 'Social trust and self-rated health in US communities: A multilevel analysis', *Journal of Urban Health*, 79(1), pp. 21–34. doi: 10.1093/jurban/79.suppl_1.s21.

Thas, J. J. (2008) 'Siddha Medicine-background and principles and the application for skin diseases', *Clinics in Dermatology*, 26(1), pp. 62–78. doi: 10.1016/j.clindermatol.2007. 11.010.

The Law Commission Revisions (2015) *The Statutes of the Republic of Singapore - COPYRIGHT ACT*.

The State Council Information Office (2016) *Traditioanal Chinese Medicine in China*. Available at: http://english.www.gov.cn/archive/white_paper/2016/12/06/content_281475509333700. htm.

Al Thiab Al Kendi, A. (2014) *Health and Medicall Care in the First Hijri Century (1–101 AH/ 622–719 AD)*. National Center for Complementary and Alternative Medicine.

Thompson, N. and Thompson, S. (2001) 'Empowering Older People', *Journal of Social Work*, 1(1), pp. 61–76.

Tiemeier, H. (2003) 'Biological risk factors for late life depression', *European Journal of Epidemiology*, 18(8), pp. 745–750. Available at: http://ovidsp.ovid.com/ovidweb.cgi?T= JS&PAGE=reference&D=emed6&NEWS=N&AN=2003347329.

Traditional and Complementary Medicine (2020) *Guidelines for Registration of Traditional and Complementary Medicine Practitioners in Brunei Darussalam, Ministry of Health Brunei*.

Traditional and Complementary Medicine Division (2007) *National Policy on Traditional/ Complementary Medicine, Malaysia.* 2nd edn.

Tse, C. (2013) 'Migration and health outcomes of left-behind elderly in rural China', *Available at SSRN 2440403.*

United Nations (2016) *ESCAP population data sheet Population and Development Indicators for Asia and the Pacific, 2012.* Available at: https://www.unescap.org/sites/default/d8files/knowledge-products/SPPS PS data sheet 2016 v15-2.pdf.

United Nations (2020) *Policy Brief: The Impact of COVID-19 on Older Person, Online2.* Available at: https://www.un.org/development/desa/ageing/wp-content/uploads/sites/24/2020/05/COVID-Older-persons.pdf (Accessed: 5 June 2021).

Uttley, L. et al. (2015) 'Systematic review and economic modelling of the clinical effectiveness and cost-effectiveness of art therapy among people with non-psychotic mental health disorders', *Health Technology Assessment*, 19(18). doi: 10.3310/hta19180.

Verghese, J. et al. (2003) 'Leisure Activities and the Risk of Dementia in the Elderly', *The New England Journal of Medicine*, 348, pp. 2508–2516.

Wang, Hongmei et al. (2009) 'The flip-side of social capital: The distinctive influences of trust and mistrust on health in rural China', *Social Science and Medicine*, 68(1), pp. 133–142. doi: 10.1016/j.socscimed.2008.09.038.

Watanabe, K. et al. (2011) 'Traditional Japanese Kampo medicine: Clinical research between modernity and traditional medicine - The state of research and methodological suggestions for the future', *Evidence-based Complementary and Alternative Medicine.* doi: 10.1093/ecam/neq067.

Water for Health (2019) *Ten Rules of Ikigai: A Blueprint for a Fuller, Healthier Life?, Online.* Available at: Water for Health (Accessed: 24 June 2021).

Wen, M., Browning, C. R. and Cagney, K. A. (2003) 'Poverty, affluence, and income inequality: Neighborhood economic structure and its implications for health', *Social Science and Medicine*, 57(5), pp. 843–860. doi: 10.1016/S0277–9536(02)00457–4.

WHO (2002) *WHO Traditional Medicine Strategy 2002–2005.* Geneva, Switzerland.

WHO (2013) *WHO Traditional Medicine Strategy.* Geneva, Switzerland.

WHO (2018) *Traditional, Complementary and Integrative Medicine, WHO TM Strategy.* Available at: https://www.who.int/health-topics/traditional-complementary-and-integrative-medicine#tab=tab_1 (Accessed: 30 August 2020).

WHO (2019) *WHO Global Report on Traditional and Complementary Medicine 2019.*

Wilms, S. (2010) 'Nurturing Life in Classical Chinese Medicine: Sun Simiao on Healing without Drugs, Transforming Bodies and Cultivating Life', *Journal of Chinese Medicine*, 93.

World Health Organization (2002) *Active Ageing: A Policy Framework.*

World Health Organization (2009) *WHO Guidelines on Hand Hygiene in Health Care.* Available at: https://www.ncbi.nlm.nih.gov/books/NBK144013/pdf/Bookshelf_NBK144013.pdf.

World Health Organization (2017) *Depression and Other Common Mental Disorders: Global Health Estimates.* Geneva, Switzerland. Available at: https://apps.who.int/iris/bitstream/handle/10665/254610/WHO-MSD-MER-2017.2-eng.pdf.

World Health Organization (2018) *Mental Health Atlas 2017.* Geneva.

World Health Organization (2020a) *COVID-19 Strategy Update, Online.*

World Health Organization (2020b) *Nutrition for Older Persons, Online.* Available at: https://www.who.int/nutrition/topics/ageing/en/index1.html.

World Health Organization (2020c) *WHO Timeline COVID-19, Online.* Available at: https://www.who.int/news/item/27-04-2020-who-timeline---covid-19 (Accessed: 24 June 2021).

Xiang, A., Jiang, D. and Zhao, Z. (2016) 'The impact of rural-urban migration on the health of the left-behind parents', *China Economic Review*, 37, pp. 126–139. doi: 10.1016/j.chieco.2015.09.007.

Yamaoka, K. (2008) 'Social capital and health and well-being in East Asia: A population-based study', *Social Science and Medicine*, 66(4), pp. 885–899. doi: 10.1016/j.socscimed. 2007.10.024.

Yang, D. (2006) *Dusk Without Sunset: Actively Aging in Traditional Chinese Medicine*. University of Pittsburgh.

Yip, W. et al. (2007) 'Does social capital enhance health and well-being? Evidence from rural China', *Social Science and Medicine*, 64(1), pp. 35–49. doi: 10.1016/j.socscimed. 2006.08.027.

Zhang, Y. (2020) 'A case of severe COVID19 cured by Qinfei Paide decoction combined with Western Medicine', *Tianjin Journal of Traditional Chinese Medicine*, pp. 1–4.

Zhao, K. et al. (2016) 'A systematic review and meta-analysis of music therapy for the older adults with depression', *International Journal of Geriatric Psychiatry*, 31(11), pp. 1188–1198. doi: 10.1002/gps.4494.

Zhong, Y. et al. (2017) 'Association between social capital and health-related quality of life among left behind and not left behind older people in rural China', *BMC Geriatrics*, 17(1), pp. 1–11. doi: 10.1186/s12877-017-0679-x.

10 Traditional Malay Ulam for Healthy Ageing

Jamia Azdina Jamal
Universiti Kebangsaan Malaysia (UKM)

Khairana Husain
Universiti Kebangsaan Malaysia (UKM)

CONTENTS

Introduction 135
    Antidiabetic Activity 136
    Antihypertensive Activity 139
    Antihyperlipidaemic Activity 141
    Anticancer Activity 142
    Protective Effect for Cognitive Decline and Dementia 143
Conclusion and Recommendation 144
References 145

INTRODUCTION

The World Health Organization defines healthy ageing as "the process of developing and maintaining the functional ability that enables wellbeing in older age". Functional ability is the capability to do something that everyone has a reason to be grateful for (WHO 2020). Ageing is commonly associated with the risk of having non-communicable chronic diseases such as cardiovascular disease, diabetes and cancer, as well as cognitive decline and dementia. It is suggested that many of these diseases can be prevented, delayed or improved by managing lifestyle factors such as diet, physical activity, education, mental activity and social activity (Quach et al. 2017; Clare et al. 2017). Poor dietary habits have a direct impact on health, often resulting in an increase in body mass index (BMI) and obesity or malnutrition.

O'Mullan (2019) found much evidence to suggest that a plant-based diet reduced BMI and improved cardiovascular disease, metabolic disorders and inflammatory conditions. Evidence for some cancers was insufficient, except for breast cancer. Eating lots of fruits, vegetables and protein-rich foods is also associated with reducing the chances of memory loss (Xu et al. 2020).

In an experimental model, cashew (*Anacardium occidentale* L.) leaves have anti-ageing properties and extend the lifespan of *Caenorhabditis elegans*, indicating potential health benefits (Duangjan et al. 2019). Numerous studies have shown that ursolic acid, a triterpene compound that occurs naturally in many fruits and

DOI: 10.1201/9781003043270-10

136 Healthy Ageing in Asia

vegetables, may be used to treat and prevent cancer, obesity, diabetes, cardiovascular disease, brain disease, liver disease and muscle wasting (sarcopenia) (Seo et al. 2018).

The Malaysian Dietary Guidelines prescribe the Malaysian Food Pyramid that recommends eating three servings of vegetables daily (National Coordinating Committee on Food and Nutrition 2010). According to the National Health and Morbidity Survey 2018 involving 6,795 pre-elderly and elderly people, the prevalence of adequate vegetable intake (at least three servings per day) was 11.4% among the pre-elderly and 10.9% among the elderly (Institute of Public Health 2019).

The Malay community in Malaysia have eaten traditional vegetables and herbs (ulam) for generations. Some of the commonly eaten ulam include jering (*Archidendron pauciflorum* (Benth.) I.C. Nielsen), papaya (*Carica papaya* L.), pegaga or Asiatic pennywort (*Centella asiatica* (L.) Urb.), ulam raja (*Cosmos caudatus* Kunth), turmeric (*Curcuma longa* L.), sambung nyawa or longevity spinach (*Gynura procumbens* (Lour.) Merr.), peria katak or bitter melon (*Momordica charantia* L.), kari or curry leaves (*Murraya koenigii* (L.) Spreng.), selom or water celery (*Oenanthe javanica* (Blume) DC) and petai or stink bean (*Parkia speciosa* Hassk.). They are eaten fresh as salads, blanched or cooked.

This chapter aims to provide a systematic review of typically consumed ulam, along with pharmacological and phytochemical studies associated with the most common diseases in the elderly. Hopefully, it will provide scientific information on the benefits of eating ulam to encourage a healthy diet to improve and maintain health and well-being.

ANTIDIABETIC ACTIVITY

Diabetes is a complex metabolic disorder caused by insulin deficiency or dysfunction. It is characterized by hyperglycaemia, polyuria and polydipsia and is the result of decreased insulin secretion and/or action. Scientific studies have shown that several traditional Malay ulam have antidiabetic properties, as evidenced by in vitro and in animal models (Table 10.1).

In 1998, Kamtchouing et al. reported the protective effect of aqueous extract of *Anacardium occidentale* leaves (175 mg/kg) administered to rats twice daily against streptozotocin-induced diabetes (Kamtchouing et al. 1998).

The best-known use of ulam for its hypoglycaemic effect is the fruit of *Momordica charantia* fruits. Ethanol extract (70%) and juice of *M. charantia* fruits administered to rats with alloxan-induced diabetes for 30 days reduced serum glucose levels ($p < 0.01$) compared to the baseline level (Batran et al. 2006; Thomas et al. 2012). Another study by Mahwish et al. (2021) reported that whole fruit powder of *M. charantia* (300 mg/kg) given to Sprague-Dawley diet-induced hyperglycaemic rats significantly reduced blood glucose and increased insulin levels after 28 and 56 days of treatment. This powder has been shown to prevent diabetes in a group of normal rats eating a diet without excess sucrose. The hypoglycaemic effects have been found to be associated with charantin and vicine content.

An in vitro study reported the potential antidiabetic activity of various organic fractions of *Carica papaya* leaves and *Cosmos caudatus* (Loh & Hadira 2011).

Juárez-Rojop et al. (2012) found that oral administration of an aqueous extract of *C. papaya* leaves (0.75 g and 1.5 g/100 mL) to male Wistar rats with streptozotocin-induced diabetes for 30 days significantly reduced serum glucose levels ($p < 0.05$) compared to untreated diabetic ones. In another study, the aqueous leaf extract (400 mg/kg/day) significantly reduced serum glucose levels ($p < 0.01$) in male and female Wistar albino rats with alloxan-induced diabetes compared to the glibenclamide (0.1 mg/kg/day)-treated group (Maniyar & Bhixavatimath 2012). Andawurlan et al. (2010; 2012) reported the presence of flavonoids (e.g. quercetin, kaempferol, apigenin, quercetin-3-*O*-rutinoside), alkaloids (e.g. carpaine), phenolic acids (e.g. caffeic acid, chlorogenic acid, ρ-coumaric acid) and cyanogenic glucoside (e.g. prunasin) in an aqueous methanol extract of *C. papaya* leaves.

An aqueous extract of *Moringa oleifera* leaves (200 mg/kg) orally administered to male Wistar rats with streptozotocin-induced diabetes significantly reduced blood glucose levels in normal rats and normalized hyperglycaemic levels in sub-diabetic and mild diabetic rats after glucose intake, but improved glucose tolerance in all groups (Jaiswal et al. 2009). In chronic diabetic rats, fasting and postprandial blood glucose levels were significantly reduced after 7, 14 and 21 days of treatment. The extract was found to be more effective than glipizide. In another study, an aqueous extract of 100 mg/kg dose, administered by oral gavage to albino mice with alloxan-induced diabetes for 14 days, significantly reduced blood sugar and increased insulin levels. Homoeostasis model assessment of insulin resistance (HOMA-IR) showed that the extract reduced insulin resistance, which was associated with antioxidant capability and insulin sensitivity (Tuorkey 2016).

Ethanol extract of *Murraya koenigii* leaves (200 mg/kg) administered to Sprague-Dawley rats with diabetes induced with streptozotocin and nicotinamide for 4 weeks also significantly reduced blood glucose levels and HOMA-IR index, which may be related to increased glutathione and decreased malondialdehyde levels (Husna et al. 2018).

Several studies have elucidated the potential hypoglycaemic effects of *Clitoria ternatea* flowers. Its aqueous extract (400 mg/kg) administered orally showed a hypoglycaemic effect in alloxan-induced diabetic rats possibly by increasing insulin secretion and enhancing glycogenesis (Daisy & Rajathi 2009). Chayaratanasin et al. (2015) demonstrated that the aqueous extract had antioxidant activity and inhibited the formation of advanced glycation end products (AGE) which is associated with mediating diabetic complications. A randomized crossover study showed that the aqueous extract (1 g/400 mL and 2 g/400 mL) given as beverage increased plasma antioxidant capacity without hypoglycaemia in the fasting state and improved postprandial glucose, insulin and antioxidant status when consumed with sucrose in healthy men (Chusak et al. 2018). In another study, methanol (95%) extract of the flower and its ethyl acetate and chloroform fractions (300 mg/kg) significantly reduced blood glucose levels, increased serum protein levels and restored serum albumin to normal levels in alloxan-induced diabetic male Wistar albino rats (Rajamanickam et al. 2015). A similar result was obtained with methanol extract (Borikar et al. 2018).

Archidendron pauciflorum fruits given orally to streptozotocin-induced diabetic rats significantly normalized blood glucose levels ($p < 0.05$) after 12 weeks. After

15 weeks of treatment, the fruits improved the oxidative status of organs and the number of active islets of Langerhans for normal and diabetic rats. However, the study had found that long-term use has toxic effects on organs of normal rats, including the heart, kidneys, liver, lungs and pancreas (Syukri et al. 2011). An aqueous extract *of Gynura procumbens* leaves (1000 mg/kg) significantly reduced fasting blood glucose ($p < 0.05$) after 14 days of treatment in male Wistar rats with streptozotocin-induced diabetes, comparable with metformin (500 mg/kg) due to uptake of glucose by rat abdominal muscle (Hasnan et al. 2010).

Aqueous extract of *Oenanthe javanica* leaves (10 and 20 g/kg/day) given orally for 2 days significantly reduced blood glucose levels in normal and alloxan-induced diabetic mice. Different doses of the extract (50, 100 and 200 g/kg) demonstrated protective effects in mice against degeneration and necrosis of islets of Langerhans cells caused by streptozotocin (Chuan-li & Xie-fen 2019). An aqueous extract of *Vitex negundo* leaves was also found to significantly reduce blood glucose levels ($p < 0.01$) in alloxan-induced diabetic rats compared to the glibenclamide-treated group (Prasanna et al. 2012).

Studies have also been conducted using organic extracts. Ethyl acetate fraction (25 mg/kg) obtained from an aqueous extract of the fruits of *Averrhoa bilimbi* was administered to diabetic-induced male Sprague-Dawley rats by intragastric route once daily after a morning meal for 60 days. It significantly lowered blood glucose levels ($p < 0.05$) and was comparable to diabetic rats treated with metformin (100 mg/kg) (Kurup 2017). Aqueous and aqueous-acetone extracts of *A. bilimbi* fruits contain proanthocyanidins, tannins, flavonoids (e.g. catechin, epicatechin) and fatty acids beneficial to human health (Ramasay 2016). In addition, *Cymbopogon citratus* sheath and stem essential oil (400 and 800 mg/kg) administered subcutaneously to male rats with poloxamer 407-induced type 2 diabetes significantly reduced glucose and insulin levels compared to diabetic control rats ($p < 0.001$). The effect may be due to the presence of monoterpenes (e.g. myrcene, oxygenated monoterpenes), terpenes (e.g. linalool), monoterpenoids (e.g. citronellal, geraniol), terpenoids (e.g. neral, geranial), bicyclic sesquiterpene (e.g. β-caryophyllene), sesquiterpenes and oxygenated sesquiterpenes (Barti et al. 2013).

A recent study reported that aqueous extracts and methanol fractions of the aqueous extracts of *Musa × paradisiaca* bract and flower (200 mg/kg/day) were given orally twice daily, resulting in a marked reduction in fasting blood glucose levels in male Wistar rats with streptozotocin-induced diabetes, better than the diabetic group treated with insulin (4 UI/kg/day). The aqueous extract of bract and methanol fraction of the aqueous extract of flower improved glucose tolerance, almost comparable with the insulin-treated diabetic group. This study suggested that the presence of flavonol glycosides and anthocyanins in the bract extracts could explain the antidiabetic effect (Vilhena et al. 2020).

An in vitro study of ethyl acetate, methanol and water fractions of *Curcuma longa* rhizome showed inhibitory activity against α-glucosidase and α-amylase, as well as antioxidant and antiglycation activities. The correlation between the curcuminoid content in the fractions and the inhibitory potential of glucosidase and formation of AGE indicates that curcuminoids may be important bioactive components contributing to antidiabetic activity of the rhizome (Lekshmi et al. 2014).

Traditional Malay Ulam for Healthy Ageing

ANTIHYPERTENSIVE ACTIVITY

Hypertension is considered a major risk factor for several cardiovascular diseases among elderly such as atherosclerosis, heart failure, stroke, coronary artery disease and renal insufficiency. Scientific investigations have shown that some traditional Malay ulam possess antihypertensive properties (Table 10.1).

TABLE 10.1
Compilation of Traditional Malay Ulam with Medicinal Values Associated with Ageing

Scientific Name	Vernacular Name in Malay	Plant Part	Form Consumed	Medicinal Properties
Alpinia galanga (L.) Willd.	Lengkuas	Stalk	Cooked	Anticancer activity
Anacardium occidentale L.	Pucuk gajus	Young leaves	Fresh	Antidiabetic activity, anticancer activity, protection against cognitive decline
Archidendron pauciflorum (Benth.) I.C. Nielsen	Jering	Seeds	Fresh, cooked	Antidiabetic activity, antihypertensive activity
Averrhoa bilimbi L.	Belimbing buloh, belimbing asam	Fruits	Fresh, cooked	Antidiabetic activity, antihyperlipidaemic activity
Barringtonia racemosa (L.) Spreng.	Putat	Young leaves	Fresh, cooked	Anticancer activity
Carica papaya L.	Betik	Young leaves	Fresh, blanched, cooked	Antidiabetic activity, antihyperlipidaemic activity
Centella asiatica (L.) Urb.	Pegaga	Leaves	Fresh	Anticancer activity, antioxidant activity, protection against cognitive decline
Cleome rutidosperma DC.	Maman	Leaves	Cooked	Anticancer activity
Clitoria ternatea L.	Kacang telang	Flowers	Fresh, cooked	Antidiabetic activity
Plectranthus rotundifolius (Poir.) Spreng.	Ubi keling	Roots	Cooked	Anticancer activity
Cosmos caudatus Kunth	Ulam raja	Leaves	Fresh	Antidiabetic activity, antihypertensive activity, anticancer activity, antioxidant activity
Curcuma longa L.	Kunyit	Rhizome	Fresh, cooked	Antidiabetic activity, antihypertensive activity, anticancer activity, antioxidant activity

(Continued)

TABLE 10.1 (*Continued*)
Compilation of Traditional Malay Ulam with Medicinal Values Associated with Ageing

Scientific Name	Vernacular Name in Malay	Plant Part	Form Consumed	Medicinal Properties
Curcuma zedoaria (Christm.) Roscoe	Temu kuning, temu putih	Rhizome	Fresh, cooked	Antihyperlipidaemic activity
Cymbopogon citratus (DC.) Stapf	Serai	Leaf sheath	Cooked	Antidiabetic activity, antioxidant activity
Gynura procumbens (Lour.) Merr	Sambung nyawa	Young leaves	Fresh	Antidiabetic activity, antihypertensive activity, anticancer activity
Manihot esculenta Crantz.	Pucuk ubi kayu	Young leaves	Blanched, cooked	Anticancer activity
Morinda citrifolia L.	Mengkudu	Leaves	Fresh	Anticancer activity
Momordica charantia L.	Peria katak	Fruits	Fresh, cooked	Antidiabetic activity
Moringa oleifera Lam.	Merunggai, kelor	Young leaves, fruits	Fresh, blanched, cooked	Antidiabetic activity, antihypertensive activity, antihyperlipidaemic activity
Murraya koenigii (L.) Spreng.	Kari	Leaves	Fresh, cooked	Antidiabetic activity, anticancer activity, anticancer activity, antioxidant activity
Musa × paradisiaca L. *Musa balbisiana* Colla	Jantung pisang	Flower	Blanched, cooked	Antidiabetic activity
Ocimum basilicum L.	Selasih, kemangi	Young leaves	Fresh, cooked	Anticancer activity
Oenanthe javanica (Blume) DC	Selom	Leaves	Fresh	Antidiabetic activity, antioxidant activity
Pachyrhizus erosus (L.) Urb.	Ubi sengkuang	Roots	Fresh, cooked	Anticancer activity
Parkia speciosa Hassk.	Petai	Seed	Fresh, cooked	Antihypertensive activity
Persicaria hydropiper (L.) Delarbre *Persicaria minor* (Hudz.) Opiz	Kesum	Leaves	Fresh, cooked	Anticancer activity, antioxidant activity
Piper betle L.	Sireh	Leaves	Fresh, cooked	Anticancer activity
Piper sarmentosum Roxb.	Kaduk	Leaves	Fresh, cooked	Anticancer activity
Sauropus androgynus (L.) Merr.	Cekur manis	Leaves	Fresh, cooked	Anticancer activity
Solanum melongena L.	Terung telunjuk	Fruits	Blanched, cooked	Anticancer activity

Traditional Malay Ulam for Healthy Ageing 141

The carefree short-lived perennial ulam *Cosmos caudatus* has a noticeable blood pressure-lowering effect. Oral pre-treatment with its aqueous extract (500 and 1000 mg/kg) to male Wistar rats prior to adrenaline induction prevented the increase in frequency of heart rate and amplitude of stroke volume comparable to atenolol (9 mg/kg). The extracts prevented the increase of stroke volume amplitude in rats treated with sodium chloride comparable to hydrochlorothiazide (0.45 mg/kg) and captopril (13.5 mg/kg). The extracts also had a significant diuretic effect ($p < 0.0001$) similar to that of furosemide (1.8 mg/kg) (Amalia et al. 2012).

In another study, an aqueous extract of *Gynura procumbens* leaves (500 mg/kg) administered orally once daily to spontaneously hypertensive rats for four weeks significantly decreased ($p < 0.05$) systolic blood pressure, lactate dehydrogenase and creatine phosphate kinase and significantly increased ($p < 0.001$) nitric oxide compared with the normal group receiving only distilled water (Kim et al. 2006).

Chen et al. (2012) reported that hexane extract (4.5 mg/kg) from *Moringa oleifera* leaves lowered pulmonary arterial pressure immediately after monocrotaline injection to induce pulmonary hypertension in male Wistar rats. The extract significantly increased superoxide dismutase activity and was found to contain niaziridin and niazirin.

In an *ex vivo* study, purified *Anacardium occidentale* leaf extract rich in flavonoid and phenolic compounds (0.5 and 1.0 mg/mL) was reported to inhibit contraction of isolated rat aorta caused by phenylephrine, which mimics the hypertensive action, and to mildly relax the aorta (Nugroho et al. 2013).

An in vitro study demonstrated that a bioactive peptide fraction (<10 kDa) from the hydrolysed *Parkia speciosa* seed inhibited angiotensin-1-converting enzyme (ACE) activity ($p < 0.05$) with a value of $80.2 \pm 2.8\%$ inhibition (Siow & Gan 2013). Fractions of ethyl acetate ($IC_{50} = 0.06\,\mu g/mL$), methanol ($IC_{50} = 0.19\,\mu g/mL$) and water ($IC_{50} = 0.38\,\mu g/mL$) of *C. longa* rhizome inhibited ACE activity more strongly than captopril ($IC_{50} = 6.28\,\mu g/mL$) (Lekshmi et al. 2014). ACE inhibitors lower blood pressure by dilating and relaxing blood vessels, demonstrating the potential antihypertensive effect of these extracts.

Antihyperlipidaemic Activity

Lipids in the body are mainly represented by cholesterol, triglycerides and phospholipids. High blood lipid levels are an important risk factor for cardiovascular, coronary artery, cerebrovascular and peripheral vascular diseases. These conditions often lead to heart attacks and strokes. A few traditional Malay ulam have been scientifically evaluated for their lipid-lowering ability (Table 10.1).

Moringa oleifera fruits (200 mg/kg/day) given to rabbits on hypercholesterolaemia diet for 120 days lowered total serum cholesterol, low-density lipoprotein (LDL) cholesterol, very low-density lipoprotein (VLDL) cholesterol, phospholipid, triglyceride, cholesterol-to-phospholipid ratio and atherogenic index, but has been found to increase the high-density lipoprotein (HDL) cholesterol and total-cholesterol-to-HDL ratio. In addition, the lipid profile of the liver, heart and aorta was decreased, and faecal cholesterol excretion was increased (Mehta el al. 2003).

Oral administration of ethanol (50%) *Curcuma zedoaria* rhizome extract (200 and 400 mg/kg) for 12 days reduced total serum cholesterol and LDL cholesterol levels in male rats with hyperlipidaemia induced by poloxamer 407, but the results were not comparable to atorvastatin (75 mg/kg). Its effect may be attributed to the alkaloid content (Srividya et al. 2012).

A previous in vitro study reported that an aqueous extract of the fruits of *Averrhoa bilimbi* inhibited cholesterol uptake by 20 to 30% into human colorectal adenocarcinoma (Caco-2) cell model of intestinal absorption. The fruits (125 mg/kg) and aqueous fruit extract (50 mg/kg) were effective in reducing lipids in rats fed with high-fat diet (Pattamadilok et al. 2010).

Aqueous extract of *Carica papaya* leaves (3 g/100 mL) significantly decreased total cholesterol and triglyceride levels ($p < 0.05$) in streptozotocin-induced diabetic male Wistar rats' serum and liver after 4 weeks of treatment compared to the untreated diabetic control group (Juárez-Rojop et al. 2012).

ANTICANCER ACTIVITY

According to the Malaysian National Cancer Registry Report 2012–2016 (Ministry of Health 2019), the incidence of cancer increased exponentially with age, with the highest age at diagnosis ranging from 60 to 64 years for men and from 55 to 59 years for women. The 10 most common cancers for Malaysians are breast cancer, colon cancer, lung cancer, lymphoma, nasopharyngeal cancer, leukaemia, prostate cancer, liver cancer, cervical cancer and ovarian cancer. Breast and colorectal cancers are most common in older people.

It has been reported that 11 methanol extracts of Malay ulam (Table 10.1) strongly inhibited tumour promoter-induced Epstein–Barr virus (EBV) activation in human B-lymphoblastoid Raji cells (Murakami et al. 2000). These include *Anacardium occidentale* leaves, *Cleome rutidosperma* leaves, *Cosmos caudatus* leaves, *Trichosanthes anguina* fruits, *Plectranthus rotundifolius* roots, *Barringtonia racemosa* leaves, *Pachyrhizus erosus* roots, *Persicaria hydropiper* leaves, *Solanum melongena* fruits, *Alpinia galanga* stalks and *Curcuma longa* rhizomes at a concentration of 200 µg/mL with 100% inhibition rate without any cytotoxicity (90% cell viability), whereas *Manihot esculenta* leaves, *Sauropus androgynus* leaves, *Ocimum basilicum* leaves, *Piper betle* leaves and *Murraya koenigii* leaves showed strong inhibition at a lower concentration (40 µg/mL). The EBV activation inhibition test can be considered as one of the most effective in vitro methods to predict chemopreventive potential in vivo.

A meta-analysis by Hou et al. (2019) found an association between a healthy diet and a reduced risk of breast cancer. However, only in vitro studies of the Malay ulam have been found in the literature. Various extracts were reported to inhibit human breast cancer (MCF-7) cell lines, including ethanol (50%) extract of *Anacardium occidentale* leaves, methanol (80%) extract of *C. asiatica*, ethyl acetate fraction of *Gynura procumbens* leaf ethanol extract and methanol extract of *Murraya koenigii* leaves (Lingaraju et al. 2008; Babykutty et al. 2009; Nurulita et al. 2012; Ghasemzadeh et al. 2014). Antiproliferative activity against the MDA-MB-231 cell line that models the triple-negative breast cancer cells was also reported for ethanol extract of *Sauropus androgynus* leaves, methanol extract of *M. koenigii* leaves and ethanol (70%) extract of *Morinda citrifolia* shoots (Rahmat et al. 2003; Noolu et al. 2013; Meli et al. 2019). Aqueous extract of *Centella asiatica* showed antimetastatic activity of voltage-gated sodium channel-expressing MDA-MB-231 cells (Mokhtar 2018). In addition, methanol extract of *C. caudatus* leaves and ethyl acetate fraction of ethanol extract of *G. procumbens* leaves demonstrated cytotoxic activity against progesterone-sensitive human T47D breast cancer cells (Pebriana et al. 2008; Nurulita et al. 2012).

Numerous studies have been reported on the anticancer potential of Malay ulam in colorectal cancer. *Ocimum basilicum* leaf powder (1%) mixed with the diet significantly (p<0.05) reduced tumour incidence by 50%, number and size in rats induced with colon tumour compared to the control group (Gajula et al. 2010). In vitro experiments have shown that aqueous extract of *Barringtonia racemosa* leaves inhibited proliferation of Caco-2 cells (Ho et al. 2020). In addition, ethanol extract of *Cosmos caudatus* leaves caused cytotoxic activity against human colorectal cancer (HCT 116) cell lines via apoptosis (Sia et al. 2020). Ethanol extract of *Musa balbisiana* inflorescence demonstrated cytotoxicity towards human colorectal cancer HT-29 cell line (Revadigar et al. 2017), whereas ethanol (70%) extract of *Morinda citrifolia* shoots also inhibited the cells via apoptosis (Meli et al. 2019).

Antiproliferative activity of several Malay ulam against various cancer cell lines has been investigated. Ethanol extracts of *Morinda citrifolia* leaves, *Persicaria minor* leaves, *Piper sarmentosum* leaves and *Cosmos caudatus* leaves were cytotoxic against human cervical epithelial adenocarcinoma (HeLa) cell lines (Ali et al. 1996; Nurhayati et al. 2018; Dwira et al. 2019). Methanol extract of *Murraya koenigii* leaves inhibited HeLa and human androgen-sensitive prostate adenocarcinoma (LNCaP) cell lines (Ghasemzadeh et al. 2014; Noolu et al. 2013; 2015). In addition, pentagalloyl glucose isolated from the ethanol extract of *Anacardium occidentale* leaves was significantly cytotoxic to HeLa cells at a concentration of 100 µg/mL due to induction of reactive oxygen species (ROS) and oxidative stress (Taiwo et al. 2020).

A recent study reported that aqueous extract of *Murraya koenigii* leaves exhibited antiangiogenesis activity by inhibiting the formation of intersegmental vessels and sub-intestinal veins in a transgenic zebrafish embryo (Dinesh et al. 2020). This model mimics the process of tumour angiogenesis in vivo for tumour progression and spread.

PROTECTIVE EFFECT FOR COGNITIVE DECLINE AND DEMENTIA

Dementia is a disorder characterized by a decrease in memory, thinking, behaviour and ability to perform daily activities (WHO 2020). The most common form of dementia is neurodegenerative Alzheimer's disease, followed by vascular dementia which is caused by reduced blood supply to the brain due to hypertension and atherosclerosis. A cross-sectional study that conveniently sampled elderly adults from low-income families who are more likely to have cognitive decline showed a positive correlation between consuming ulam and working memory and cognitive flexibility (You et al. 2019). Eating at least one serving of ulam per day improves nutritional status, mood and cognitive abilities (You et al. 2020).

Ageing often reduces the removal of ROS, such as reactive oxygen ion superoxide and hydrogen peroxide, and increases ROS activity, leading to oxidative stress. New research evidence suggests that antioxidants may reduce oxidative stress in neurodegenerative diseases. Water extracts of *Persicaria minus*, *Murraya koenigii*, *Centella asiatica*, *Cosmos caudatus* and *Oenanthe javanica* (Table 10.1) showed antioxidant activities in the reducing antioxidant power, ferric thiocyanate (FTC), thiobarbituric acid (TBA), 2,2-diphenyl-1-picrylhydrazyl (DPPH) radical scavenging and reducing ferric ion antioxidant power (FRAP) assays (Huda-Faujan et al. 2007; Reihani & Azhar 2012). Ethanol (95%) extracts of *Curcuma longa*, *Cymbopogon citratus* and *C. asiatica* significantly reduced oxidative stress-induced rabbit erythrocyte haemolysis when compared to the positive control, ascorbic acid (Rafat et al. 2011). In the same study, Rafat et al. reported that the ethanol (95%) extracts of *C. caudatus* gave strong free radical scavenging activity of 86.87% and 86.86%, respectively, compared to the positive control, butylated hydroxytoluene (94.86%), while ethanol (95%) extracts of *C. caudatus* (98.56%), *C. citratus* (91.54%), *C. longa* (89.60%) and *O. javanica* (73.51%) inhibited superoxide dismutase activity (SOD), compared with ascorbic acid (99.20%). Antioxidative studies of the ulam could support their potential use to reduce oxidative stress in cognitive decline and dementia associated with ageing.

Puttarak et al. (2017) performed a systematic review and meta-analysis of the effect of *Centella asiatica* on cognitive abilities. A quantitative synthesis of 11 related papers found no conclusive evidence to support the effect of *C. asiatica* on overall cognitive performance improvement. However, *C. asiatica* could improve working memory. When mixed with other herbs, it could improve attentiveness and focus, executive functioning skills and information processing speed. In vitro and in vivo studies conducted by Hafiz et al. (2020) have reported that an ethanol extract (95%) of *C. asiatica* inhibits acetylcholinesterase, LPS-induced neuroinflammation and oxidative stress. Neuroinflammation is associated with neurodegenerative diseases such as Alzheimer's disease (AD) and cognitive dysfunction. Agathisflavone isolated from 80% methanol extract of *Anacardium occidentale* leaves inhibits neuroinflammation in BV2 microglia via activation of immune-related NF-κB signalling pathway (Velagapudi et al. 2018).

CONCLUSION AND RECOMMENDATION

Healthy diet and lifestyle can slow the ageing process, reduce the risk of ageing-associated chronic diseases and increase lifespan. This review provides scientific information on the medicinal properties of 34 Malay ulam. Many in vitro and in vivo studies have been conducted to demonstrate their activities against diabetes, hypertension, hypercholesterolaemia, cancer and cognitive decline. The findings give preliminary data on the potential health benefits of ulam that can be used to recommend a healthy lifestyle change by regular intake of ulam. However, further studies in animals and humans are needed to confirm their long-term therapeutic value. Consuming three servings of a variety of ulam in the daily diet can provide the body with more phytonutrients and antioxidants, while increasing fibre intake and reducing calories. Most of the ulam can be grown in the home garden or even on the balcony in pots. Home-grown ulam should be encouraged to make it easily accessible and consumed on a regular basis in order to promote healthy ageing and longevity.

REFERENCES

Ali, A. M., Mackeen, M. M., El-sharkawy, S. H., Hamidi, J. A., Ismail, N. H., Ahmad, F. H. and Lajis, N. H. (1996) Antiviral and cytotoxic activities of some plants used in Malaysian indigenous medicine, *Pertanika Journal of Tropical Agricultural Science*, 19(2/3), pp. 129–136.

Amalia, L., Anggadiredja, K., Sukrasno Fidrianny, I. and Inggriani, R. (2012) Antihypertensive potency of wild Cosmos (*Cosmos caudatus* Kunth, Asteraceae) leaf extract. *Journal of Pharmacology and Toxicology*, 8, 359–368.

Andarwurlan, N., Batri, R., Sandrasari, D.A., Bolling, B. and Wijaya, H. (2010) Flavonoid content and antioxidant activity of vegetables from Indonesia. *Food Chemistry*, 121, 1231–1235.

Andarwulan, N., Kurniasih, D., Apriady, R. A., Rahmat, H., Roto, A. V. and Bolling, B. W. (2012) Polyphenols, carotenoids and ascorbic acid in underutilized medical vegetables. *Journal of Functional Foods*, 4, 339–347.

Babykutty, S., Padikkala, J., Sathiadevan, P., Vijayakurup, V., Azis, T., Srinivas, P. and Gopala, S. (2009) Apoptosis induction of *Centella asiatica* on human breast cancer cells. *African Journal of Traditional, Complementary and Alternative Medicines*, 6(1), 9–16.

Bharti, S. K., Kumar, A., Prakash, O., Krishnan, S. and Gupta, A. K. (2013) Essential oil of *Cymbopogon citratus* against diabetes: Validation by in vivo experiments and computational studies. *Journal of Bionalysis and Biomedicine*, 5(5), 194–203.

Borikar, S. P., Kallewar, N. G., Mahapatra, D. K. and Dumore, N. G. (2018) Dried flower powder combination of *Clitoria ternatea* and *Punica granatum* demonstrated analogous anti-hyperglycemic potential as compared with standard drug metformin: in vivo study in Sprague Dawley rats. *Journal of Applied Pharmaceutical Science*, 8, 75–79.

Chayaratanasin, P., Barbieri, M. A., Suanpairintr, N. and Adisakwattana, S. (2015) Inhibitory effect of *Clitoria ternatea* flower petal extract on fructose-induced protein glycation and oxidation-dependent damages to albumin in vitro, *BMC Complementary and Alternative Medcine*, 15(27), 1–9.

Chen, K. H., Chen, Y. J., Yang, C. H., Liu, K. W., Chang, J. L., Pan, S. F., Lin, T. B. and Chen, M. J. (2012) Attenuation of the extract from *Moringa oleifera* on monocrotaline-induced pulmonary hypertension in rats. *Chinese Journal of Physiology*, 55, 22–30.

Chuan-li, L. and Xiu-fen, L. (2019) A review of *Oenanthe javanica* (Blume) DC. as traditional medicinal plant and its therapeutic potential, *Evidence-Based Complementary and Alternative Medicine*, Article ID 6495819, pp. 1–17.

Chusak, C., Thilavech, T., Henry, C. J. and Adisakwattana, S. (2018) Acute effect of *Clitoria ternatea* flower beverage on glycemic response and antioxidant capacity in healthy subjects: a randomized crossover trial, *BMC Complementary and Alternative Medcine*, 18, pp. 1–11.

Clare, L., Wu, Y. T., Teale, J. C., MacLeod, C., Matthews, F., Brayne, C. and Woods, B. (2017) Potentially modifiable lifestyle factors, cognitive reserve, and cognitive function in later life: A cross-sectional study. *PLOS Medicine*, 14(3), e1002259. doi.org/10.1371/journal. pmed.1002259.

Daisy, P. and Rajathi, M. (2009) Hypoglycemic effects of *Clitoria ternatea* Linn. (Fabaceae) in alloxan-induced diabetes in rats, *Tropical Journal of Pharmaceutical Research*, 8, 393–398.

Dinesh, D., Nanjappa, D. P., Chakraborty, G. and Chakraborty, A. (2020) Evaluation of toxicity and antiangiogenic activity of *Murraya koenigii* leaf extracts in zebrafish, *Journal of Health and Allied Sciences NU*, 10(2), pp. 79–85.

Duangjan, C., Rangsinth, P., Gu, X., Wink, M. and Tencomnao, T. (2019) Lifespan extending and oxidative stress resistance properties of a leaf extracts from *Anacardium occidentale* L. in *Caenorhabditis elegans*, *Oxidative Medicine and Cellular Longevity*, 2019, Article ID 9012396. doi.org/10.1155/2019/9012396.

Dwira, S., Fadhillah, M. R., Fadilah, F., Azizah, N. N., Putrianingsih, R. and Kusmardi, K. (2019) Cytotoxic activity of ethanol and ethyl acetate extract of kenikir (*Cosmos caudatus*) against cervical cancer cell line (HELA), *Research Journal of Pharmacy and Technology*, 12(3), pp. 1225–1229.

El Batran, S. A. E. S., El Gengaihi, S. E. and El Shabrawy, O. A. (2006) Some toxicological studies of *Momordica charantia* L. on albino rats in normal and alloxan diabetic rats. *Journals of Ethnopharmacology*, 108, pp. 236–242.

Gajula, D., Verghese, M., Boateng, J., Shackelford, L., Mentreddy, S. R., Sims, C., Asiamah, D. and Walker, L. T. (2010) Basil (*Ocimum basilicum* and *Ocimum tenuiflorum*) reduces azoxymethane induced colon tumors in Fisher 344 male rats. *Research Journal of Phytochemistry*, 4, pp. 136–145.

Ghasemzadeh, A., Jaafar, H. Z., Rahmat, A. and Devarajan, T. (2014) Evaluation of bioactive compounds, pharmaceutical quality, and anticancer activity of curry leaf (*Murraya koenigii* L.). *Evidence-Based Complementary and Alternative Medicine*, 2014, Article ID 873803, pp. 1–8.

Hafiz, Z. Z., Mohd Amin, M. A., James, R. M. J., Teh, L. K., Salleh, M. K. and Adenan, M. I. (2020) Inhibitory effects of raw-extract *Centella asiatica* (RECA) on acetylcholinesterase, inflammations, and oxidative stress activities via in vitro and in vivo, *Molecules*, 25, p. 892, doi:10.3390/molecules25040892.

Hassan, Z., Yam, M. F., Ahmad, M. and Yusof, A. P. (2010) Antidiabetic properties and mechanism of action of *Gynura procumbens* water extract in streptozotocin-induced diabetic rats. *Molecules*, 15(12), 9008–9023.

Ho, I. Y. M., Abdul Aziz, A. and Mat Junit, S. (2020) Evaluation of anti-proliferative effects of *Barringtonia racemose* and gallic acid on Caco-2 cells, *Scientific Reports*, 10, p. 9987, doi.org/10.1038/s41598-020-66913-x.

Hou, R., Wei, J., Hu, Y., Zhang, X., Sun, X., Chanrdasekar, E. K. and Voruganti, V. S. (2019) Healthy dietary patterns and risk and survival of breast cancer: a meta-analysis of cohort studies, *Cancer Causes Control*, 30, pp. 835–846.

Huda-Faujan, N., Noriham, A., Norrakiah, A. S. and Babji, A. S. (2007) Antioxidative activities of water extracts of some Malaysian herbs. *ASEAN Food Journal*, 14(1), pp. 61–68.

Husna, F., Suyatna, F. D., Arozal, W. and Poerwaningsih, E. H. (2018) Anti-diabetic potential of *Murraya koenigii* (L) and its antioxidant capacity in nicotinamide-streptozotocin induced diabetic rats. *Drug Research (Stuttg)*, 68, pp. 631–636.

Institute for Public Health (IPH), National Institutes of Health, Ministry of Health Malaysia. (2019) National Health and Morbidity Survey (NHMS) 2018: Elderly Health. Vol. II: Elderly Health Findings, 2018, p. 182.

Jaiswal, D., Rai, P. K., Kumar, A., Mehta, S. and Watal, G. (2009) Effect of *Moringa oleifera* Lam. leaves aqueous extract therapy on hyperglycemic rats, *Journal of Ethnopharmacology*, 123, 392–396.

Juárez-Rojop, I. E., Díaz-Zagoya, J. C., Ble-Castillo, J. L., Miranda-Osorio, P. H., Castell-Rodríguez, A. E., Tovilla-Zárate, C. A., Rodríguez-Hernández, A., Aguilar-Mariscal, H., Ramón-Frías, T. and Bermúdez-Ocaña, D. Y. (2012) Hypoglycemic effect of *Carica papaya* leaves in streptozotocin-induced diabetic rat, *BMC Complementary and Alternative Medicine*, 12, p. 236. https://doi.org/10.1186/1472–6882–12–236.

Kamtchouing, P., Sokeng, D. S., Moundipa, P. F., Pierre, W., Jatsa, B. H. and Lontsi, D. (1998) Protective role of *Anacardium occidentale* extract against streptozotocin-induced diabetes in rats. *Journal of Ethnopharmacology*, 62, pp. 95–99.

Kim, M. J., Lee, H. J., Wiryowidago, S. and Kim, H. K. (2006) Antihypertensive effects of *Gynura procumbens* extract in spontaneously hypertensive rats, *Journal of Medicinal Food*, 9(4), pp. 587–590.

Kurup, S. B. and Saraswathy, M. (2016) *Averrhoa bilimbi* fruits attenuate hyperglycaemia-mediated oxidative stress in streptozotozin-induced diabetic rats, *Journal of Food and Drug Analysis*, 25(2), pp. 360–365.

Lekshmi, P. C., Arimboor, R., Nisha, V. M., Menon, A. N. and Raghu, K. G. (2014) *In vitro* antidiabetic and inhibitory potential of turmeric (*Curcuma longa* L) rhizome against cellular and LDL oxidation and angiotensin converting enzyme, *Journal of Food Science and Technology*, 51(12), pp. 3910–3917.

Lingaraju, S. M., Keshavaiah, K. and Salimath, B. P. (2008) Inhibition of *in vivo* angiogenesis by *Anacardium occidentale* L. involves repression of the cytokine VEGF gene expression, *Drug Discoveries & Therapeutics*, 2(4), pp. 234–244.

Loh, S. P. and Hadira, O. (2011) In vitro inhibitory potential of selected Malaysian plants against key enzymes involved in hyperglycaemia and hypertension, *Malaysian Journal of Nutrition*, 17(1), pp. 77–86.

Mahwish Saeed, F., Sultan, M. T., Riaz, A., Ahmed, S., Bigiu, N., Amarowicz, R. and Manea, R. (2021) Bitter melon (*Momordica charantia* L.) fruit bioactives charantin and vicine potential for diabetes prophylaxis and treatment, *Plants*, 10(4), p. 730. doi.org/10.3390/plants10040730.

Maniyar, Y. and Bhixavatimath, P. (2012) Antihyperglycemic and hypolipidemic activities of aqueous extract of *Carica papaya* L. leaves in alloxan-induced diabetic rats, *Journal of Ayurveda and Integrated Medicine*, 3(2), pp. 70–74.

Mehta, K., Balaraman, R., Amin, A. H., Bafna, P. A. and Gulati, O. D. (2003) Effect of fruits of *Moringa oleifera* on the lipid profile of normal and hypercholesterolaemic rabbits, *Journal of Ethnopharmacology*, 86, pp. 191–195.

Meli, M. A. A., Shafie, N. H., Loh, S. P. and Rahmat, A. (2019) Anti-proliferative and apoptosis-inducing effects of *Morinda citrifolia* L. shoot on breast, liver, and colorectal cancer cell lines, *Malaysian Journal of Medicine and Health Sciences*, 15(SP1), pp. 129–135.

Ministry of Health Malaysia. (2019) Malaysia National Cancer Registry Report (MNCR) 2012–2016. Ministry of Health Malaysia, Putrajaya, p. 100.

Mokhtar, N. F. (2018) *Centella asiatica* aqueous extract inhibits motility of VGSCs-expressing MDA-MB-231 cells without affecting cell growth, *Journal of Medicinal Plants Studies*, 6(1), pp. 67–70.

Murakami, A., Ali, A. M., Mat-Salleh, K., Koshimizu, K. and Ohigashi, H. (2000) Screening for the in vitro antitumor promoting activities of edible plants from Malaysia, *Bioscience, Biotechnology and Biochemistry*, 64, pp. 9–16.

National Coordinating Committee on Food and Nutrition, Ministry of Health Malaysia (2010) Malaysian Dietary Guidelines. Ministry of Health Malaysia, Kuala Lumpur, p. 220.

Noolu, B., Ajumeera, R., Chauhan, A., Nagalla, B., Manchala, R. and Ismail, A. (2013) *Murraya koenigii* leaf extract inhibits proteasome activity and induces cell death in breast cancer cells, *BMC Complementary and Alternative Medicine*, 13(1), 7. doi.org/10.1186/1472-6882-13-7.

Noolu, B. and Ismail, A. (2015) Anti-proliferative and proteasome inhibitory activity of *Murraya koenigii* leaf extract in human cancer cell lines. *Discovery Phytomedicine*, 2, pp. 1–9.

Nugroho, A. E., Malik, A. and Pramono, S. (2013) Total phenolic and flavonoid contents and in vitro anti-hypertension activity of purified extract of Indonesian cashew leaves (*Anacardium occidentale* L.), *International Food Research Journal*, 20, pp. 299–305.

Nurhayati, B., Rahayu, I. G., Rinaldi, S. F., Zaini, W. S., Afifah, E., Arumwardana, S., Kusuma, H. S. W., Rizal and Widowati, W. (2018) The antioxidant and cytotoxic effects of *Cosmos caudatus* ethanolic extract on cervical cancer, *The Indonesian Biomedical Journal*, 10(3), pp. 243–249.

Nurulita, N.A., Meiyanto, E., Sugiyanto Matsuda, E. and Kawaichi, M. (2012) *Gynura procumbens* modulates the microtubules integrity and enhances distinct mechanism on doxorubicin and 5-flurouracil-induced breast cancer cell death, *Oriental Pharmacy and Experimental Medicine*, 12, pp. 205–218.

O'Mullan, A. (2019). Can a wholefood plant-based diet affect healthy ageing?, *Age & Ageing*, 48(3), Supplement, iii17.

Pattamadilok, D., Niumsakul, S., Limpeanchob, N., Ingkaninan, K. & Wongsinkongman, P. (2010) Screening of cholesterol uptake inhibitor from Thai medicinal plant extracts, *Journal of Traditional Thai and Alternative Medicine*, 8, pp. 146–151.

Pebriana, R.B., Wardhani, B. W. K. and Widayanti, E. (2008) Pengaruh ekstrak metanolik daun kenikir (*Cosmos caudatus Kunth.*) terhadap pemacuan apoptosis sel kanker payudara, *Pharmacon*, 9(1), pp. 21–28.

Prasanna, R. P., Sivakumar, V. and Riyazullah, M. S. (2012) Antidiabetic potential of aqueous and ethanol leaf extracts of *Vitex negundo*, *International of Pharmacognosy and Phytochemical Research*, 4(2), pp. 38–40.

Puttarak, P., Dilokthornsakul, P., Saokaew, S., Dhippayom, T., Kongkaew, C., Sruamsiri, R., Chuthaputti, A. and Chaiyakunapruk, N. (2017) Effects of *Centella asiatica* (L.) Urb. on cognitive function and mood related outcomes: A systematic review and meta-analysis, *Scientific Reports*, 7, p. 10646. doi: 10.1038/s41598-017-09823-9.

Quach, A., Levine, M. E., Tanaka, T., Lu, A. T., Chen, B. H., Ferrucci, L., Ritz, B., Bandinelli, S., Neuhouser, M. L., Beasley, J. M., Snetselaar, L., Wallace, R. B., Tsao, P. S., Absher, D., Assimes, T. L., Stewart, J. D., Li, Y., Hou, L., Baccarelli, A. A., Whitsel, E. A. and Horvath, S. (2017) Epigenetic clock analysis of diet, exercise, education, and lifestyle factors, *Aging (Albany NY)*, 9(2), pp. 419–437.

Rafat, A., Philip, K. and Muniandy, S. (2011) Antioxidant properties of indigenous raw and fermented salad plants, *International Journal of Food Properties*, 14(3), pp. 599–608.

Rahmat, A., Kumar, V., Fong, L. M., Endrini, S. and Abdullah Sani, H. (2003) Determination of total antioxidant activity in three types of local vegetables shoots and the cytotoxic effect of their ethanolic extracts against different cancer cell lines. *Asia Pacific Journal of Clinical Nutrition*, 12(3), pp. 292–295.

Rajamanickam, M., Kalaivanan, P. and Sivagnanam, I. (2015) Evaluation of anti-oxidant and anti-diabetic activity of flower extract of *Clitoria ternatea* L, *Journal of Applied Pharmaceutical Science*, 5, pp. 131–138.

Ramasay, A. and Mueller Harvey, I. (2016) Proanthocynidins from *Averrhoa bilimbi* fruits and leaves, *Journal of Food Composition and Analysis*, 16, pp. 16–20.

Reihani, S. F. S. and Azhar, M. E. (2012) Antioxidant activity and total phenolic content in aqueous extracts of selected traditional Malay salads (*Ulam*), *International Food Research Journal*, 19(2), pp. 409–416.

Revadigar, V., Al-Mansoub, M. A., Asif, M., Hamdan, M. R., Abdul Majid, A. M. S., Asmawi, M. Z. and Murugaiyah, V. (2017) Anti-oxidative and cytotoxic attributes of phenolic rich ethanol extract of *Musa balbisiana* Colla inflorescence, *Journal of Applied Pharmaceutical Science*, 7(5), pp. 103–110.

Seo, D. Y., Lee, S. R., Heo, J. W., No, M. H., Rhee, B. D., Ko, K. S., Kwak, H. B. & Han, J. (2018) Ursolic acid in health and disease, *Korean Journal of Physiology and Pharmacology*, 22(3), pp. 235–248.

Shukri, R., Mohamed, S., Mustapha, N. M. and Hamid, A. A. (2011) Evaluating the toxic and beneficial effects of jering beans (*Archidendron jiringa*) in normal and diabetic rats, *Journal of the Science of Food and Agriculture*, 91(14), pp. 2697–2706.

Sia, Y. S., Chern, Z. W., Hii, S. P., Tiu, Z. B. and Arifin, M. A. (2020) Antimicrobial activity against pathogenic bacteria, antioxidant and cytotoxic activity of *Cosmos caudatus*, *International Journal of Engineering Technology and Sciences*, 7(1), pp. 32–43.

Srividya, A. R., Dhanabal, S. P., Yadav, K. A., Kumar, S. M. N. and Vishnuvarthan, V. J. (2012) Phytopreventive antihyperlipidemic activity of *Curcuma zedoaria*, *Bulletin of Pharmaceutical Research*, 2(1), pp. 22–25.

Siow, H. L. and Gan, C. Y. (2013) Extraction of antioxidative and antihypertensive bioactive peptides from *Parkia speciosa* seeds, *Food Chemistry*, 141(4), pp. 3435–3442.

Taiwo, B. J., Popoola, T. D., van Heerden, F. R. and Fatokun, A. A. (2020) Pentagalloyl glucose, isolated from the leaf extract of *Anacardium occidentale* L., could elicit rapid and selective cytotoxicity in cancer cells, *BMC Complementary Medicine and Therapies*, 20, p. 287. doi.org/10.1186/s12906-020-03075-3.

Thomas, C., Reddy, P. and Devanna, N. (2012) Impact of cooking on charantin estimated from bitter melon fruits using high performance thin layer chromatography. *International Research Journal of Pharmacy*, 3(6), pp. 149–154.

Tuorkey, M. J. (2016) Effects of *Moringa oleifera* aqueous leaf extract in alloxan-induced diabetic mice, *Interventional Medicine and Applied Science*, 8, pp. 109–117.

Velagapudi, R., Ajileye, O. O., Okorji, U., Jain, P., Aderogba, M. A. and Olajide, O. A. (2018) Agathisflavone isolated from *Anacardium occidentale* suppresses SIRT1-mediated neuroinflammation in BV2 microglia and neurotoxicity in APPSwe-transfected SH-SY5Y cells, *Phytotherapy Research*, 32(10), pp. 1957–1966.

Vilhena, R. O., Figueiredo, I. D., Baviera, A. M., Silva, D. B., Marson, B. M., Oliveira, J. A., Peccinini, P. G., Borges, I. K. and Pontarolo, R. (2020) Antidiabetic activity of *Musa × paradisiaca* extracts in streptozotocin-induced diabetic rats and chemical characterization by HPLC-DAD-MS, *Journal of Ethnopharmacology*, 254, 112666. doi.org/10.1016/j.jep.2020.112666.

WHO (2020) Ageing: Healthy ageing and functional ability. https://www.who.int/westernpacific/news/q-a-detail/ageing-healthy-ageing-and-functional-ability

WHO (2020) Dementia. https://www.who.int/news-room/fact-sheets/detail/dementia

Xu, X., Ling, M., Inglis, S. C., Hickman, L. and Parker, D. (2020) Eating and healthy ageing: a longitudinal study on the association between food consumption, memory loss and its comorbidities, *International Journal of Public Health*, 65, pp. 571–582.

You, Y. X., Shahar, S., Haron, H., Yahya, H. M. and Che Din, N. (2020) High traditional Asian vegetables (ulam) intake relates to better nutritional status, cognition and mood among aging adults from low-income residential areas, *British Food Journal*, 122(10), pp. 3179–3191.

You, Y. X., Shahar, S., Mohamad, M., Yahya, H. M., Haron, H. and Abdul Hamid, H. (2019) Does traditional Asian vegetables (ulam) consumption correlate with brain activity using fMRI? A study among aging adults from low-income households, *Journal of Magnetic Resonance Imaging*, 51, pp. 1142–1153.

11 The Value of TCM in Health Preservation in Healthy Ageing

Zhang Qin
Sichuan University

CONTENTS

A Good Quality and Sufficient Sleep 152
Eat on Time and Eat Local and Seasonal Food 153
Good Conjugal Love for Health and Longevity 153

As everyone knows, we are facing an ageing era, and healthy ageing is now one of the most important subjects to all human beings around the world. People are living longer and longer, at the same time, health and ageing problems are growing much more serious than ever before, and many countries face much more of these challenges. So, this conference is held in proper time. As Asian people, especially Japanese, Chinese, South-East Asians, are getting to the ageing era faster than the rest of the world, this conference being held in Malaysia is held in proper place, too.

I'm a professor as well as a practitioner of the traditional Chinese Daoist Health preservation; I have been studying and practising in this field for more than 30 years since I was an undergraduate student of Chinese philosophy in Sichuan University in 1983. I began to learn and practice Qigong and Taiji Quan at that time.

According to Chinese tradition, "There are nine Daoists among ten famous doctors, and there are nine doctors among ten famous Daoists", As for me, because I'm a scholar of Daoism, especially a scholar of Daoist health preservation, so, 15 years ago when I became a professor of Daoism in Sichuan University, I decided to learn Acupuncture and Tuina of TCM, systematically, at the Chengdu university of TCM. From then on, I have some background about TCM.

It is my honour to be invited to take part in this conference and I thank the organizers so much.

I'm very happy to be here to share some opinions and experiences of this exact topic with you.

According to WHO's definition, health is a state of complete physical, mental and social well-being and not merely the absence of disease or infirmity. This helps us have a wider and deeper understanding of health. And when we face healthy ageing,

DOI: 10.1201/9781003043270-11

we can get some enlightenment in a wide range from this definition. Looking back on Chinese traditional medical theories and methods, we can find some very useful data that value us to get a healthy ageing today.

In my opinion, healthy ageing has two meanings: one is to live healthily into old age, and the other is to remain healthy in old age. The first is an ongoing state, which is a process; the second is an outcome state, which refers to the healthy old age, and it's still a process, too.

On the first meaning, namely how to live a healthy life into old age, TCM has a comprehensive and in-depth theoretical and practical system. In terms of modern people's lifestyle and many physical and mental states of chronic diseases, TCM's practical help can be provided from the following three aspects.

A GOOD QUALITY AND SUFFICIENT SLEEP

According to the classic Chinese health guidelines: our sleep should follow the season's change and adjust the length of sleeping time accordingly. For example, the time to go to bed should not exceed at the local time of 23:00 O'clock in summer, and the wake-up time should not exceed at the local time of 7:00 O'clock. In winter, the time of going to bed should not exceed 22:00 O'clock and the wake-up time should not be earlier than 8:00 O'clock (The time can vary slightly depending on the individual, but the basic principles are the same.) According to my in-class survey of public lectures over the past 20 years, less than 25% of Chinese adults follow these sleep principles; that shows how most modern Chinese people are short of sleep. This really has brought a lot of healthy problems in their everyday life.

Both ancient and modern data show that good sleep quality and sufficient sleep time are the foundation of health. But in many parts of the world at present, because of capital era's value orientation, modern people always work overtime and enjoy excess entertainment and incur the compression of sleep time. So, inferior sleep quality, sleep disorder and even long-term insomnia increase in large areas and bring a series of health problems and diseases. Many research reports show that the shortage and poor quality of sleep are always the causes of a lot of health problems. So, there is a popular saying in China: if you want to be healthy, you must sleep well first.

According to the classical thoughts of Chinese medicine and Daoism, going to bed and getting up on time following seasonal changes is very important and it is the basic of health maintenance principles. Briefly speaking, these are:

- early to bed and early to rise in spring;
- late to bed and early to rise in summer;
- late to bed and late to rise in autumn;
- Early to bed and late to rise in winter.

Of cause I must say that people who live in equatorial places or polar areas do not belong to this principle; their daily life time is rarely influenced by seasonal change as other places, as there are rarely no seasonal changes.

The Value of TCM in Health Preservation 153

EAT ON TIME AND EAT LOCAL AND SEASONAL FOOD

Three meals a day is a longtime human habit, which is the most healthy daily life-style, but for a variety of reasons, many modern people no longer have such a rhythmic habit. Modern medical investigations of diseases show that many digestive tract diseases are caused by malnutrition and not eating regularly. People have a variety of reasons to not eat on time, so their body has a variety of diseases to fight back this wayward behaviour.

According to the tradition of TCM and Chinese Daoism, the best foods for people are local, seasonal and abundant grains, vegetables, fruits and meats. But as a result of today's progress of globalization and logistics developments, as well as the progress of planting technology and the appearance of greenhouses, people can easily get different area's foods and different seasonal foods. It seriously challenges the human gastrointestinal function; unseasonal and endemic food will no doubt bring difficulties of physiological adaptability, cause a lot of physical and mental problems and even diseases.

So, to live a healthy life, we need to have a deep and comprehensive understanding of our food and its effects on our body and mind. With the guidance of TCM and Chinese Daoism, it will bring some convenience to our further research and practices of the wisdom of eating.

How to find good foods for our everyday life? There is a very simple but practical method: go to any supermarket, you will always find that a lot of cheaper vegetables and meats are local. So just buy them; they are often nutritional as well as economical. If you want to keep health, just keep this habit. Remember: the simpler, the better. This is the wisdom of TCM.

GOOD CONJUGAL LOVE FOR HEALTH AND LONGEVITY

Couple life is an important part of family life. Thousands of years ago, Chinese doctors and health experts have paid great attention to this content of life, produced more than ten schools and created more than a hundred methods to cure diseases, strengthen the body and get health and longevity. This knowledge of Chinese medicine and health care can contribute to the wisdom of the whole human sexual life. Many of these principles and methods can enlighten and guide modern people.

To follow these principles, a moderate couple life is needed. From this, both can enjoy the pleasures as well as maintain health and longevity. To achieve such a satisfactory effect requires systematic physical and mental training, and mutual cooperation and support in the couple life. For systematic information on this subject, you can read some Chinese bed chamber Classic such as "White Madam Jing" (Su NV Jing), "The Pengzu sutra", as well as the modern works like "The Sexology of Tao", etc.

As for the second meaning of healthy ageing, namely, to keep an elderly healthy life, there are also two important contents in TCM besides the three above that are very useful as follows:

1. "Motion to keep in shape, rest to tranquilize the mind"

   Retired people have completed their contribution to the society and started their retirement life at home or in a nursing home. In Chinese culture, this time is the golden autumn of life and is the season of enjoying old age. In order to live a long and healthy life, it is advisable for old people to plan out enough time and energy to keep fit.

   As we know, old people's blood vessels and energy supplies have weakened, so appropriate sports are good, but do not do too intense sports and activities in competitive sports games. At present in China, Taijiquan, Baduanjin and other Daoist exercises are recommended for the old people, as well as some exercises such as meditation, softening tendons and doing self-massage. The promotion of these exercises will make good use for the physical and mental health. In this regard, China's experience is worth for other countries' health care institutions.

2. "Have multiple practices for longevity"

   More than 1,700 years ago, there was a famous Chinese pharmacologist, chemist and health care expert, Mr. Ge hong. He said: "Use the combination of all techniques to live long". The first of his teachings is that health and longevity are determined by people themselves. This view fully affirms and enhances people's confidence in their health and longevity pursuing.

   The second point is to tell people to learn more, see more and practice more for health maintenance; do not persist in and rely on a single part of them. Many traditional Chinese health care theories and methods have been accumulated since thousands of years ago; it's really a great work!

For example, the internal cultivation system of Daoism in China over a thousand years is a good way for people to improve the energy of body and mind, upgrade the life system and achieve a healthy ageing. If you have a chance to learn authentic theories and its methods and have done continuous practices, you will really have a very successful and healthy life. This has been proved by many masters from one generation to another for thousands of years. If you or your friends really want to learn, you can go to China to find a real master and practice hard. I believe you will have a rich harvest.

Health maintenance is indeed a very large systematic engineering. To live healthy into old age and to keep a healthy body and mind in old age really involve the multilayer relationships between human and nature, between human and society and between human and himself or herself (That is to say, between his or her body and soul). And it is really very difficult for us to handle this comprehensive process. According to the theories and methods of TCM and Chinese Daoism, it is necessary to grasp some basic principles and practice them persistently under guidance. If so, you can achieve the ideal result: "die a natural death". That is to say: One at last can die without any illness at the end of one's natural life.

If the above theories and methods can be used in your everyday life, then you really can benefit a lot from it.

The Value of TCM in Health Preservation

Modern lifestyle has two breaches of natural law.

a. Sleep too late;
b. Eat too much.

Hope everyone who have read or heard the above words can find something useful and practical from TCM and Chinese Daoism. And from now on have a good sleep and eat a good meal!

We really can find much valuable enlightenment from TCM when we face healthy ageing! Wish everyone of this secular world have a real healthy ageing!

Thank you very much!

12 The Value of Disease Prevention and Health Promotion of Hua Tuo Five-Animal Play with Traditional Chinese Medicine

Yang Yu
First Affiliated Hospital of Guangxi
University of Chinese Medicine

CONTENTS

Conduction Exercise (Dao Yin) and Hua Tuo Five-Animal Play 158
    Connotation in TCM 158
    Connotation in Modern Medicine 159
    Connotation in TCM 159
    Connotation in Modern Medicine 159
    Connotation in TCM 159
    Connotation in Modern Medicine 160
    Connotation in TCM 160
    Connotation in Modern Medicine 160
    Connotation in TCM 160
    Connotation in Modern Medicine 161
Practising Essentials of Hua Tuo Five-Animal Play 161

Wu Qin Xi(five-animal play), also known as Hua Tuo Five-Animal Play, was created by the legendary Chinese Physician and Surgeon Hua Tuo who had lived during the Late Eastern Han Dynasty more than 1,800 years ago. It incorporates the theory of Yin Yang, five elements, "Zang Xiang" (visceral manifestation), meridian lines, and qi (internal harvested energy) to move the limbs and spine as well as massages along the meridian lines, following a set of traditional guided health techniques created for promoting good health as well as for the prevention and treatment of diseases.

DOI: 10.1201/9781003043270-12

Hua Tuo Five-Animal Play is the oldest-known guided healthcare technique in China. It consists of five sets of stances, namely, the tiger's stance, the deer's stance, the bear's stance, the monkey's stance and the crane's stance. Each action mimics the corresponding animal's movements in Nature. The stances combine dynamic and static movements, some rigid while others flexible, performed in tandem with proper controlled breathing techniques. Hua Tuo Five-Animal Play is the predecessor to many exercise techniques in the later generations and has great significance in the history of traditional healthcare in China or even the whole world.

The content of this section is based on the book *Health Qigong Tuo Five-Animal Play*, published by the People's Sports Press in 2003 in collaboration with the Health Qigong Management Center of the State General Administration of Sports.

CONDUCTION EXERCISE (DAO YIN) AND HUA TUO FIVE-ANIMAL PLAY

Hua Tuo Five-Animal Play is a type of TCM exercise. Conduction exercise (Dao Yin) – "Dao" is to guide the Qi (internal harvested energy) through breath exercises, whereas "Yin" is to move the body and limbs in a soft and swift motion to promote the softening of joints movement through exercises. "Dao Yin" is often being mentioned together with "An Qiao" (a type of massage) as both originated from the "*The Yellow Emperor's Canon of Medicine*: first complete summary of ancient Chinese medicine". The movements of the tiger, deer, bear, monkey and stoerk reflects the five elements – wood, water, earth, fire and gold which corresponds to the five vital internal organs in the human namely the liver, kidney, spleen, heart and lungs. By imitating the movements and morphological characteristics of these five animals, the practitioner can move the qi to open the blocked pressure points through a self-massage method and re-adjust the internal organs' meridian lines, joint mobility and other aspects of the internal body to achieve preventive and therapeutic effects.

The Corresponding Principles and Health Connotation of Hua Tuo Five-Animal Play, Five Elements and Five Internal Organs

2.1 *The Tiger's stance belongs to the wood element in the five elements and it represents the "Gan" (liver) which functions to store blood and is related to the tendons in our body.*

CONNOTATION IN TCM

In the tiger's stance, the hand is to mimic the tiger's claw. The tendons are stretched, and this enhanced the grip strength of the practitioner. By contracting and relaxing the grip four times, it promotes qi and blood flow producing a warm sensation in the upper limbs. Simultaneously, toxins from the liver is evacuated. The upper limb should be stretched as far as possible while the practitioner breathes with deep and shallow breathes. At the same time, both eyes must be made to rotate all around which helps to improve eyesight as well as for cleansing of the liver because the eyes are related to the liver. During this exercise, the whole body's bones and muscles are stretched to promote the flow of qi along the meridians.

The Value of Disease Prevention

CONNOTATION IN MODERN MEDICINE

In the tiger's stance, perfusion of blood to the heart and the peripheral circulation are promoted which helps to protect the heart's function. It also helps in the spine and joints mobility and extensibility. By stretching the whole body, the muscles surrounding the spine can be strengthened for better mobility of the spine and to prevent spinal diseases, especially cervical spondylosis, lumbar spine degenerative changes, thoracic facet joint disorders and others.

2.2 *The deer's stance is associated with the water element and corresponds to the organ "Shen" (kidneys), which functions to absorb qi and is related to all the bones of the body.*

CONNOTATION IN TCM

In the deer's stance, the focus is on rotation movement and lateral flexion of the waist. Exercises on the waist has the same effect of massaging the "Shen" and nourishing the "Shen" as well as strengthening the bones. While twisting the waist, the arms are placed like the antlers of a deer, one limb is kept on the waist, and while the other limb is propped up to the head / by alternating the limbs, the "Xin" (heart) and "Xin Boa" (pericardium) meridians can be stretched and exercised. This stance helps to condition the heart and blood. In the deer stance, initially the arms are rotated forward, the body's centre of gravity and abdomen being pushed backward. When the body is relaxed, the centre of gravity is moved forward. This movement rejuvenates the "Du" Meridian which has the effect of invigorating the male reproductive organ and the "Shen".

CONNOTATION IN MODERN MEDICINE

In the deer's stance, the focus is on waist rotation, lateral flexion and twisting. These help to strengthen the waist muscles and lumbar spine and to prevent accumulation of waist fat caused by obesity. In addition, it helps in the adjustment of lumbar facet joints. In the deer's stance, the arms are rotated forward to exercise the muscles of the shoulders and the back. It helps to alleviate pain and soreness caused by cervical and peri-shoulder diseases.

2.3 *The bear's stance belongs to the earth element and corresponds to "Pi" (spleen) and is related to muscles of the body.*

CONNOTATION IN TCM

In bear's stance, the waist and abdomen are rotated clockwise and anticlockwise, producing a good dredge effect on the "Pi" (spleen) and "Wei" (stomach) meridians. With the waist and abdomen as axes, the practitioner draws a circle on the abdomen with both palms, starting from the "Ren" meridian's Guanyuan acupoint, passing through the "Wei" (stomach) meridian's Tianshu acupoint, the "Pi" (spleen) meridian's Dahuang acupoint, and the "Ren" meridian's Zhongwan acupoint. These actions can strengthen the intra-abdominal Qi and blood movement. The self-massage on the abdomen and ribs enhances the digestive function of the "Pi" (spleen) and "Wei" (stomach), which can help to treat indigestion, abdominal flatulence, anorexia and constipation. When the limbs are stretched from side to side, it will facilitate the body to shake from side to side, which not only promotes the movement of the ribs, but also soothes the "Gan" (liver), regulates qi and fortifies the "Pi" (spleen).

CONNOTATION IN MODERN MEDICINE

In the bear's stance, the clockwise and anticlockwise rotation of the waist and abdomen helps in the relaxation of the waist and in the prevention and treatment of strain-induced waist disease. The clockwise rubbing of the abdomen can promote gastrointestinal motility and treat constipation as well as promote digestion and absorption of food whereas the anti-clockwise movement can slow gastrointestinal peristalsis and can be used as a therapeutic way to treat diarrhoea. Exertion on the hips while training will also enhance the muscle strength of the hip joint and this can help to improve the balancing of the human body.

2.4 *Monkey's stance belongs to the fire element and corresponds to the "Xin" (heart) and is related to the blood vessel.*

CONNOTATION IN TCM

In the monkey's stance, as the practitioner inhales, he shrugs his shoulders, lift his abdomen and anus, contracts his neck muscles and lift his heels. During exhalation, all muscles are relaxed. The tightening and loosening of muscles help to massage the heart and keeps the blood vessels unobstructed and the qi and blood to run smoothly. A two-way regulation effect of removing "Xin" (heart) fire and raising "Xin" (heart) blood is achieved. The monkey's picking movement is easy and flexible, and the upper and lower limbs are well coordinated. It enables the mind to be nurtured and helps to refresh and resuscitate the brain.

CONNOTATION IN MODERN MEDICINE

In the monkey's stance, inhalation and exhalation squeezes the thoracic cavity and helps in the proper function of the heart and lungs. It helps the practitioner to breathe better and increases blood supply to the heart which directly improves symptoms such as palpitation and chest tightness. The actions of shrugging the shoulders, abdomen, raising the anus, raising the neck, etc., enhances the sensitivity of the local nerves and effectively relieves neck and shoulder pains. Monkey's stance mimics the entire process of a monkey picking peaches. These movements are easy and flexible, which can effectively relieve mental stress, improve sleep and balance.

2.5 *Crane's stance which belongs to metal element and corresponds to the "Fei" (lungs) and is related to breathing the skin.*

CONNOTATION IN TCM

In the Crane's stance, breathing coordination is the most important factor. When practiseing this stance, the practitioner inhales with his arms stretched forward and

The Value of Disease Prevention

exhales with his arms downward, then inhale with the back swing and retract the breath. These actions do not only stimulate the "Fei" (lungs) meridian but helps to produce deep and even breathings. It enhances lungs function and effectively relieves lung diseases. This exercise also helps in moisturizing the skin. In the crane's stance, the legs are straightened and raised backwards, which helps to unblock the qi, blood flow and meridians in the chest and back and strengthens the blood-qi circulation into the legs. Swinging the arms up and down, combining with deep breathing can adjust the "San Jiao" movement. By squeezing the thoracic cavity, this exercise plays a role in massaging the heart and lungs, and a two-way adjustment of the heart and lungs.

CONNOTATION IN MODERN MEDICINE

In the Crane's stance, the use of deep and uniform breathing exercises and body movements helps to improve lung capacity, blood oxygen exchange and cardio pulmonary function and enhances human immunity. It can effectively relieve chest tightness, shortness of breath, etc. By alternately standing on left and then right foot, it helps in balancing of the human body and has the power of strengthening the brain. The deep and long breathings have a calming effect and helps in relieving stress.

PRACTISING ESSENTIALS OF HUA TUO FIVE-ANIMAL PLAY

The stance is simple, relaxing and the breathing is natural. Although the "figure" of Hua Tuo Five-Animal Play is displayed outside, it has a related inner meaning. The shape of the movement should not only imitate the characteristics of the five animals, but also strive to contain its charm during practice. The natural posture and body's comfort should be kept if possible while maintaining the correct posture required by the exercises. Only when the limbs are free and natural and the breathing is at ease, can the qi be generated continuously and consciously to smoothen the flow of blood and qi, thus enhancing the physique.

Extending the limbs and moving the joints: During the practice of Hua Tuo Five-Animal Play, we must pay attention to both the standardization of the practice and the individuality of the practice. We must adjust the scope of the exercise according to different groups and physical fitness. It is also necessary to comprehensively exercise according to the characteristics of each animal, using the waist as the main axis and hub to drive the upper and lower limbs to move in all directions, pay attention to the spine and "Du" meridian exercises. Special attention must be paid to the movements of small joints such as fingers and toes and other unusual parts of the body to ventilate blood, exercise the joints and strengthen the body.

Step-by-step perseverance: The exercise of Hua Tuo Five-Animal Play should not be rushed or over-trained. Follow a step-by-step exercise requirement to develop a personalized exercise plan. Hua Tuo states that

> "The human body desires labour but avoid improper use. Hua Tuo Five-Animal Play has a distinctive feature in TCM as it practices both the exercise and mind cultivation in prevention and treatment of disease. You cannot give up at will. Only by perseverance and perseverance alone can one truly achieve the goal of good health and longevity".

To sum up, Hua Tuo five-animal play is a distinctive conduction exercise for TCM. Based on the "four diagnosis" of TCM, it is the dialectical basis for differentiating diseases. Exercise guidance for different diseases and symptoms is the ultimate application mode. Hua Tuo also stated that "If you have unpleasant feelings, start practising an animal's action. You can practise some of them when your body is uncomfortable. Then, you can either perform corrective exercises based on the different five elements and "'Zang Xiang'"(visceral manifestation) attributes, or use the theory of traditional Chinese medicine as the basis, and use the "'four diagnosis'" of Chinese medicine as the evaluation method to individualize and personalize the exercise guidance for different diseases and symptoms". Preliminary studies have confirmed its feasibility, but the sample size is relatively small and a complete theoretical system has not been formed. Henceforth, from the perspective of evidence-based medicine, a comparative study of larger sample and a multi-centre random method should be used to further improve the construction of this theoretical system of Hua Tuo Five-animal Play.

13 An Ayurvedic Approach for Healthy Ageing

Gopesh Mangal
National Institute of Ayurveda

CONTENTS

Introduction 163
    Ayurvedic Aspect 164
    Ayurveda- An Answer to Healthy Ageing 165
Conclusion 168
References 168

INTRODUCTION

Nowadays, the term "premature ageing" is something no one is unaware of. Though the sedentary lifestyle and faulty food habits have comforted our lives to an extent they also have cursed us with the signs of its consequence known as premature ageing where for some individuals the symptoms of ageing are more pronounced and arrive much earlier. The signs of premature skin ageing are sometimes visible and can be very distressing as they are unforeseen. Premature greying of hair, wrinkles over the skin, untimely ailments that were thought to accompany ageing are a few concerns of this big issue. It is a well-known fact that everybody ages, everybody dies, and there is no turning back the clock, but "healthy ageing" is what everyone desires. Holding on to youth and delaying ageing is a universal desire.

Physiological influence of ageing [1]:

Physiological changes occur in all organs and body as age advances:

- The cardiac output decreases, blood pressure increases and arteriosclerosis develops.
- The lungs display a decrease in vital capacity and impaired gas exchange which also results in slower expiratory flow rates.
- The creatinine clearance declines with ageing even though the serum creatinine level remains relatively constant. This can be due to a proportionate age-related diminution in the production of creatinine.
- Functional changes like changed motility patterns, changes with old age in the gastrointestinal system like atrophic gastritis and altered hepatic drug metabolism are visible in the aged.

DOI: 10.1201/9781003043270-13

164   Healthy Ageing in Asia

- There is a gradual and progressive elevation in blood glucose levels with age on a multifactorial basis.
- Osteoporosis and low bone mineral density is frequently seen because of a linear decline in bone mass after the fourth decade.
- Due to changes in the collagen and elastin, the skin tone and elasticity is lost and there occur skin atrophies with ageing.
- The lean body mass declines with age which may be mainly due to loss and atrophy of muscle cells.
- There are degenerative changes in multiple joints and this, when united with the loss of muscle mass, hinders the motion in an elderly patient.

These changes with age have significant practical consequences on the clinical management of elderly patients.

AYURVEDIC ASPECT

Jara is a term which indicates the declining phase, especially old age or the ageing process [2]. He describes it of two types, *Kalaja Jara* (timely ageing) and *Akalaja Jara* (premature ageing). *Kalaja Jara* or timely ageing should be healthy and *Akalaja Jara* or premature ageing should be prevented. In the case of *Kalaja Jara*, the symptoms of ageing appear at the appropriate time. It involves the simultaneous occurrence of chronological ageing and biological ageing. Whereas, in *Akalaja Jara*, ageing occurs before its due time owing to ignorance and not taking care of the body by following *Swasthavritta* (good health conduct) and *Sadvritta* (good conduct/social behavior).

Ayurveda describes the sequential value lost in ageing as an interesting scheme of loss of different biological factors during life as a function of ageing [3]. During the approximate hundred years of the total span of life, an individual loses different values in different decades of life in the following sequence:

TABLE 13.1
Showing Value Lost According to Decade

Decade of Life	Value Lost
First	*Balya* (Childhood)
Second	*Vriddhi* (Growth)
Third	*Chavi* (Beauty)
Fourth	*Medha* (Intellect)
Fifth	*Tvaka* (Health of Skin)
Sixth	*Drushti* (Vision)
Seventh	*Shukra* (Sexual competence)
Eighth	*Vikramam* (Strength)
Ninth	*Buddhi* (Wisdom)
Tenth	*Karmendriya* (Active senses)

An Ayurvedic Approach for Healthy Ageing

But in today's era of faulty lifestyle, these values do not wait for their respective decade to end them. Loss of healthy skin, vision, strength etc., can be seen decreasing at a comparatively early age, inviting premature ageing.

AYURVEDA- AN ANSWER TO HEALTHY AGEING

Ayurveda, being the science of life and medicine, efforts to protect life from disease and ageing. The concept of *Vayasthapana* which deals with conserving the youthfulness of the body regardless of its age and restricting headway towards old age, along with development of longevity, brainpower, physical and mental strength and prevention from diseases is unique to *Ayurveda*.

Ayurveda, being too vast, was divided into eight subjects, known as *Ashtanga Ayurveda* to facilitate learning. Among the *Ashtanga Ayurveda*, *Jara/Rasayana Chikitsa* finds mention that reflects the importance of measures to avoid ageing or bring about healthy ageing. Healthy ageing involves two aspects – prevention of diseases that otherwise might affect the older individual and cure of the diseases elderly people suffer from.

Ayurveda holds enormous measures for longevity and healthy ageing: *Dincharya* (Daily regimen), *Ritucharya* (Seasonal regimen), *Naveganndharniya* (not to withhold natural urges) are a few of the measures to achieve the same.

Brahm Muhurta (Pre-dawn wake up): *Ayurveda* proposes that one who desires for a healthy life should wake up in *Brahm Muhurta* (before sunrise, after digestion of previous meal) [4]. *Brahm* means knowledge. The time apt for perceiving knowledge is known as *Brahm Muhurta*. *Brahm Muhurta* is 1 hour 36 minutes before sunrise. It is believed that a high level of *Prana* or vital life energy is abundantly present in the atmosphere during the *Brahm Muhurta*. Scientific research has determined that in *Brahm Muhurta*, the oxygen level in the atmosphere is the most (~41%), which is beneficial to the lungs. Studies prove that early risers generally have lower body mass index (BMI) and consequently are less likely to suffer from obesity. According to the same study, early risers are less likely to develop diabetes or suffer from depression or insomnia. Turning our biological clock to the rising and setting of the sun is the best way to reversing the ageing process.

Usha Pana: According to *Acharya Vagbhata*, one who drinks eight *Prasriti* water before sunrise (1 *Prasriti* = Volume that occupies cupped palm) is saved from diseases and untimely ageing. It boosts up metabolism. A study shows that dehydration can cause the body to build up more fat. It also makes one tired; water helps transport oxygen and other important nutrients to different parts of the body and flushes out impurities. It keeps skin healthy – keeps the body hydrated throughout the day. Moreover, it boosts the immune system; drinking water after waking up improves the efficiency of the lymphatic system, which in turn makes the immune system stronger.

Vyayama (exercise): Physical exercise that is favourable to the mind and increases strength and firmness of the body is known as Vyayamain Ayurveda. It should be continued till half of the strength is exhausted. It is believed that one who regularly exercises does not get afflicted by untimely ageing [5]. A study compared a group of older people who have exercised all of their lives, with a group of similarly aged adults and younger adults who do not exercise regularly. The results presented that those who have exercised regularly have resisted the ageing process, have higher immunity, muscle mass and cholesterol levels as that of a young person [6].

Snana (Bathing) is said to promote health and longevity. It is said to impart strength to the body. According to *Ayurveda,* the body above the neck should be subjected to normal/ mild cold water whereas the body below should be bathed with lukewarm water. Excessive hot water for bathing can diminish strength [7].

Dharniya (suppressible urges) – **Adharniya Vega** (non-suppressible urges): To avoid diseases, one should strictly follow the concept of *Dharaniya* and *Adharaniya Vega.* Suppression halts the elimination of waste products and creates various disorders of the nervous system, which leads to illnesses. One should neither suppress natural urges nor should forcibly induce urges.

Dharaniya Vega includes *Krodha* (Anger), *Moha* (Affliction), *Lobha* (Greed) etc. These urges should be suppressed and mastered over. *Adharaniya Vega* are the urges that one should not withhold, and these should be attended to immediately. It includes 13 types of urges viz. *Vata Vega* (urge of passing flatus), *Purisha* (feces), *Mutra* (urine), *Kshavathu* (sneeze), *Trishna* (thirst), *Kshudha* (hunger), *Nidra Vega* (sleep), *Kasa* (Coughing urge), *Shrama-Shwas* (breathe heavily on exertion), *Jrumbha* (yawn), *Ashru* (urge to cry), *Chardi* (urge to vomit) and *Shukra* (discharge seminal fluid) [10].

Nidra (sleep): Sleep is said to influence the body in terms of health, emaciation, strength, *Vrishta* (fertility) and life [8]. Proper sleep promotes a healthy life. Withholding the urge to sleep leads to excessive yawning, body ache, headache, drowsiness and heaviness in eyes [9].

Ahara (Diet): one should take a light meal in the evening [10]. One should always eat in an amount less than hunger. The optimum amount of meal promotes strength, complexion and healthy life [11]. Withholding the hunger leads to emaciation, weakness, body ache, dislike towards food, fainting etc. [12]

Ayurveda has mentioned some conducts regarding diet [13]:

- Not taking a meal leads to diminished lifespan.
- Milk is said to be the best among *Jeevaniya Dravya* (which promotes life)
- Regular use of milk and Ghrita is said to be the best *Rasayana* (Rejuvenation).

Vayasthapana Gana: A list of drugs that are believed to delay ageing includes *Amrita* (Tinospora cordifolia), *Abhaya* (Terminalia chebula), *Dhatri* (Phyllanthus emblica), *Mukta (Rasna- Chakrapani*, Pluchea lanceolata), *Shweta* (Clitoria ternatea), *Jeevanti* (Leptadenia reticularis), *Shatavari* (Asparagus racemosus), *Madukparni* (Centella asiatica), *Sthira* (Desmodium gangeticum) and *Punarnava* (Boerrhavia diffusa) [14]. *Guggulu* (Commiphora mukul) also is said to possess *Rasayana* properties [15].

Rasayana, a treasure of *Ayurveda*, has its importance in promoting longevity and healthy ageing. *Rasayana* is defined as a drug that destroys Jara/ageing [16]. Thus, any measure that delays ageing promotes health and longevity is termed as *Rasayana*, but a purification of the body (*Panchkarma*) is an essential prerequisite for the administration of *Rasayana* (Rejuvenation therapy). Rejuvenation

An Ayurvedic Approach for Healthy Ageing

can only be possible if all the channels of the body remain free from any obstruction or toxins.

Panchkarma is a therapeutic way of eliminating toxic elements from the body. It includes five detoxification processes used to treat diseases as well as to maintain health including healthy ageing.

1. *Vamana* (Medicated emesis),
2. *Virechana* (Medicated purgation),
3. *Basti* (Medicated enema),
4. *Nasya* (Medication through the route of the nose),
5. *Rakta mokshan* (Bloodletting)

Panchkarma therapy reduces the chances of reappearance of the diseases and helps in developing positive health by rejuvenating body tissues. The process of bio-purification thus delays the process of ageing. *Ritu Shodhan* (seasonal *Panchkarma*) is the safe way to stay healthy and avoid illnesses.

Ayurveda is a science of life, and it narrates a simple regimen to be followed daily that provides health benefits in the long run, popularly characterized as *Dincharya* (daily regime) as:

Nasya (Nasal drops or instillation): *Nasya* is a *Panchakarma* therapy that involves nasal administration of medicine or medicated oil. According to *Ayurveda*, one who performs *Nasya* daily does not get afflicted by visual disorders; olfactory and auditory power remain intact; hairs do not turn grey; and falling of hairs is also prevented. Moreover, it also helps to prevent tremors in the head, which is a symptom of Parkinsonism usually associated with old age. The signs of ageing are not reflected by performing *Nasya* daily [17]. *Nasya* with *Anutaila* (*Ayurveda* oil preparation) daily helps in subsiding wrinkles, greying of hairs and pigmentation over the face [18]. These indeed are signs of ageing that are prevented through *Nasya*.

Gandusha (oil pooling): The process of keeping *Sneha* (oil) in the mouth in an amount that does not allow rinsing of mouth is called *Gandusha*. It provides strength to the jaw and improves voice. It clears the tongue off impurities that improves the taste perception which is hampered in old age. It furthermore strengthens the teeth and checks their falling [19]

Karnapoorana (Ear pooling): *Karnapoorana* refers to filling of medicated oil into the ears for a prescribed time. It is recommended regularly to prevent from hearing loss or any other aliments of the ear due to *Vata Dosha* [20].

Abhyanga (Massage): Application of oil externally is simply termed as *Abhyanga*. It is practiced as a part of daily routine in healthy individuals. *Abhyanga* slows down the ageing process. It controls *Vata* which is vitiated in old age. Just asan earthen pot gets reinforced and durable after oleation, similarly *Abhyanga* imparts longevity and makes the skin devoid of wrinkles [21]

Massage promotes quick removal of waste products and renewal of the nutritive elements. The improved arterial blood flow after massage takes more oxygen and other nutritive elements. It also causes quick oxygenation of the blood. These changes make the exchange of waste products between the blood and the tissue at the cellular level more efficiently. This may improve overall the trophic condition of the part being massaged [22]

Shiroabhyanga (Head massage): Head massage delays the process of ageing; it reduces fatigue and controls *Vata* [23]

Padabhyanga (Foot massage): It comes under *Abhyanga* but has been separately mentioned because of its specific virtues. *Padabhyanga*, when performed daily, is said to be beneficial for eye, induces sleep, cures insomnia, one of the issues almost all elderly suffer and gives a feeling of wellbeing [24]

Basti (Medicated enema) is one of the important therapies of *Panchkarma*, *Basti* is said to arrest premature old age and the progress of white hair [25] It sustains age [26] and provides firmness [27]. It can be counted as a standalone therapy to arrest premature ageing.

Among the other health benefits of *Basti* are that it improves intellectual power and clarity of sense organs, induces sound sleep [28] invigorates eyesight [29] provides strength by increasing muscle power, delays degenerative changes, imparts optimum functioning of organs, and increases strength and lifespan. These functions attributed to *Basti* make it an unavoidable choice of therapy in elderly patients who desire healthy ageing.

CONCLUSION

Ageing is a subject of concern since time immemorial. *Ayurvedic* texts have clearly emphasized *Dincharya* or the regime to be followed regularly for a healthy living and healthy ageing devoid of diseases. *Panchakarma* owing to its preventive as well as curative aspect can be a boon for the aged population and *Rasayana* for sustainable health and longevity. As WHO advocates, it is not just important to add years to life but add life to the years one lives.

REFERENCES

1. Boss GR, Seegmiller JE. (1981). Age-related physiological changes and their clinical significance. *Western J. Med.*, 135(6), 434–440. https://www.who.int/news-room/factsheets/detail/ageing-and-health [Last accessed on 2019 May].
2. *Vachaspatyam (Brihat Sansritabhidhanam) - Compiled by Sri Taranatha Tarkavachaspati.* Vol. 4. Chowkhamba Sanskrit series office, Varanasi, 1962; P. 3058.
3. Sharangdhara, Sharangdhara Samhita, Purvakhanda, 6/19, with Hindi commentary by Shailja Srivastava, Chaukhamba Orientalia, Varanasi, Reprint 2013; P.54.
4. Vriddha Vagbhata, Ashtanga Sangraha, Sutrasthana, Dincharya adhyay, 3/3, with Hindi commentary by Kaviraj Atridev Gupta Chowkhambha Krishnadas Academy, Varanasi; P.20.
5. Vriddha Vagbhata, Ashtanga Sangraha, Sutrasthana, 3/62–64, with Hindi commentary by Kaviraj Atridev Gupta, Chowkhamba Krishnadas Academy, Varanasi; P. 31.
6. https://www.sciencedaily.com/releases/2018/03/180308143123.htm.

An Ayurvedic Approach for Healthy Ageing   169

7. Vriddha Vagbhata, Ashtanga Sangraha, Sutrasthana, Dincharya adhyay, 3/68–71, with Hindi commentary by Kaviraj Atridev Gupta Chowkhambha Krishnadas Academy, Varanasi; P. 33.

8. Vriddha Vagbhata, Ashtanga Sangraha, Sutrasthana, Viruddhanna Vigyaneeya adhyay, 9/41, with Hindi commentary by Kaviraj Atridev Gupta Chowkhambha Krishnadas Academy, Varanasi; P. 99.

9. Charaka, Charaka Samhita, Sutra Sthana, Naveganndharaniya adhaya, 7/23, edited by Pt. Rajeswara Datta Shastri, Chaukhamba Bharati Academy, Varanasi, 2008; P. 157.

10. Vriddha Vagbhata, Ashtanga Sangraha, Sutrasthana, Dincharya adhyay, 3/120, with Hindi commentary by Kaviraj Atridev Gupta Chowkhambha Krishnadas Academy, Varanasi; P. 38.

11. Charaka, Charaka Samhita, Sutra Sthana, Matrashitiya adhaya, 5/8, edited by Pt. Rajeswara Datta Shastri, Chaukhamba Bharati Academy, Varanasi, 2008; P. 105.

12. Charaka, Charaka Samhita, Sutra Sthana, Naveganndharaniya adhaya, 7/20, edited by Pt. Rajeswara Datta Shastri, Chaukhamba Bharati Academy, Varanasi, 2008; P. 155.

13. Charaka, Charaka Samhita, Sutra Sthana, Yajjahpurushiya adhaya, 25/40, edited by Pt. Rajeswara Datta Shastri, Chaukhamba Bharati Academy, Varanasi, 2008; PP. 467–469.

14. Charaka, Charaka Samhita, Sutra Sthana, Shadvirechanashatashritiyadhaya, 4/18/50, edited by Pt. Rajeswara Datta Shastri, Chaukhamba Bharati Academy, Varanasi, 2008; P. 98.

15. Vriddha Vagbhata, Ashtanga Sangraha, Sutrasthana, Vividhaushadha Vigyaneeya adhyay, 12/74, with Hindi commentary by Kaviraj Atridev Gupta Chowkhambha Krishnadas Academy, Varanasi; P. 126.

16. Chakrapani, Chakradatta, Rasayanadhikara/1, edited and commentary by Pt. Sadanand Sharma, Meherchand Lachhmandas Publications, New Delhi, reprint March, 2000; P.411.

17. Charaka, Charaka Samhita, Sutra Sthana, Matrashiteeyadhaya, 5/56–63, edited by Pt. Rajeswara Datta Shastri, Chaukhamba Bharati Academy, Varanasi, 2008; P.123.

18. Vriddha Vagbhata, Ashtanga Sangraha, Sutrasthana, Dincharya adhyay, 3/29, with Hindi commentary by Kaviraj Atridev Gupta Chowkhambha Krishnadas Academy, Varanasi; P.25.

19. Charaka, Charaka Samhita, Sutra Sthana, Matrashiteeyaadhaya, 5/78–81, edited by Pt. Rajeswara Datta Shastri, Chaukhamba Bharati Academy, Varanasi, 2008; P. 127.

20. Charaka, Charaka Samhita, Sutra Sthana, Matrashitiyaiya adhaya, 5/84, edited by Pt. Rajeswara Datta Shastri, Chaukhamba Bharati Academy, Varanasi, 2008; P. 128.

21. Vriddha Vagbhata, Ashtanga Sangraha, Sutrasthana, Dincharya adhyay, 3/56–57, with Hindi commentary by Kaviraj Atridev Gupta Chowkhambha Krishnadas Academy, Varanasi; P. 28.

22. Principles and practices of therapeutic massage. P. 13.

23. Vagbhata, Ashtanga Hridya, Sutrasthana, Dincharya adhyay, 2/8, with Hindi commentary by Kaviraj Atridev Gupta, Chaukhamba Prakashan, Varanasi, Reprint 2012; P. 24.

24. Sushruta, Sushruta Samhita, Chikitsasthana, Anagatabadhpratishedh adhyaya, 24/70, edited by Kaviraja Ambikadutta Shastri, ChaukhambaSanskrit Sansthan, Varanasi, Reprint, 2010; P. 136.

25. Sushruta, Sushruta Samhita, Chikitsasthana, Netrabastiprmanapravibhagcikitsa adhyaya, 35/3, edited by Kaviraja Ambikadutta Shastri, ChaukhambaSanskrit Sansthan, Varanasi, Reprint, 2010; P. 189.

26. Charaka, Charaka Samhita, Siddhisthana, Kalpnasiddhi adhaya, 1/27, edited by Pt. Rajeswara Datta Shastri, Chaukhamba Visvabharati, Varanasi, Reprint 2009; P. 968.

27. Charaka, Charaka Samhita, Siddhisthana, Kalpnasiddhi adhaya, 1/28, edited by Pt. Rajeswara Datta Shastri, Chaukhamba Visvabharati, Varanasi, Reprint 2009; P. 969.

28. Charaka, Charaka Samhita, Siddhisthana, Kalpnasiddhi adhaya, 1/44, edited by Pt. Rajeswara Datta Shastri, Chaukhamba Visvabharati, Varanasi, Reprint 2009; P. 972.
29. Sushruta, Sushruta Samhita, Chikitsasthana, Netrabastiprmanapravibhagcikitsa adhyaya, 35/3, edited by Kaviraja Ambikadutta Shastri, ChaukhambaSanskrit Sansthan, Varanasi, Reprint, 2010; P. 189.

14 Principles and Practice of Yoga for Rejuvenation

Gunjan Garg
Mahatma Jyotiba Fule Ayurveda Mahavidhayala

CONTENTS

Introduction 171
What Is *Yoga* 172
Astanga Yoga 172
   Yama and Niyama 172
Role of *Yama* and *Niyama* in Rejuvenation 173
Asana 173
How *Asana* Rejuvenates 175
Pranayama (*Yogic* Breathing Technique) 176
Physiology of *Puraka-Kumbhaka-Rechaka* 177
How *Pranayama* Rejuvenates 177
Pratyahara (Sensorial Transcendence) 177
How *Pratyahara* Rejuvenates 177
Dharana (Concentration), *Dhyana* (Meditation), and
Samadhi (Super-Conscious Stage/Enlightenment) 178
How Meditation Helps in Rejuvenation 178
Conclusion 178
References 178

INTRODUCTION

Rejuvenation means "to make or feel young again". It can be defined as delaying or reversing the ageing process. It is a phenomenon of vitality and restoration of youthful condition which requires a strategy of repairing or replacement of damaged tissue with new tissue, which is associated with ageing. Complete rejuvenation is the combination of physical, mental, sensorial, intellectual and spiritual rejuvenation as well.

From ancient to modern times, human beings always have an urge to live, a desire for youthfulness, distaste for old age and quest for rejuvenation. As age advances, every cell and tissue of the body changes. It is thus necessary to rejuvenate the body system for a better harmony of body, mind and soul (Sharma, Anand and Gupta, 2017). *Yoga* is a traditional Indian system of medicine that has given great emphasis to the promotion of health. It is a great way to cleanse our body channels, heal the damaged tissue and maintain the body's subtle energy and thus, create rejuvenation – physically and psychologically.

DOI: 10.1201/9781003043270-14

WHAT IS *YOGA*

The word "*Yoga*" comes from the *Sanskrit* root "*Yuj*" which means "to join" or "union", i.e. union of body, mind and soul for healthy living or the union of individual consciousness with the universal consciousness (Garg, 2014). It is originated from *Veda*, the oldest Indian scripture (5000 B.C.), and systematically compiled by sage *Patanjali* in the text "*Yogsutra*" around 150 B.C. It is a spiritual discipline involving the union, balance and harmony of our mind, body and soul. Gradual and continuous practice of *Yoga* promotes power, stamina and flexibility and facilitates characteristics of friendliness, sympathy, self-control and ultimately well-being. *Yoga* combines different yogic techniques for rejuvenation of body, mind, senses and spirit.

ASTANGA YOGA

The *Astanga Yoga* (the eight-fold practice of *Yoga*) is described in the *Yogsutra* of *Patanjali* (Singh, 2014, p. 300). They are *Yama, Niyama, Asana, Pranayama, Pratyahara, Dharana, Dhyana* and *Samadhi*. The first four are the external methods of purification whereas the three in the last are considered as internal methods of purification of the mind. *Pratyahara* acts as the bridge between both external and internal pathways.

Yama and Niyama

(Singh, 2014, p. 302)
   Yama (Restraints) – It is a group of five social disciplines

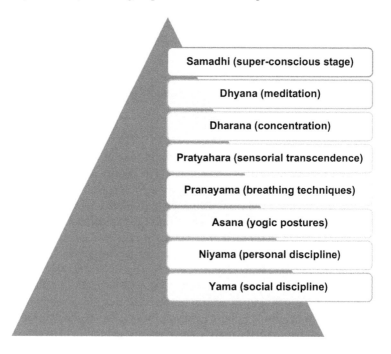

FIGURE 14.1   The Astanga yoga.

Principles and Practice of Yoga for Rejuvenation

1. *Ahimsa* (Non-violence, harmlessness)
2. *Satya* (Truthfulness, honesty)
3. *Asteya* (Non-Stealing, honesty)
4. *Brahmacharya* (control of continence)
5. *Aparigraha* (non-possessiveness, non-greed, non-selfishness)

Niyama (Observances) – It is a group of five personal disciplines

1. *Saucha* (Cleanliness of body, mind and spirit)
2. *Santosh* (Attitude of contentment)
3. *Tapa* (Self-discipline)
4. *Swadhyaya* (Inner exploration, self-study, spiritual study)
5. *Ishwara Pranidhana* (Devotion or surrender to the supreme creator)

ROLE OF *YAMA* AND *NIYAMA* IN REJUVENATION

These practices constitute a code of living that revitalizes thoughts, behavior, mental and emotional state towards us and society and promotes self-healing and awareness. It helps to attain harmony and a perfect equilibrium between body, mind and soul. Epigenetic research shows that cellular rejuvenation can be stimulated by our positive thoughts, behaviour, and emotional state which can be achieved by practising *Yama* and *Niyama*.

ASANA

(*Yogic* postures)

It is defined as "*Sthiram shukham asanam*" (Garg, 2014) meaning steady and comfortable body posture. While performing *Asana*, the body is kept in various postures in such a way that the activity of internal organs and glands becomes more efficient, resulting in the improvement of their functions. They have immense physical

Asana for Heathy Thyroid

(a)
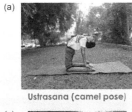
Ustrasana (camel pose)

(b)
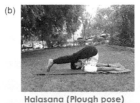
Halasana (Plough pose)

(c)
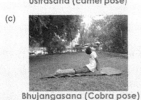
Bhujangasana (Cobra pose)

(d)
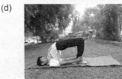
Setubandhasana (Bridge pose)

FIGURE 14.2 Asana for thyroid gland (a) Ustrasana (Camel Pose) (b) Halasana (Plough Pose) (c) Bhujangasana (Cobra pose) (d) Setubandhasana (Bridge Pose).

and mental benefits and are the simplest and easiest ways to rejuvenate the body at a cellular level.

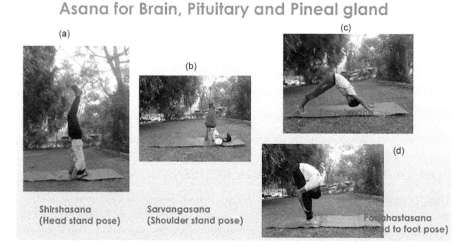

FIGURE 14.3 Asana for brain, pituitary and pineal gland (a) Shirshasana (Headstand pose) (b) Sarvangasana (Shoulder stand pose) (c) Parvatasana (Mountain pose) (d) Padahastasana (Hand-to-foot pose).

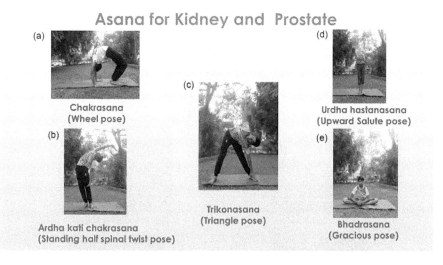

FIGURE 14.4 Asana for kidney and prostate (a) Chakrasana (wheel pose) (b) Ardha katichakrasana (standing half spinal twist pose) (c) Trikonasana (Triangle pose) (d) Urdha hasatasana (upward salute pose) (e) Bhadrasana (Gracious pose).

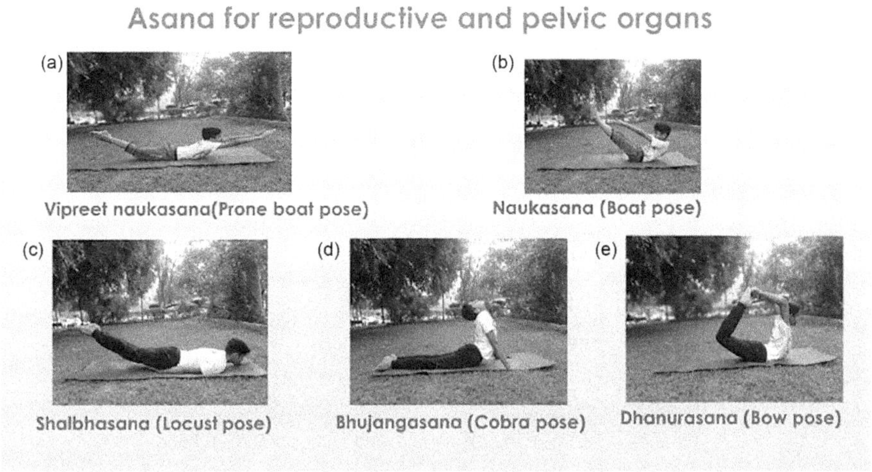

Principles and Practice of Yoga for Rejuvenation 175

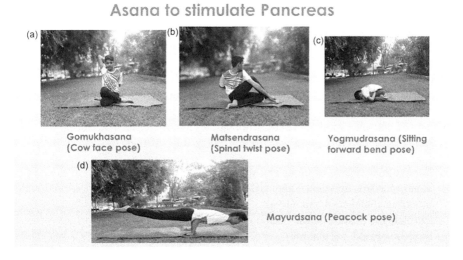

FIGURE 14.5 Asana for reproductive and pelvic organs (a) Vipreet naukasana (prone boat pose) (b) Naukasana (boat pose) (c) Shalbhasana (locust pose) (d) Bhujangasana (Cobra pose) (e) Dhanurasana (Bow pose).

FIGURE 14.6 Asana to stimulate pancreas (a) Gomukhasana (cow-face pose) (b) Ardha matsendrasana (half spinal twist pose) (c) Yogmudrasana (sitting forward bend pose) (d) Mayurasana(peacock pose).

HOW *ASANA* REJUVENATES

The primary motor cortex is involved in awareness of the posture, soon needs to focus on stressed areas, different joints and muscles while holding the *Asana*. It helps in increasing the blood flow and nervous system activity in that area. Good blood circulation is the key to staying energized and active as body cells get enough nutrients

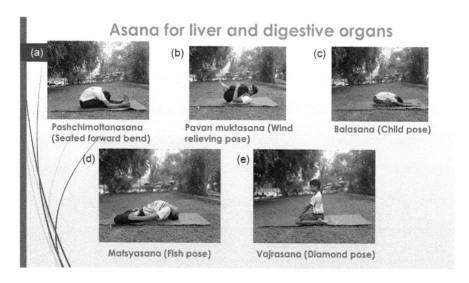

FIGURE 14.7 Asana for liver and digestive organs. (a) Pashchimottanasana (seated forward bend pose) (b) Pavan muktasana (wind relieving pose) (c) Balasana (child pose) (d) Matsyasana (fish pose) (e) Vajrasana (diamond pose).

and oxygen. It saves the tissues from getting stagnant. *Yoga* poses pressurize and stretch various endocrine glands, affecting the secretion of hormones and improving metabolism. Internal organs are also pressurized and squeezed, get more oxygenated blood and become more efficient and stronger. *Yoga* poses exert pressure on the heart, making it strong, draining impure blood from various parts of the body and thus affecting the entire circulatory system positively. Different static poses make breathing more efficient and increase lung capacity. Red muscle fibers become more active and consume more fats and carbohydrates and increase endurance.

Benefits of *Asana* (Cowen and Adams, 2005; Ray, 2010, p. 384)

Enhances flexibility of joints and spinal cord
Tones muscles, ligaments, and cartilages
Stretches spinal cord and nerves
Corrects the posture of the body
Improves blood circulation
Maintains the alignment of the body
Strengthens internal organs
Stimulates endocrine glands
Increases vitality
Strengthens the immune system
Promotes strength and stamina

PRANAYAMA (YOGIC BREATHING TECHNIQUE)

Pranayama is comprised of two words as "*Prana*" means "life force or vital energy (oxygen/ breath)" and "*Ayama*" means "expansion or regulation". Thus, it means expansion

Principles and Practice of Yoga for Rejuvenation

of life force or regulation of breath. It includes various rhythmic breathing techniques. Regular practising of *Pranayama* regulates the flow of energy into the 72,000 *Nadis* [channels through which consciousness flows] in the body, which helps to improve inner wellbeing. *Pranayama* extends life by rejuvenating the body. The main aspects of *Pranayama* are *Puraka* (deep inhalation), *Kumbhaka* (Retention of breath) and *Rechka* (exhalation). The ideal ratio of *Puraka: Kumbhaka: Rechaka* is 1:4:2 seconds (Sen, 2005).

PHYSIOLOGY OF *PURAKA-KUMBHAKA-RECHAKA*

During *Puraka,* the heart rate becomes slow, the diastole period gets prolonged, heart muscles get relaxed and the chamber of the heart is better filled with blood. Thus, more blood is pushed into circulation with a better force during the systole.

During *Kumbhaka,* no new air enters the lungs and the oxygen level in the blood gets reduced, which leads to cerebral anoxia. The brain is sensitive to lowered oxygen tension, and so it tries to get more blood and leads to cerebral vasodilation (more capillaries opening up). This increases blood circulation in different systems of the body.

During *Rechaka,* more carbon dioxide and other toxins are expelled out of the body. Thus, it helps to purify the blood. Slow and deep exhalation also maintains the elasticity of the lungs.

HOW *PRANAYAMA* REJUVENATES

Pranayama strengthens the lungs and increases their capacity. More fresh oxygenated air enters the lungs during deep inhalation and more carbon dioxide and other toxins are expelled out of the body during deep exhalation. It helps the heart to pump blood more efficiently; thus it improves and regulates the circulation of blood. *Prana* or vital energy (oxygen) reaches all parts of the body, so tissues get nourished. It enhances rejuvenation of the cells and stimulates the nervous system, endocrine glands and other vital organs for their optimal functioning by a supply of oxygenated blood.

PRATYAHARA (SENSORIAL TRANSCENDENCE)

Pratyahara, the fifth limb of *Astanga Yoga*, is the withdrawal or sensory transcendence. It is a very important but least practised limb of yoga. These are conscious efforts to draw our awareness away from the external world and outer stimuli. The practice of *Pratyahara* helps to control or withdraw senses from sensory objects (Sen, 2005).

HOW *PRATYAHARA* REJUVENATES

It brings supreme control over senses and helps to control desires. It reduces the effects of negative influence on life and helps to avoid environmental disturbances. It allows us to observe habits that are unfavourable for our health and are possibly responsible to interfere with inner growth. *Pratyahara* withdraws our mind from unhealthy food and other practices as well and creates awareness towards a healthy lifestyle.

DHARANA (CONCENTRATION), *DHYANA* (MEDITATION), AND *SAMADHI* (SUPER-CONSCIOUS STAGE/ENLIGHTENMENT)

These are advanced practices of meditation. *Dharana* is to focus attention at one point. *Dhyana* is the uninterrupted or constant flow of concentration. *Samadhi* is a superconscious stage of merging consciousness with the object of meditation.

Meditation means cessation of the thought process. It is described as a state of consciousness when the mind is unrestricted of scattered thoughts and different patterns. The observer (one who is doing meditation) appreciates that all the activity of the mind is reduced to one. Meditation is like watching your breath, listening to the birds. As long as these activities are free from any other distraction to the mind, it is effective meditation.

HOW MEDITATION HELPS IN REJUVENATION

It stimulates the parasympathetic nervous system and reduces the activation level of the brain. This relaxation response decreases metabolism, lowers blood pressure, heart rate, breathing rate and brain waves. It also reduces the catabolic process of cell deterioration which eventually relaxes the mind and brain and promotes self-healing.

CONCLUSION

Yoga affects every cell of the body. It brings better neuro-effector communication. It improves the strength and stamina of the body. It also increases the optimum functioning of all organ systems. It relaxes the mind and senses. It brings tranquility, balance and a positive attitude. It nourishes and rejuvenates all body tissues.

REFERENCES

Cowen, V. and Adams, T. (2005) 'Physical and perceptual benefits of Yoga Asana practice; Result of a pilot study', *Journal of Bodywork and Movement Therapies*, 9, pp. 211–19.

Garg, G. (2014) *Patanjali Yogsutra - Jagdish Sanskrit Pustkalaya*. Jagdish Sanskrit Pustakalaya, Jaipur. ISBN 9789383452385.

Ray, B. (2010) 'Swasthavritt Vigyan', in *Chowkhamba2*. Varanasi, India, p. 378.

Sen, G. (2005) *Pranayama: A Conscious Way of Breathing*. New Delhi: New Age Book.

Sharma, M., Anad, P. and Gupta, R. (2017) 'Rejuvenation and geriatric consideration in preventive, promotive, and social concept of health care', *International Journal of Ayurveda and Pharma Research*, 5(3), pp. 88–91.

Singh, R. (2014) *Swastahavritta*. Chowkhamba Surbharati, Varanasi, p. 300. https://parsspiritual. wordpress.com/2017/05/05/meditation-towards-a-stress-free-life/.

15 Rapid Ageing in Thailand and Implications for Thai Traditional Medicine

Anchalee Chuthaputti
Ministry of Public Health

Khwanchai Wisithanon
Ministry of Public Health

CONTENTS

The Ageing Society of Thailand 179
Thai Traditional Medicine.. 180
    The Role of Thai Traditional Medicine for the Health Care of the Elderly 182
        Traditional and Herbal Medicines 182
        Nuad Thai (Traditional Thai Massage) 183
        Hot Herbal Compress 184
        Herbal Poultice for Knee Osteoarthritis 185
        Health Promotion Activities 185
Conclusion 186
References 186

THE AGEING SOCIETY OF THAILAND

Thailand is one of the ten Member States of the Association of Southeast Asian Nations with 66.56 million inhabitants, of which 65,614,157 are Thais and 944,778 are non-Thais (Office of Central Registration, 2020). The life expectancy of Thais is 77.7 years for both sexes; 81.3 years for females and 74.2 years for males (Worldometers, no date). In 2005, Thailand entered the ageing society with 6.6 million people aged over 60, reaching 10% of the total population (Prasartkul, 2016). As Thailand has become a rapidly ageing country, such proportion rose to 16.54% in 2016, and for the first time in the country's history, the proportion of the elderly aged 60 and over surpassed the proportion of children aged under 15 in 2018. It is expected that Thailand will become an aged society (>20% of the population aged 60 and over) in 2021 (Prasartkul, 2016).

The Fifth National Health Examination Survey conducted in 2014 in 7,365 people who are 60 years of age or over showed that the top three health problems of the elderly were body movement problem (57.8%), hearing and communication (23.8%)

DOI: 10.1201/9781003043270-15

and eyesight (19.2%), and these problems worsened as they got older (Aekplakorn, 2016). The prevalence of chronic diseases of the elderly found in this survey were hypertension (53.2%), metabolic syndrome (46.8%), knee osteoarthritis (KOA) (22.5%), cataract (22.3%), hypercholesterolaemia (19%), diabetes (18.1%), dementia (18.1%), gout (5.6%), ischaemic heart disease (4.8%), asthma (4.6%), depression (2.9%), stroke (2.7%) and emphysema/chronic obstructive pulmonary disease (1.6%) (Aekplakorn, 2016). Regarding major causes of death of Thai people, the mortality rates per 100,000 population in 2016 were 117.7 from all types of cancer, 48.7 from stroke, 32.3 from ischaemic heart disease and 22.3 from diabetes (Pokpermdee, 2017). As most elder people have more than one disease or symptom, 'polypharmacy' or administration of multiple drugs at the same time is common among Thai elderly as well, leading to decreased drug compliance, increased medication expense and chances of adverse drug reactions and drug interaction (Ruangritchankul, 2018).

THAI TRADITIONAL MEDICINE

Thai traditional medicine (TTM), a part of the health service system of Thailand, is a holistic healthcare and natural medicine that plays a role in the health care and way of life of Thai people of all ages. The main philosophy of TTM is related to Buddhism and aims for people to stay in balance and in harmony with nature. The balance of the four basic dhatus of the body – namely earth, wind, water and fire – is the key for each individual to achieve and maintain a healthy status. If the irregularity or imbalance of the four dhatus occurs, i.e. deficit, excess, or impaired, a person will become ill (Subcharoen, 2001).

In addition to dhatu imbalance, in TTM, the following factors can also influence our health and cause sickness, i.e. (Subcharoen, 2001)

- Seasonal weather: Temperature and dampness during different seasons obviously affect human health.
- Age: Based on the principle of TTM, during different periods of life, people are more prone to become ill from the influence of different dhatu, e.g. wind is the main cause of illnesses in the elderly, while the health of the young is mostly affected by water.
- Geographic location where one lives: As the geographic location influences the weather and the environment, it can affect one's health.
- Time: As the attraction force between the sun, the moon and the earth changes during different periods of time in a day, it influences body dhatu and health.
- Inappropriate behaviours and temper that can be the causes of ailments according to TTM are as follows:
  - Inappropriate eating habits, e.g. eating too much or too little, eating unfamiliar food, food that has gone bad or food unsuitable for one's underlying disease.
  - Imbalanced postures while sitting, standing, walking or sleeping can cause disequilibrium of the body structure and needless worsening of health.
  - Exposure to extreme weather or polluted air.

Rapid Ageing and Its Implications in Thailand 181

- Being deprived of food, water or sleep.
- Delayed urination or defaecation.
- Overwork, over-exercise or excessive sexual activity.
- Deep sorrow or extreme exhilaration.
- Extreme anger, lack of equanimity

The treatment of diseases or symptoms by TTM aims to correct dhatu imbalance using different forms of TTM practice to complement each other, i.e. TTM herbal formulas, traditional pharmacy, Nuad Thai or traditional Thai massage, hot herbal compress and herbal steam baths. Various treatment modalities in traditional midwifery are used for the health care of pregnant women, post-partum care and child care, and the practice of meditation is also promoted for mental health and support (Institute of Thai Traditional Medicine, 2014).

A TTM health-promotion approach is also used to achieve good health by correcting the unhealthy behaviours mentioned above and practising 'Dhammanamai' in a TTM way (Subcharoen, 2001) which is comprised of:

- *Kayanamai* (healthy body) which can be achieved by, i.e.
  - Eat healthy food, especially indigenous nutritious fruits and vegetables that are compatible with one's own-based dhatu or underlying disease, and take traditional medicines or food that can correct the imbalance of body dhatu to maintain good health
  - Exercise, e.g. practise *'Ruesi Dadton'*, which is different postures of Thai traditional stretch exercise (similar to the yoga of India). Health benefits of all 127 postures of Ruesi Dadton were poetically described in the classical record on Ruesi Dadton. The Institute of Thai Traditional Medicine selected 15 postures suitable for all ages to be promoted for health promotion as it helps increase body agility, muscle coordination, and joint mobility, stimulate blood circulation and promote good concentration (Subcharoen, 2001; Institute of Thai Traditional Medicine, 2014). Training of patients and the elderly to be able to practise Ruesi Dadton is one of the activities of TTM clinics in public health service facilities.
- *Chittanamai* (healthy mind), e.g.
  - Practise *Buddhist meditation* to develop mental strength, concentration and mindfulness, or
  - Practise *SKT meditation* developed by Assoc. Prof. Somporn K. Triamchaisri, Faculty of Public Health, Mahidol University, who created seven techniques of new meditation therapy. The principles and practices of SKT were formulated by combining the knowledge of meditation, yoga, qigong, stretch exercise, breathing technique of meditation, and the control of the senses, especially sight and hearing. Different SKT techniques are useful for different purposes, i.e. techniques 1 & 2 are for health promotion, disease prevention and symptomatic relief, techniques 3, 4 & 5 are meant for patients to reverse existing disorders back to normal states and techniques 6 & 7 are for palliative care and rehabilitative purpose for patients in more serious

conditions or terminally ill patients to improve their health and quality of life (Triamchaisri, 2013; Institute of Thai Traditional Medicine, 2016b; Kaweekorn et al., 2016).

- *Jivitanamai* (healthy lifestyle and behaviours), e.g. live one's life in the 'Middle Path' of Buddhism, observe the five precepts or five rules of morality and follow dhamma or the teaching of Lord Buddha, live in a clean and healthy environment and have healthy behaviours (Subcharoen, 2001).

THE ROLE OF THAI TRADITIONAL MEDICINE FOR THE HEALTH CARE OF THE ELDERLY

TTM services in the healthcare system are covered by the three health security systems of Thailand, namely Universal Health Coverage Scheme (UHC), Social Security Scheme and Civil Servant Medical Benefit Scheme (CSMBS). In the fiscal year 2020, 21.35% of outpatient department (OPD) visits in the hospitals under the Office of the Permanent Secretary, the Ministry of Public Health (MoPH) in all provinces, except Bangkok, received TTM and alternative medicine services (Ministry of Public Health, 2020). TTM service has played an important role in the care of Thai people of all ages and it is well-liked by most patients, esp. the elderly, partly because most TTM treatment modalities are manual therapies providing personal care and touch for each patient by TTM doctors or TTM assistants for a considerable amount of time per session. Department of Thai Traditional and Alternative Medicine (DTAM) has developed clinical practice guidelines for the treatment, rehabilitation and health promotion of various diseases and symptoms (Institute of Thai Traditional Medicine, 2016b, 2016a; Tanasilangkoon and Sitthitanyakij, 2016; Tanasilangkoon, 2018), including those commonly found in the elderly, e.g. KOA (Subcharoen, 2001; Tanasilangkoon and Sitthitanyakij, 2016), paralysis & paraplegia (Subcharoen, 2001) and wind-associated symptoms (Tanaskilankoon and Sitthitanyakij, 2019). The followings are TTM services commonly given to elder patients.

Traditional and Herbal Medicines

Currently, there are 94 items of traditional and herbal medicines (61 traditional medicine formulas and 33 single herbal medicines) available in the National List of Essential Herbal Medicines (NLEHM) for common and minor illnesses or symptoms. The selection of traditional medicines and herbal medicines into NLEHM is based on the history of safe and effective use, e.g. those in the MoPH List of Traditional Household Remedies, those in Traditional Hospital Formularies of some hospitals with more than 10 years of continuous production and use in not less than 1,000 cases and those with clinical research evidence to support efficacy and safety (Committee on the Development of the National Medicine System, 2021a, 2021b, 2021c).

Symptoms and some traditional and herbal medicines commonly prescribed for the elderly are as follows:

- *Symptoms associated with wind dhatu* commonly found in the elderly (e.g. dizziness, fainting and nausea): the group of traditional medicine preparations called 'yahom', e.g. Yahom Dhebhachit, Yahom Nawakot (Tanaskilankoon and Sitthitanyakij, 2019)

- Gastrointestinal disorders
  - Indigestion, flatulence: turmeric capsule, ginger capsule, cinnamon stomachic (Tanasilangkoon, 2018)
  - Diarrhea: Ya Lueng Pidsamut, *Andrographis paniculata* capsule (Government of Thailand, 2019)
  - Constipation: *Senna alata* infusion, *Senna alexandrina* tablet (Tanasilangkoon and Sitthitanyakij, 2016)
  - Haemorrhoid: *Cissus quadrangularis* traditional medicine preparations (Tanasilangkoon, 2018)
- Fever: Chantaleela capsule (Government of Thailand, 2019)
- Respiratory symptoms and diseases
  - Cough: Emblic myrobalan (*Phyllanthus emblica*)-containing traditional medicine antitussives, Triphala (equal proportion of fruits of *Terminalia chebula, Terminalia bellirica, Phyllanthus emblica*) capsule, pill or infusion (Tanasilangkoon, 2018)
  - Common cold: *Andrographis paniculata* capsule, Ya Prab Chompu Taweep (Tanasilangkoon, 2018)
  - Musculoskeletal symptoms
  - Muscle ache: Plai (*Zingiber montanum*) cream, Plai oil, Sahassatara capsule, Ya Toranee Santakat, *Derris scandens* capsule and *Derris scandens*-containing traditional medicine preparations (Tanasilangkoon, 2018)
  - KOA: hot herbal compress, Plai cream or oil, herbal knee poultice preparations, *Derris scandens* capsule (Subcharoen, 2001; Tanasilangkoon and Sitthitanyakij, 2016)

Nuad Thai (Traditional Thai Massage)

Nuad Thai is the most important part of manual therapy of TTM that was inscribed in the UNESCO's Representative List of the Intangible Cultural Heritage of Humanity in December 2019 (United Nations, 2019). Nuad Thai has long been a common self-care practice among family members and within communities in all regions of Thailand. The practice of Nuad Thai is based on 'Sen Prathan Sib' or '10 principal body lines' and sen pressure points associated with Sen Prathan Sib (Tantipidok and Jaidee, 2016). The obstruction of the flow of the wind along the sen lines is believed to be the cause of musculoskeletal pain and massage on the sen pressure points associated with the sen lines will relieve the pain by normalising the wind flow along the sen lines. The knowledge of Nuad Thai was systematised and inscribed on marble tablets placed in 'Wat Pho' Buddhist temple in Bangkok during the reign of King Rama III (1824–1851) and codified in the classical TTM textbook entitled 'Tamra Vejasaj Chaba Luang King Rama V' (literally means 'Medical Textbook Royal Edition King Rama V') in 1871 (Tantipidok and Jaidee, 2016).

Nuad Thai plays a major role as a manual therapy in the TTM service. In the fiscal year 2019, there were over 9.8 million OPD visits in public hospitals under MoPH receiving Nuad Thai treatment (Ministry of Public Health, 2019). Nuad Thai can effectively cure or relieve several symptoms, e.g. muscle pain of different organs (Thepsongwatt et al., 2006; Iampornchai et al., 2009; Netchanok

184 Healthy Ageing in Asia

et al., 2012), myofascial pain syndrome (Kumnerddee, 2009), KOA (Peungsuwan et al., 2014), scapulocostal pain syndrome (Buttagat et al., 2012), frozen shoulder (Tankitjanon, 2019), tension headache (Kruapanich et al., 2012; Sooktho et al., 2012) and migraine (Sooktho et al., 2012). In addition, Nuad Thai is usually given together with physiotherapy (PT) for the rehabilitative purposes to help prevent disability in post-stroke patients with satisfactory results (Thanakiatpinyo et al., 2014; Chartsuwan, 2016). Moreover, the provision of Nuad Thai service is also delivered to post-stroke and bedridden patients at home through regular home visits by TTM practitioners from the nearest hospitals or health centres where patients live. In the fiscal year 2019, there were 305,763 visits of Nuad Thai services for patients provided outside health service facilities (Ministry of Public Health, 2019). Family members or caregivers of stroke and bedridden patients are also taught basic Nuad Thai techniques and rehabilitative methods using basic home-made PT equipment, e.g. shoulder pulley, so that patients can properly have a daily exercise for better treatment outcomes.

At the community level, different types of folk massage in different regions of the country, e.g. Nuad Tok Sen or wooden hammer massage of the north, also play a role in the health care of community people including the elderly, and currently there are 719 DTAM-certified folk massage healers nationwide. They usually earn their respect from community people for their community service and effective treatment at a very low treatment fee. Folk massage is well-accepted as it is congruent to the way of life and the local culture of people and easily accessible as it is usually provided at the homes of folk massage healers.

The teaching and learning of Nuad Thai can be classified into different levels depending on the learning methods and hours and curricula, i.e. professional level (for therapeutic and rehabilitative purposes) (not less than 800 hours.) (Professional Commission of Thai Traditional Medicine, 2007), TTM assistant level (330–<800 hours.) (Institute of Thai Traditional Medicine, 2010b) and Nuad Thai for health promotion level (150– <330 hours.) (Institute of Thai Traditional Medicine, 2010a). Professional Nuad Thai practice is a part of TTM services available at all levels of public health service facilities. TTM practitioners, TTM practitioners in Nuad Thai and TTM assistants are available for providing Nuad Thai for therapeutic and rehabilitative purposes in all provincial and general hospitals and community hospitals and in about 17% of primary public health service facilities. Meanwhile, Nuad Thai for health promotion is offered at private Nuad Thai and spa establishments throughout the country and has generated a large income for the country via health tourism and wellness business. Nowadays, Nuad Thai is recognised as one of the most popular massage therapies among non-Thais as well and Nuad Thai services have spread to major cities around the world.

Hot Herbal Compress

The application of 'Luk Prakob' or hot herbal compress is one of the TTM treatment modalities that is given alone, or usually after Nuad Thai, for the relief of pain, myofascial pain syndrome or KOA as well as for post-partum care (Chiranthanut, Hanprasertpong and Teekachunhatean, 2014; Srithupthai, 2014; Dhippayom et al.,

2015; Wongwan, Chitirabaib and Kamontum, 2018; Boonruab et al., 2019). In 2019, hot herbal compression was given to more than 8.3 OPD visits in public health service facilities under MoPH (Ministry of Public Health, 2019).

The most commonly used Luk Prakob formula contains several herbs in the family Zingiberaceae with well-established anti-inflammatory activity, i.e. Plai (*Zingiber montanum,* synonym *Z. cassumunar*) (Pongprayoon et al., 1997), turmeric (*Curcuma longa*) (Jacob et al., 2007) and Khamin Oi (*Curcuma* sp. "Khamin Oi"). Luk Prakob is steamed prior to the application on the affected areas of the body. The heat helps increase the regional blood flow and release volatile oil and active ingredients from turmeric & Plai to exert the anti-inflammatory action. Researches show that Luk Prakob is effective for the treatment of KOA and myofascial pain syndrome.

Growing herbs used in Luk Prakob and the preparation of Luk Prakob for hospital use and even for export to spa business abroad is currently one of the community activities that generate jobs and extra income for people including the elderly in several communities all over the country.

Herbal Poultice for Knee Osteoarthritis

KOA is a joint disease commonly found in the elderly affecting about one-third of people over 60. It causes pain, stiffness, loss of function, disability and deformity and reduces the quality of life. KOA is one in ten diseases that cause disability in the Thai elderly (Kuptniratsaikul et al., 2002; Nimit-arnun, 2014).

The treatment of knee OA by TTM is composed of Nuad Thai, hot herbal compress, oral and topical traditional medicine preparations and single herbal medicines mentioned above and exercise (Subcharoen, 2001; Tanasilangkoon and Sitthitanyakij, 2016). During the past 10 years, herbal poultice has gained wider acceptance by TTM doctors as another treatment modality for knee OA. One of the formulas was developed by a folk healer and it has been tested and used in Khun Han Community Hospital in Sisaket province (Wanthong, 2016). Later on, TTM doctors in other hospitals have also developed hospitals' formulas of knee herbal poultice comprising of a mixture of local herbs with anti-inflammatory activity with different methods to keep the poultice preparation over the knee while patients can move during the application of the poultice and researches have been conducted to prove the efficacy of their preparations (Department of Thai Traditional and Alternative Medicine, 2018; Poonsuk et al., 2018). DTAM is now in the process of submitting the necessary information to the National Health Security Office to request for the inclusion of knee herbal poultice in the TTM service coverage of UHC.

Health Promotion Activities

As previously mentioned, in addition to providing TTM service for the treatment and rehabilitative purposes, community people including the elderly are also trained by TTM doctors on how to use Thai traditional and complementary medicine approach for health promotion, e.g. follow the principle of Dhammanamai, taking foods that suit one's based dhatu and help balance dhatu or suit one's underlying disease, practise Buddhist meditation or SKT meditation to strengthen concentration and develop mindfulness and exercise by practicing Ruesi Dadton.

CONCLUSION

As Thailand has become an aged society since 2021, the public health service system should therefore use an integrative approach to take care of the health of the elderly so that they stay healthy as long as possible and reap the benefit of having TTM as a part of health service system to maximise the use of TTM for health promotion, treatment of diseases and symptoms and rehabilitation of elder patients. TTM doctors should use the strength of TTM to fill the gap of the service system and conduct more clinical researches on the efficacy and safety of new herbal medicines and their treatment modalities to gain enough clinical evidence to support the selection into NLEHM and to be covered by the National Health Security Systems of the country. This will not only benefit the health of Thai people but also help reduce the national health expenditure in the future.

REFERENCES

Aekplakorn, W. (2016) *The Fifth National Health Examination Survey of Thai Population.* Nonthaburi: Health System Research Institute, pp. 219–76.

Boonruab, J. et al. (2019) 'Effectiveness of hot herbal compress versus topical diclofenac in treating patients with myofascial pain syndrome', *Journal of Traditional and Complementary Medicine*, 9(2), pp. 163–7.

Buttagat, V. et al. (2012) 'Therapeutic effects of traditional Thai Massage on pain, muscle tension and anxiety in patients with scapulocostal syndrome: A randomized single-blinded pilot study', *Journal of Body Movement Therapy*, 16(1), pp. 57–63.

Chartsuwan, J. (2016) *Comparative Study on Efficacy of Physiotherapy and Physiotherapy Combined with Thai Massage on Rehabilitation Outcome and Quality of Life of Ischemic Stroke Patients.* Bangkok: Thammasat University.

Chiranthanut, N., Hanprasertpong, N. and Teekachunhatean, S. (2014) 'Thai massage, and Thai herbal compress versus oral ibuprofen in symptomatic treatment of osteoarthritis of the knee: A randomized controlled trial', *BioMed Research International*, 2014, pp. 1–13, Article ID 490512.

Committee on the Development of National Medicine System. (2021a) *National List of Essential Herbal Medicines B.E.2564*. Government Gazette. Vol. 139 Special Section 41 Ngor. 18 Feb 2022. p. 47 and 12 pages of attachment list.

Committee on the Development of National Medicine System. (2021b) *National List of Essential Herbal Medicines B.E. 2564*. Government Gazette. Vol 138. Special Section 103 Ngor. 14 May 2021. p. 60 and 3 pages of attachment list.

Committee on the Development of National Medicine System. (2021c) *National List of Essential Herbal Medicines B.E. 2564*. Government Gazette. Vol 138. Special Section 120 Ngor. 4 Jun 2021. pp. 46–7 and 2 pages of attachment list.

Department of Thai Traditional and Alternative Medicine. (2018) 'Journal of Thai Traditional Medicine, Alternative Medicine and Folk Medicine', in *13th Annual National Conference in Thai Traditional Medicine, Indigenous Medicine and Alternative Medicine.*

Dhippayom, T. et al. (2015) 'Clinical effects of Thai herbal compress: A systematic review and meta-analysis', *Evidence-Based Complementary and Alternative Medicine*, pp. 1–14, Article ID 942378.

Iampornchai, S. et al. (2009) 'Court-type traditional Thai massage and hot herbal compress: Effectiveness in relieving early postpartum backache', *Journal of Thai Traditional Alternative Medicine*, 1(2–3), pp. 181–8.

Institute of Thai Traditional Medicine. (2010a) *Training Manual of Nuad Thai for Health 150 Hours*. Bangkok: War Veterans Organization Printing Mill.

Institute of Thai Traditional Medicine. (2010b) *Training Manual of Thai Traditional Medicine Assistant 372 Hours*. Bangkok: War Veterans Organization Printing Mill.

Institute of Thai Traditional Medicine. (2014) *Thai Traditional Exercise: 15 Postures of Basic Ruesi Dadton*, YouTube. Available from: https://www.youtube.com/watch?v=fddNO4nsokE

Institute of Thai Traditional Medicine. (2016a) *Clinical Practice Guidelines for Patient Care Using Thai Traditional Medicine for Pilot Thai Traditional Medicine Hospitals*. Bangkok: Samcharoen Panich.

Institute of Thai Traditional Medicine. (2016b) *Clinical Practice Guidelines of Thai Traditional and Alternative Medicine in Complete Traditional and Alternative Medicine Service Clinics*. Bangkok: Sam Charoen Panich.

Jacob, A. et al. (2007) 'Mechanism of the anti-inflammatory effect of curcumin: PPAR-gamma activation', *PPAR Research*, pp. 1–5, Article ID 89369.

Kaweekorn, P. et al. (2016) 'SKT meditation therapy model by SKT trainers for controlling blood pressure in hypertensive patients, Yasothon province', *Journal of Preventive Medicine Association of Thailand*, 6(3), pp. 231–9.

Kruapanich, C. et al. (2012) 'The immediate effects of traditional Thai massage for reducing pain on patients related with episodic tension-type headache', *Journal of Medical Technology Physical Therapy*, 24(2), pp. 220–34.

Kumnerddee, W. (2009) 'Effectiveness comparison between Thai traditional massage and Chinese acupuncture for myofascial back pain in Thai military personnel: A preliminary report', *Journal of Medical Association Thailand*, Suppl 1, pp. 117–23.

Kuptniratsaikul, V. et al. (2002) 'The epidemiology of osteoarthritis of the knee in elderly patients living an urban area of Bangkok', *Journal of Medical Association Thailand*, 85(2), pp. 154–61.

Ministry of Public Health. (2019) OPD Services Nuad Thai, herbal steam bath, hot herbal compress in Fiscal Year B.E. 2562, HDC Report. Available at: https://hdcservice.moph.go.th/hdc/reports/report.php?source=pformated/format1.php&cat_id=30bc6364fc06a33a7802e16bc596ac3b&id=9615f70d993b1b673fbe65ae958a59fc (Accessed: 31 March 2020).

Ministry of Public Health. (2020) *Percentage of OPD Visits Receiving Thai Traditional and Alternative Medicine Services Including Traditional Chinese Medicine but Excluding Health Promotion Services*. Available from: https://hdcservice.moph.go.th/hdc/reports/report.php?source=pformated/format1.php&cat_id=30bc6364fc06a33a7802e16bc596ac3b&id=50980b81323b2978d9ed4c4b353c58bc (Accessed 29 January 2022)

Netchanok, S. et al. (2012) 'The effectiveness of Swedish massage and traditional Thai massage in treating chronic low back pain: A review of the literature', *Complementary Therapy Clinical Practice*, 18(4), pp. 227–34.

Nimit-arnun, N. (2014) 'The epidemiological situation and risk assessment of knee osteoarthritis among Thai people', *Journal of the Royal Thai Army Nurses*, 15(3), pp. 185–94.

Office of Central Registration. (2020) 'Number of Inhabitants in the Kingdom based on civil registration evidence', *Government Gazette*, 137(24D), pp. 17–9.

Peungsuwan, P. et al. (2014) 'The effectiveness of Thai exercise with traditional massage on the pain, walking ability and QOL of older people with Kneww osteoarthritis: A randomized controlled trial in the community', *Journal of Physical Therapy Science*, 26(1), pp. 139–44.

Pokpermdee, P. (2017) *Health at a Glance - Thailand 2017*. Nonthabury: Division of Strategy and Planning, Office of the Permanent Secretary, Ministry of Public Health, pp. 15–9.

Pongprayoon, U. et al. (1997) 'Topical antiinflammatory activity of the major lipophilic constituents of the rhizome of Zingiber cassumunar', *Phytomedicine*, 3(4), pp. 319–22.

Poonsuk, P. et al. (2018) 'Effectiveness of herbal poultice for knee pain relief in patients with osteoarthritis of knee', *Thammasart Medical Journal*, 18(1), pp. 104–10.

Prasartkul, P. (2016) *Situation of the Thai Elderly 2014*. Edited by P. Prasartkul. Bangkok: Foundation of Thai Gerontology Research and Development Institute.

Professional Commission of Thai Traditional Medicine. (2007) *Professional Curriculum of Thai Traditional Medicine in the Branch of Nuad Thai*. Available from: https://thaimed.or.th/home/wp-content/uploads/2017/05/%E0%B8%AB%E0%B8%A5%E0%B8%B1%E0%B8%81%E0%B8%AA%E0%B8%B9%E0%B8%95%E0%B8%A3%E0%B8%81%E0%B8%B2%E0%B8%A3%E0%B8%99%E0%B8%A7%E0%B8%94%E0-%B9%84%E0%B8%97%E0%B8%A2.pdf

Ruangritchankul, S. (2018) 'Polypharmacy in the elderly', *Ramathibodi Medical Journal*, 41(1), pp. 95–104.

Sooktho, S. et al. (2012) 'Immediate effects of traditional Thai massage for reducing pain in patients with chronic-tension type headache and migraine', *Journal Medical Technology Physical Therapy*, 24(2), pp. 220–34.

Srithupthai, K. (2014) 'Herbal formulas developed to reduce maternal postpartum breast engorgement. *SNRU Journal of Science and Technology*, 7(2), pp. 33–9.

Subcharoen, P. (2001) *Thai Traditional Medicine: Holistic Medicine*. 2nd edn. Bangkok: E.T.O. Printing.

Tanasilangkoon, B. (2018) *Clinical Practice Guidelines in Thai Traditional Medicine to Promote the Use of Herbal Medicines in the Health Service System Vol 1*. Edited by B. Tanaskilankoon. Nonthaburi: Institute of Thai Traditional Medicine.

Tanasilangkoon, B. and Sitthitanyakij, K. (2016) *Ways to examine, diagnose and treat knee osteoarthritis with Thai traditional medicine*. Edited by B. Tanasilangkoon and K. Sitthitanyakij. Nonthaburi: Institute of Thai Traditional Medicine. pp. 1–85.

Tanaskilankoon, B. and Sitthitanyakij, K. (2019) *Clinical Practice Guidelines in Thai Traditional Medicine to Promote the Use of Herbal Medicines in the Health Services System* Vol. 2. Edited by B. Tanasillangkoon and K. Sitthitanyakij. Nonthaburi: Institute of Thai Traditional Medicine. pp. 1–93.

Tankitjanon, P. et al. (2019) 'Court-Type Traditional Thai Massage Efficacy on Quality of Life among Patients with Frozen Shoulder: A Randomised Controlled Trial', *Journal of Medical Association Thailand*, 102 (8), p. 19.

Tantipidok, Y. and Jaidee, S. (2016) *Textbook of Thai Massage* Vol 1. 5th edn. Bangkok: Health and Development Foundation.

Thanakiatpinyo, T. et al. (2014) 'The efficacy of traditional Thai massage in decreasing spasticity in elderly stroke patients', *Clinical Intervention Aging*, 9, pp. 1311–9.

Thepsongwatt, J. et al. (2006) 'Effectiveness of the royal Thai traditional massage for relief of muscle pain', *Siriraj Medical Journal*, 58, pp. 702–4.

Triamchaisri, S. (2013) Change meditation therapy SKT - new alternative to be healthy, Mahidol channel. Available at: https://www.youtube.com/watch?v=lPAPUhVqMHQ (Accessed: 31 March 2020).

United Nations. (2019) Nuad Thai traditional Thai massage, United Nations educational, scientific, and cultural organization. Available at: https://ich.unesco.org/en/RL/nuad-thai-traditional-thai-massage-01384 (Accessed: 31 March 2020).

Wanthong, P. (2016) 'Efficacy of knee poultice (Thai Traditional Medicine Center Formula) for the relief of knee pain in the elderly with knee osteoarthritis, Khun Han Hospital, Khun Han District, Srisaket Province', in *13th Annual National Conference in Thai Traditional Medicine, Indigenous Medicine and Alternative Medicine*.

Wongwan, S., Chitirabaib, S. and Kamontum, T. (2018) 'Effect of massage with moist herbal ball hot compression in postpartum primiparous women', *Journal of Nursing Health Science*, 12(4), pp. 61–72.

Worldometers (no date) Thailand demographics. Available at: https://www.worldometers.info/demographics/thailand-demographics/ (Accessed: 31 March 2020).

16 Health Benefits of Exercise for Older People
The Research Evidence and Approaches to Maximize Participation

Keith Hill
Monash University

CONTENTS

Introduction 189
Evidence, Gaps and Future Research 190
Conclusion 193
References 194

INTRODUCTION

While ageing populations are a demographic reality worldwide, there is a substantial difference in the trajectory of ageing and the point in that trajectory that various countries are at. Countries are considered to have a young aged population when 7% of their population is aged over 65 years and to have an aged population when 14% or more of their population is aged over 65 years. Some countries like France and the United States have taken a long period (115 and 69 years respectively) to transition from seven to 14% of their population to be aged over 65 years. This reasonably long period for this demographic change to occur allows time for health, social and care policies and services to adjust to the population demographic change (although this still requires significant focus and change, which countries have responded to with varying approaches and success). However, for many 'young' ageing countries, although their current population demonstrates a profile with only a small percentage of their population aged over 65, projections indicate many of these countries are on a rapidly ageing trajectory and will transition from 7% to 14% of their population aged over 65 years within a 15–20-year period (e.g. Vietnam, Malaysia, Indonesia and Brazil) (The World Bank, 2015). These countries need to be planning and resourcing

DOI: 10.1201/9781003043270-16

changes to their health, social and care systems to be able to accommodate this rapid demographic change.

A number of countries have transitioned through and in some cases well beyond the point of 14% of their population being aged over 65 years. Japan is the world's oldest country, with 26.6% of its population aged over 65 (He, Goodkind and Kowal, 2016). In the Asia–Oceania region, Australia has progressed to have 15% of its population aged over 65 years (Australian Institute of Health and Welfare, 2018). Some of the strategies adopted by these 'older' aged countries in their transition may help inform changes as the 'young' ageing populations adjust to their rapidly ageing populations.

Ageing populations have the potential for rapid increases in the incidence of health problems associated with ageing, such as falls, dementia, osteoporosis and osteoarthritis. An essential change of focus that is required with population ageing is to resource and support prevention approaches, which mean that the future ageing population will age more well than the current older population. Health promotion and prevention programs also have the potential to support older people with multiple comorbidities to age well within the context of their existing health problems. So, health promotion and prevention approaches are essential across the full spectrum of the health of older populations.

Exercise is one health promotion and prevention approach that has the excellent potential to support ageing populations to age well. While the focus of this paper is on exercise for older populations, exercise should be considered in a lifespan context, with a focus on exercise through childhood, adolescence, adulthood as well as older age being required to optimise the potential benefits for ageing populations (Viña et al., 2016).

EVIDENCE, GAPS AND FUTURE RESEARCH

There are many health benefits of exercise for older people, including reduced risk of coronary and cardiac disease, diabetes, obesity, some cancers such as colorectal cancer and reduced risk of falls (Sims et al., 2006). In addition to reducing the risk of many health conditions and chronic disease, there is strong research evidence that exercise can result in improved physical performance (balance, strength, mobility and function), improved mental health (improved mood and reduced depression) and improved quality of life (Sims et al., 2006). Although there are some generic benefits of exercise irrespective of the type of exercise undertaken (for example most exercise approaches can result in improved mood or psychological well-being), different exercise types may also have different effects (termed specificity of training). An important example of this is the type of exercise that will be likely to reduce falls risk. An essential element of exercise to reduce the risk of falls is that it needs to have moderate-to-high challenge to balance (Sherrington et al., 2017). Walking programs and resistance training programs in isolation, that do not have a challenge to balance included, are not likely to reduce falls risk (Voukelatos et al., 2015; Sherrington et al., 2017), although these types of programs do have important other health benefits (Liu and Latham, 2011). Physical activity guidelines for older people recommend multi-modal programs, that incorporate balance, strength training, cardiovascular fitness

Health Benefits of Exercise for Older People

training and flexibility exercises, (Sims et al., 2010) either within a single session (e.g. a group exercise program that targets each of these exercise types) or by mixing the type of sessions during the week to meet the 150-minute recommendation for moderate-to-vigorous exercise levels (for example, separate strength, cardiovascular and balance training sessions).

The older population is diverse in terms of their health, function and well-being; however, exercise can be appropriate and effective in achieving positive physical and mental health outcomes, even for very old people, and those with high levels of frailty, sarcopenia or dysmobility syndrome, (Theou et al., 2011; Hill et al., 2017; Beckwée et al., 2019) and including those with cognitive impairment (Suttanon et al., 2013; Burton et al., 2015). However, with increasing frailty and comorbidities, there is an increased need for health professional guidance to ensure that appropriate and safe exercise is undertaken. Physiotherapists and exercise physiologists are health professionals with extensive training in providing safe and appropriate exercise programs for older people, even those with advanced health problems.

The World Health Organisation has defined a health fitness gradient, which includes three broad subgroups to consider in exercise prescription (WHO, 1997). These include (i) the physically fit and healthy; (ii) the physically unfit and unhealthy but independent (including a moderate proportion of the population who do insufficient levels, intensity or types of exercise to maintain health but have not yet developed significant health problems); and (iii) the physically unfit, frail, unhealthy and dependent (which generally includes the component of the population often seeing multiple health practitioners to address their comorbidities). Each of these population subgroups can benefit from exercise.

There are many different forms of exercise, and even within a single type of exercise, there can be important differences that mean that care may need to be used in prescribing a particular form of exercise for older people with differing levels of health and comorbidities. For example, tai chi is an excellent form of exercise for older people, that has been shown to result in improved strength, balance, function, balance confidence, and improvement in some cardiovascular measures (Sun and Buys, 2013; Huang and Liu, 2015; Huang et al., 2017), even in the presence of health problems such as lower limb osteoarthritis. However, some forms of tai chi are more challenging (e.g. from a balance or fitness perspective) and therefore are most suitable for more well older people (e.g. Yang style), while other forms of tai chi such as the Sun style, including Tai Chi for Arthritis (Song, 2007; Huang et al., 2017) are more suitable and safe for people with comorbidities such as lower limb arthritis or reduced balance. Similarly, the widely researched and practiced Otago exercise program (Robertson et al., 2002) appears to be most effective for older people with moderate levels of balance or functional impairments, but to perhaps not be challenging enough for older people with only mild balance dysfunction, minor falls or near falls. In the latter case, an 'Otago Plus' program that incorporated elements of the Otago program, but also some higher levels of balance challenging exercises, has been shown to improve balance, strength and function in those with mild balance dysfunction (Yang et al., 2012). Almost a quarter of this sample (who all were classified as 'outside of normal balance performance' at the commencement of the study) returned to being within the normal balance performance range after this 6-month home exercise programme with intermittent physiotherapy home visits (Yang et al., 2012). The addition of a focus on turning exercises together with the Otago program has also been shown to improve turning ability and balance performance in older people with turning difficulty (Ashari et al., 2016).

Resistance training is another excellent form of exercise for older people, which can be undertaken in a variety of ways, including using specialised equipment (e.g. at a gymnasium) or in-home or group settings incorporating functional exercises that use body weight for loading (e.g. sit to stand, stairs) or elastic resistance bands or weights/ cuffs. Resistance training has been shown to result in important health-related outcomes even in the presence of moderate health problems, for example in older people with chronic obstructive pulmonary disease (Liao et al., 2015) and knee osteoarthritis (Li et al., 2016) and in prostate cancer patients (Hasenoehrl et al., 2015). Resistance training and high-impact-type exercise have been shown to also improve bone strength and reduce fracture risk. (Giangregorio et al., 2015; Gillespie et al., 2012).

Exercise is the most researched intervention approach to reduce falls in older people, with a recent Cochrane review, reporting the outcomes of 108 randomised controlled exercise interventions (23,407 participants, 25 countries), aiming to reduce falls for older people living in the community setting (Sherrington et al., 2017). The review concludes that 'exercise programmes reduce the rate of falls and the number of people experiencing falls in older people living in the community (high certainty)'. Programmes that included a combination of balance and strength training, or tai chi, were shown to be effective. The review authors noted that they were uncertain of the effect on reducing falls of programmes that primarily focussed on resistance training. A focus on moderate challenge balance exercises appears to be an essential component of exercise programmes that are effective in reducing falls (Sherrington et al., 2017).

Exercise has also been shown to result in psychological benefits as well as physical performance benefits. Exercise approaches have been shown to improve falls efficacy (Kumar et al., 2016), 30 as well as reduce depression (Blake et al., 2009).

An approach to exercise for older people that has not been the focus of much research until recently is exercising outdoors. Exercising outdoors can provide the same benefits as exercising indoors, but may have additional benefits, such as improved social interaction and mood (Rogerson et al., 2016; Krinski et al., 2017) and sunlight exposure to improve vitamin D levels. A recent randomised trial found that exercise at a seniors' exercise park (purpose-built outdoor exercise park that is designed to improve balance, strength, flexibility, fitness and function for older people) (Levinger et al., 2018) resulted in improved physical performance (Sales et al., 2017) and high levels of enjoyment associated with the programme (Sales et al., 2017).

Despite the strong research evidence supporting a range of exercise modalities to be associated with important physical and psychological health benefits, in general, the uptake and sustained participation in exercise interventions by older people has been limited (Hughes et al., 2019). Some frequently cited barriers to resistance training include pain, injury and illness, looking too muscular and thinking that participation increased the risk of having a heart attack, stroke or death (Burton, Farrier, et al., 2017; Burton, Lewin, et al., 2017). Additional barriers to other forms

Health Benefits of Exercise for Older People

of exercise or physical activity that have been reported include environmental factors, resources, social influences, need for reinforcement and assistance in managing changes (Spiteri et al., 2019) and difficulty making exercise a habit (Morgan et al., 2016). Strategies are required to improve the knowledge of older people about the benefits of exercise and the variety of exercise options available that can have health benefits. Health practitioners should regularly discuss the subject of exercise in their consultations with older people. Positive language about the benefits of exercise (for example focussing more on benefits associated with greater independence and well-being than on preventing falls) may also be important in influencing some older people to participate in interventions (Yardley et al., 2007; Barker et al., 2019). In many cases, now there are several exercise types or options available for older people with specific health problems or specific desired health outcomes. An example is to provide choices between home- and centre-based exercises – both can be beneficial, but some older people will prefer to exercise in groups, while others will prefer to exercise alone (Jansons et al., 2018). Group dynamics and opportunities for social interaction after exercise sessions (e.g. a cup of tea and a chat) can also help build relationships among exercise participants and be an important factor in sustaining participation (McPhate et al., 2016). Exercising alone does often require a greater level of self-discipline to sustain longer-term participation.

Although there is strong evidence about the benefits of exercise for older people generally, the research evidence in some areas is less well developed. An emerging area of research in exercise for falls prevention is exercise targeting people with dementia. There is growing evidence from a small number of studies with small sample sizes that both home- and group-based exercises that incorporate balance and strength training (with carer training and support or home-based programmes) can reduce the risk of falls (Lam et al., 2018). Another gap is in residential care settings, where the conclusion from the 2018 review that included 13 exercise-related randomised controlled trials was that there was no effect of exercise on falls and the number of fallers (Cameron et al., 2018). However, a randomised trial published just after this Cochrane review has demonstrated a 55% significant reduction in falls among older people living in residential care (with almost 50% of the sample having cognitive impairment) (Hewitt et al., 2018), which provides promising new evidence in this area.

CONCLUSION

Exercise is an excellent modality for improving health outcomes for older people, irrespective of age, comorbidities and level of frailty. However, different exercise approaches can be more appropriate for differing functional or health statuses of individuals and to achieve different outcomes. Older people with health problems should receive advice from their doctors and experienced exercise practitioners (e.g. physiotherapists or exercise physiologists) to ensure that the appropriate type and level of exercise are undertaken safely. Health practitioners need to embrace behavioural change approaches to support increased uptake and sustained participation in exercise by older people.

REFERENCES

Ashari, A. et al. (2016) 'Effectiveness of individualized home-based exercise on turning and balance performance among adults older than 50 yrs: A randomized controlled trial', *American Journal of Physical Medicine and Rehabilitation*, 95(5), pp. 355–365. doi: 10.1097/PHM.0000000000000388.

Australian Institute of Health and Welfare. (2018) *Older Australia at a Glance.* Available at: https://www.aihw.gov.au/reports/older-people/older-australia-at-a-glance/contents/demographics-of-older-australians/australia-s-changing-age-and-gender-profile 2018.

Barker, A. et al. (2019) 'Evaluation of RESPOND, a patient-centred program to prevent falls in older people presenting to the emergency department with a fall: A randomised controlled trial', *PLoS Medicine*, 16(5), pp. 1–18. doi: 10.1371/journal.pmed.1002807.

Beckwée, D. et al. (2019) 'Exercise interventions for the prevention and treatment of sarcopenia. A systematic umbrella review', *Journal of Nutrition, Health and Aging*, 23(6), pp. 494–502. doi: 10.1007/s12603-019-1196–8.

Blake, H. et al. (2009) 'How effective are physical activity interventions for alleviating depressive symptoms in older people? A systematic review', *Clinical Rehabilitation*, 23(10), pp. 873–887. doi: 10.1177/0269215509337449.

Burton, E. et al. (2015) 'Effectiveness of exercise programs to reduce falls in older people with dementia living in the community: A systematic review and meta-analysis', *Clinical Interventions in Aging*, 10, pp. 421–434. doi: 10.2147/CIA.S71691.

Burton, E., Farrier, K., et al. (2017) 'Motivators and barriers for older people participating in resistance training: A systematic review', *Journal of Aging and Physical Activity*, 25(2), pp. 311–324. doi: 10.1123/japa.2015-0289.

Burton, E., Lewin, G., et al. (2017) 'Identifying motivators and barriers to older community-dwelling people participating in resistance training: A cross-sectional study', *Journal of Sports Sciences*, 35(15), pp. 1523–1532. doi: 10.1080/02640414.2016.1223334.

Cameron, I. D. et al. (2018) 'Interventions for preventing falls in older people in care facilities and hospitals', *Cochrane Database of Systematic Reviews*, 2018(9). doi: 10.1002/14651858.CD005465.pub4.

Giangregorio, L. M. et al. (2015) 'Too Fit To Fracture: outcomes of a Delphi consensus process on physical activity and exercise recommendations for adults with osteoporosis with or without vertebral fractures', *Osteoporosis International*, 26(3), pp. 891–910. doi: 10.1007/s00198-014-2881-4.

Gillespie, L. et al. (2012) 'Interventions for preventing falls in older people living in the community (Review)', *Cochrane Database of Systematic Reviews*, 2019(2). doi: 10.1002/14651858.CD013258.

Hasenoehrl, T. et al. (2015) 'The effects of resistance exercise on physical performance and health-related quality of life in prostate cancer patients: a systematic review', *Supportive Care in Cancer*, 23(8), pp. 2479–2497. doi: 10.1007/s00520-015-2782-x.

He, W., Goodkind, D. and Kowal, P. (2016) *An Aging World: 2015 (International Population Reports, P95/16-1).* Washington, DC.

Hewitt, J. et al. (2018) 'Progressive resistance and balance training for falls prevention in long-term residential aged care: A cluster randomized trial of the sunbeam program', *Journal of the American Medical Directors Association*, 19(4), pp. 361–369. doi: 10.1016/j.jamda.2017.12.014.

Hill, K. D. et al. (2017) 'Dysmobility syndrome: Current perspectives', *Clinical Interventions in Aging*, 12, pp. 145–152. doi: 10.2147/CIA.S102961.

Huang, Y. and Liu, X. (2015) 'Improvement of balance control ability and flexibility in the elderly Tai Chi Chuan (TCC) practitioners: A systematic review and meta-analysis', *Archives of Gerontology and Geriatrics*, 60(2), pp. 233–238. doi: 10.1016/j.archger.2014.10.016.

Health Benefits of Exercise for Older People

Huang, Z. et al. (2017) 'Systematic review and meta-analysis: Tai Chi for preventing falls in older adults.', *BMJ Open*, 7(2).

Hughes, K. J. et al. (2019) 'Interventions to improve adherence to exercise therapy for falls prevention in community-dwelling older adults: Systematic review and meta-analysis', *Age and Ageing*, 48(2), pp. 185–195. doi: 10.1093/ageing/afy164.

Jansons, P. S. et al. (2018) 'Barriers and enablers to ongoing exercise for people with chronic health conditions: Participants' perspectives following a randomized controlled trial of two interventions', *Archives of Gerontology and Geriatrics*, 76(July 2017), pp. 92–99. doi: 10.1016/j.archger.2018.02.010.

Krinski, K. et al. (2017) 'Let's walk outdoors! Self-paced walking outdoors improves future intention to exercise in women with obesity', *Journal of Sport & Exercise Psychology*, 39(2), pp. 145–157.

Kumar, A. et al. (2016) 'Exercise for reducing fear of falling in older people living in the community: Cochrane systematic review and meta-analysis', *Age and Ageing*, 45(3), pp. 345–352. doi: 10.1093/ageing/afw036.

Lam, F. M. et al. (2018) 'Physical exercise improves strength, balance, mobility, and endurance in people with cognitive impairment and dementia: a systematic review', *Journal of Physiotherapy*, 64(1), pp. 4–15. doi: 10.1016/j.jphys.2017.12.001.

Levinger, P. et al. (2018) 'Outdoor physical activity for older people—the senior exercise park: Current research, challenges and future directions', *Health Promotion Journal of Australia*, 29(3), pp. 353–359. doi: 10.1002/hpja.60.

Li, Y. et al. (2016) 'The effects of resistance exercise in patients with knee osteoarthritis: A systematic review and meta-analysis', *Clinical Rehabilitation*, 30(10), pp. 947–959. doi: 10.1177/0269215515610039.

Liao, W. H. et al. (2015) 'Impact of resistance training in subjects with COPD: A systematic review and meta-analysis', *Respiratory Care*, 60(8), pp. 1130–1145. doi: 10.4187/respcare.03598.

Liu, C. and Latham, N. (2011) 'Progressive resistance strength training for improving physical function in older adults', *International Journal of Older People Nursing*, 6(3), pp. 244–246. doi: 10.1111/j.1748-3743.2011.00291.x.

McPhate, L. et al. (2016) '"Are Your Clients Having Fun?"' *Journal of Aging and Physical Activity*, 24(1), pp. 129–138.

Morgan, F. et al. (2016) 'Adherence to exercise referral schemes by participants - What do providers and commissioners need to know? A systematic review of barriers and facilitators', *BMC Public Health*, 16(1), pp. 1–11. doi: 10.1186/s12889-016-2882-7.

Robertson, M. C. et al. (2002) 'Preventing injuries in older people by preventing falls: A meta-analysis of individual-level data', *Journal of the American Geriatrics Society*, 50(5), pp. 905–911. doi: 10.1046/j.1532-5415.2002.50218.x.

Rogerson, M. et al. (2016) 'Influences of green outdoors versus indoors environmental settings on psychological and social outcomes of controlled exercise', *International Journal of Environmental Research and Public Health*, 13(4). doi: 10.3390/ijerph13040363.

Sales, M. et al. (2017) 'A novel exercise initiative for seniors to improve balance and physical function', *Journal of Aging and Health*, 29(8), pp. 1424–1443. doi: 10.1177/0898264316662359.

Sherrington, C. et al. (2017) 'Exercise to prevent falls in older adults: An updated systematic review and meta-analysis', *British Journal of Sports Medicine*, 51(24), pp. 1749–1757. doi: 10.1136/bjsports-2016-096547.

Sims, J. et al. (2006) *National Ageing Recommendations for Older Australians : Discussion Document*. Available at: https://pdf4pro.com/view/national-ageing-research-institute-288e45.html.

Sims, J. et al. (2010) 'Physical activity recommendations for older Australians', *Australasian Journal on Ageing*, 29(2), pp. 81–87. doi: 10.1111/j.1741-6612.2009.00388.x.

Song, L. et al. (2007) 'Effects of a sun style Tai Chi exercise on arthritic symptoms, motivation and performance of health behaviours in women with osteoarthritis', *Taehan Kanho Hakhoe chi*, 37(2), pp. 249–256.

Spiteri, K. et al. (2019) 'Barriers and motivators of physical activity participation in middle-aged and older-adults-a systematic review', *Journal of Aging and Physical Activity*, pp. 1–80. Available at: http://www.jfmpc.com/article.asp?issn=2249-4863;year=2017;volume=6;issue=1;spage=169;epage=170;aulast=Faizi.

Sun, J. and Buys, N. (2013) 'Health benefits of Tai Chi: What is the evidence?', *Health Promotion: Community Singing as a Vehicle to Promote Health*, 62, pp. 39–57.

Suttanon, P. et al. (2013) 'Feasibility, safety and preliminary evidence of the effectiveness of a home-based exercise programme for older people with Alzheimer's disease: A pilot randomized controlled trial', *Clinical Rehabilitation*, 27(5), pp. 427–438. doi: 10.1177/0269215512460877.

The World Bank. (2015) *Live Long and Prosper: Aging in East Asia and Pacific*. The World Bank. doi: 10.1596/978-1-4648-0469-4.

Theou, O. et al. (2011) 'The effectiveness of exercise interventions for the management of frailty: A systematic review', *Journal of Aging Research*, 2011. doi: 10.4061/2011/569194.

Viña, J. et al. (2016) 'Exercise: The lifelong supplement for healthy ageing and slowing down the onset of frailty', *Journal of Physiology*, 594(8), pp. 1989–1999. doi: 10.1113/JP270536.

Voukelatos, A. et al. (2015) 'The impact of a home-based walking programme on falls in older people: The easy steps randomised controlled trial', *Age and Ageing*, 44(3), pp. 377–383. doi: 10.1093/ageing/afu186.

WHO. (1997) 'The Heidelberg guidelines for promoting physical activity among older persons.pdf', *Journal of Aging and Physical Activity*, pp. 1–8.

Yang, X. J. et al. (2012) 'Effectiveness of a targeted exercise intervention in reversing older people's mild balance dysfunction: A randomized controlled trial', *Physical Therapy*, 92(1), pp. 24–37. doi: 10.2522/ptj.20100289.

Yardley, L. et al. (2007) 'Recommendations for promoting the engagement of older people in activities to prevent falls', *Quality and Safety in Health Care*, 16(3), pp. 230–234. doi: 10.1136/qshc.2006.019802.

17 Discussion on Principles and Methods of Tai Chi Qigong in Preventing Falling Among the Elderly

Xie Yuhong
Chinese Doctor Clinic

INTRODUCTION

In the aging process from middle age to old age, there are some phenomena, such as decreased range of motion of joints, decreased ligament elasticity, and muscle weakness. The causes of these phenomena are mainly associated with decreased joint flexibility and vision and decreased vestibular function.

Why do older people fall more often? Due to muscular weakness, known as Rou Wei (肉痿) in Chinese medicine. Following the Chinese medicine theory, the kidney governs bone, spleen governs muscle, and liver governs sinew. The root of muscle weakness is in the spleen. Strengthening the spleen can delay muscle weakness. The reason why old people do not have energy is due to the inefficiency of the liver. The reason why bones and tissues are not strong enough is because of kidney and liver weakness.

In order to strengthen the spleen, nourish the liver, and strengthen the kidney, I created a set of Tai Chi Qigong for the elderly to improve these origins' function.

1. **Qi Shi Tiao Xi** (起势调息) **The Beginning Stance**
   - When inhaling, with the palms facing down, raise the arms to the front slowly until they are a little bit higher than the shoulder level.
   - When exhaling, squat down slowly and press the palms down gently to the navel level while keeping the upper body straight and the knees behind the tip of the toes (while looking down).
   - Practice the above movements six times. Then, bring the hands to the sides of the body. Intention. The continuous rising and falling are like a fountain.

DOI: 10.1201/9781003043270-17

2. **Kai Kuo Xiong Huai** (开阔胸怀) **Widening the Chest**
   - Lift the hands at the navel level upward to the front of the chest. Meanwhile, straighten the knees gradually and change the palm posture from facing down to facing each other. Then, inhale and, at the same time, pull the hands sideward to the maximum, thus expanding the chest.
   - Move the hands simultaneously and horizontally to the middle of the chest. Then, change the palm posture from facing each other to facing downward and press them down. While doing this, squat down and exhale.
   - One cycle of practice includes inhalation and exhalation. Repeat six times. Intention. Imagine you are standing on a high mountain and seeing faraway sights.

3. **Ma Bu Yun Shou** (马步云手) **Cloud Hands in Horse Stance**
   - After pushing with the left palm, move it to the eye level, facing inward. Push forward with the right palm facing to the left and at the level of the navel. Along with inhaling, turn the waist to the left and move the hands horizontally leftward.
   - When turning the waist leftward to the maximum, raise the right hand with the palm facing inward and at the eye level and push downward with the left palm with the palm facing to the right and at the level of the navel. While turning the waist to the right, move the hands horizontally and rightward and breathe out at the same time.
   - One cycle of practice includes one inhalation and one exhalation. Repeat six times. Essentials. Keep the movements mild and the eyes following the upper hand. Intention. This is an exercise integrating spirit and body.

4. **Ta Bu Pai Qiu** (踏步拍球) **Bouncing a Ball While Stepping**
   - While inhaling, raise the left leg and, at the same time, press the right hand down as if bouncing a ball in front of the right shoulder.
   - While exhaling, raise the right leg and, at the same time, press the left hand down as if bouncing a ball in front of the left shoulder.
   - One time of practice includes one ball-bouncing movement by the left hand and one by the right hand. Repeat six times.
   Intention Practice with delight and with a childish heart.

5. **Ma Bu Zhan Zhuang** (马步站桩) **Horse Stance Stake Exercise**
   - Stand erect and in a relaxed manner with the feet–shoulder width apart.
   - Drop the arms naturally with the palms facing inward and the eyes looking straight-ahead.
   - Raise the arms in the front slowly to shoulder level while keeping the palms facing each other.
   - Turn over the palms to let them face upward, flex the elbows, and withdraw the hands. Move the arms across the waist, then backward, outward, and forward in a curve.

Discussion on Principles and Methods of Tai Chi Qigong

- Turn over the palms. Withdraw the arms slightly, place them in front of the body, bend the knees, and squat down to posture the horse stance stake posture, but keep the knees behind the toes.
- Grasp the ground with the toes moderately.
- Tuck in the abdomen and lift the anus.
- Round the crotch area and relax the waist and hips.
- Sink the chest and straighten the back.
- Suspend the head and relax the neck.
- Touch the tip of the tongue to the roof of the mouth.
- The line connecting the tip of the nose and the navel should be perpendicular to the ground.
- The line connecting DU 20 (bǎi huì) with RN 1 (huì yīn) should be perpendicular to the ground.
- Relax the armpits.
- Relax the shoulders and drop the elbows.
- The forearms should be parallel to the ground.
- The forearms should be parallel to each other.
- The middle finger and the forearm need to be in a line.
- The palms should be bent like tiles.
- The fingers are echeloned; the thumbs and index fingers look like a duck's beak.
- Keep the upper body insubstantial and the lower body substantial, put a smile on the face, and breathe naturally.

6. **Hu Ju** (虎举) **Raising the tiger's paws**
- Let the arms hang loosely, with both palms turned to face the ground and the 10 fingers spread and flexed, like the paws of a tiger. Fix the eyes on the backs of the hands.
- Turn the palms outward, flex the little finger first then the other four one by one to make fists, and raise the fists slowly along the front of the body to shoulder height. Unclench the fists and raise the hands as high as possible above the head. Then form the tiger's paws again. Fix the eyes on the backs of the hands.
- Clench the fists once more, turning the palm sides to face each other. Keep the eyes fixed on the fists.
- Lower the fists to shoulder level and unclench the fists. Lower the hands with the palms down and the fingers extended to the front of the abdomen. Keep the eyes fixed on the backs of the hands.
- Let the hands hang naturally at the sides of the thighs. Look straight-ahead.
- Key points: Concentrate the strength in the fingers as they are spread, bent to assume the tiger's paws, and turned outward to form fists. When raising the palms, throw out the chest and contract the abdomen to stretch the body, as if lifting a heavyweight. When lowering the palms, contract the chest and relax the abdomen to drive Qi into Dantian. The eyes should always follow the movements of the hands. Inhale as the palms are raised and exhale as they are lowered.

- Functions and effects: Clear air is inhaled when the palms are raised, and stale air is exhaled when they are lowered, so the circulation of Qi in Sanjiao (occupying the thoracic and abdominal cavities) is promoted and its functions adjusted. Forming a tiger's paw before making a fist reinforces the grip power and propels the blood circulation to the distal joints of the arm.

7. **Zan Quan Nu Mu Zeng Qi Li** (攒拳怒目增气力) **Clenching the Fists and Glaring Fiercely to Increase Qi and Strength**
   - Move the body weight to the right. Move the left foot one step to the left, to adopt the horse stance. Clench the fists at the sides of the waist, with the thumbs up. Look straight-ahead.
   - Slowly thrust the clenched left fist forward to shoulder level, with the thumb-side up. Make the eyes glare while looking at the left fist.
   - Turn the left arm inward. Loosen the left fingers and point the thumb down. Look at the left palm. Turn the left arm outward, its elbow slightly bent. Meanwhile, twist the left hand to the left, palm up, and clench the fingers. Look at the left fist.
   - Bend the left elbow to withdraw the fist to the side of the waist, with the thumb-side up. Look straight-ahead.
   - Then move the body weight to the right and withdraw the left foot to stand straight, with the feet together. Unclench the fists and let the arms hang loose. Look straight-ahead.
   - Key points: When assuming the horse stance, squat down as low as possible. Make the eyes glare at the clenched fist when it is thrust out. Try to grasp the floor with the toes, twist the waist, and apply strength along the shoulder to the fist. Twist the wrist when withdrawing the arm and clench fingers forcefully.
   - Functions and effects: In traditional Chinese medicine, the liver is believed to control the tendons and sinews and is directly connected with the eyes. Making the eyes glare can stimulate the liver channels so as to improve blood circulation and help cultivate vital energy. Squatting, clenching the floor with the toes, clenching the fists, twisting the wrists, and holding the claw hands with force can stimulate the meridians such as Dumai and the acupuncture points Shuxue on the back, as well as Sanyin and Sanyang meridians of both the hands and feet.

8. **Hu zi Jue** (呼字诀) **Hū-Sound Exercise**
   - After pushing out the hands in the last routine, turn the palms inward to face the navel, with the fingers apart and tilted toward each other, and the palms apart as distant from the navel as from each other. Look forward and down.
   - Slowly straighten the knees to stand up and slowly move the hands together to a position some 10 cm in front of the navel.
   - Slightly squat down, and at the same time, move the hands out as distant from the navel as from each other to form a circle. Pronounce "HU," looking forward and down.

Discussion on Principles and Methods of Tai Chi Qigong

- Slowly straighten the knees to stand up, at the same time bringing the palms slowly toward the navel.
- Key points: The pronunciation of "HU" is assisted by the throat. In the process of exhalation and pronunciation, curve the sides of the tongue up, thrust the lips forward to form a round opening, and exhale through the opening. Inhale while moving the hands closer to the navel and exhale to pronounce "HU" when moving the hands out.
- Functions and effects: The theory of traditional Chinese medicine holds that the spleen will respond when the sound "HU" is pronounced and that the exhalation and pronunciation of "HU" help get rid the spleen and stomach of turbid Qi and regulate their functions. Moving the hands close to and away from the navel helps refresh the internal circulation, contraction, and extension of the abdominal cavity. It helps massage the intestines and stomach, strengthen the spleen and stomach, and cure indigestion.

9. **Tiao Li Pi Wei Xu Dan Ju** (调理脾胃须单举) **Holding One Arm Aloft to Regulate the Functions of the Spleen and Stomach**
   - Slowly straighten the knees, to stand straight, with the feet apart. Meanwhile, raise the left hand past the face, while turning the left arm inward, to a position above the head on the left side, with the elbow slightly bent. Apply strength at the base of the palm that faces upward, the fingers pointing to the right. At the same time raise the right hand a little and then press it down to the side of the right hip, with the elbow slightly bent, strength applied at the base of the palm that faces downward, and fingers pointing forward. Hold this position, looking straight-ahead.
   - Move the bodyweight slowly down and bend the knees slightly, with the waist relaxed and hips down. Meanwhile, bend the left elbow and move the left hand down past the face to a position in front of the abdomen, with the palm up. Move the right hand up to a position level with the left hand, both palms up and the fingers pointing to each other about 10 cm apart. Look straight-ahead.
   - The movements are to be done three times each, left and right.
   - During the last repetition, bend the knees slightly and press the right hand down at the side of the right hipbone, with the palm down and the fingers pointing forward. Look straight-ahead.
   - Key points: Expand the chest and body, loosen and stretch the waist, and keep the shoulders relaxed and down. Apply strength at the base of the palms when pressing them up and down.
   - Functions and effects: The raising and lowering of the arms in opposite directions have a stretching effect on the abdominal cavity and thus massage such organs as the spleen and stomach. Moreover, the channels and collaterals around the abdomen and ribs and such points as Shuxue along the spine are stimulated, thereby regulating the circulation of energy along the channels and collaterals among the organs.

10 **San Pan Luo Di** (三盘落地) **Three Dishes Falling to the Ground**
- Take a big step leftward with the left foot and stand with the feet apart slightly wider than shoulder-width. Raise the arms to the front of the body to the shoulder level, with the palms up and the arms shoulder-width apart and stretched out.
- While turning the palms inward to let them face downward and extending the elbows outward, bend the knees to posture a horse stance. Press the palms downward and position them over the knees.
- Raise the hands slowly from the knees and, at the same time, turn the palms upward and raise them to the shoulder level. Then, squat down and, at the same time, turn the palms downward and press them down to the sides of the knees.
- Rise from the knees slowly and, at the same time, turn the palms upward and raise them to the shoulder level. Then, squat down and, at the same time, turn the palms downward and press them down to the middle parts of the sides of the calves, the eyes looking straight-ahead.
- Closing form: First, inhale deeply. When exhaling slowly, rise from the knees slowly, turn the palms upward, raise them to the shoulder level, turn over them again, lower them slowly to the sides of the body, bring back the left foot, and stand upright with the feet together.
- Essentials: Raise the palms as if holding a weighty object. Then, press downward with the palms as if pressing on a floating ball.
- Effects: This exercise is effective for treating pain in the waist and lower extremities as well as pelvic inflammation. The movements mainly exercise the quadriceps and the iliopsoas muscles.

11. **Chui Zi Jue** (吹字诀) **Chuī-Sound Exercise**
- Extend the hands, relax the wrists, and point the fingers forward, with the palms down.
- Move the arms apart and hold them level with the shoulders, with the palms tilted backward and fingers pointing outward.
- Turn the arms inward. Move the palms in a curve to the back of the waist, with the palms gently touching the Yaoyan points on the back near the spine and the fingers tilted down. Look forward and down.
- Slightly bend the knees to squat down, at the same time moving the palms down along the back of the waist, hips, and thighs. Bend the elbows to lift the arms from the back of the body to the front for a hollow holding position in front of the navel, with the palms facing inward and fingers pointing toward each other. Look forward and down. Exhale to pronounce "CHUI" when moving the hands down from the back of the waist.
- Slowly straighten the knees to stand up, and at the same time withdraw the palms to gently touch the abdomen, with the fingers tilted down at an angle and the thumbs pointing toward each other. Look forward and down.
- Move the hands backward along the waist.

Discussion on Principles and Methods of Tai Chi Qigong   **203**

- Move the hands to the back of the waist, with the palms slightly touching the Yaoyan points on the back of the waist near the spine and with fingers pointing down at an angle. Look forward and down.
- Slowly straighten the knees to stand up and lift the elbows and the hands to a position in front of the chest. Raise the hands to face level and then curve them outward to a holding position distant from the head, with the palms angled upward. Look forward and up.
- Key points: The pronunciation of "CHUI" is assisted by the lips. In the process of exhalation and pronunciation, pull back the tongue and the corners of the mouth, make the back teeth parallel, draw the lips back to a stretched state, and exhale the air from the throat through the sides of the tongue and between the stretched lips. Exhale and pronounce "CHUI" when moving the hands down the back of the waist and lifting them to a hollow holding position in front of the abdomen. Inhale through the nose when moving the hands backward along the waist.
- Functions and effects: The theory of traditional Chinese medicine holds that the kidneys will respond when the sound "CHUI" is pronounced and that the exhalation and pronunciation of "CHUI" help get rid of turbid Qi of the kidneys and regulate their function. The theory holds that the waist is the home of the kidneys. As they are located on the sides of the spine, the function of the waist is closely linked with the functional activities of the kidneys. Hand massage of the waist and abdomen strengthens the waist and kidneys, improves their functions, and prevents aging.

12. **Niao Fei** (鸟飞) **Flying like a bird**
- This exercise is continuously performed from the last position of the above exercise. Adopt a semi-squatting stance and allow the arms to hang in front of the abdomen with the palms facing each other. The eyes should look straight-ahead and downward.
- The right leg is straightened and the left leg is bent and lifted so that it forms a right angle, with the toes pointing down. At the same time, the arms are lifted together at the sides so that the hands, palms down, are located slightly higher than the shoulders. The eyes look straight-ahead.
- In a semi-squatting posture, place the tips of the toes of the left foot on the ground beside the right foot. At the same time, both hands are moved to the front of the abdomen with the palms facing each other. The eyes look straight-ahead and down.
- Straighten the right leg and lift the left leg to form a right angle, with the toes pointing down. At the same time, both hands are raised upward over the top of the head until their backs almost touch, with the fingertips pointing up. The eyes look straight-ahead.
- Land the left foot beside the right foot, the sole of both feet flat on the ground to assume a semi-squatting posture, while returning the hands to their place in the first position. The eyes look straight-ahead and down.
- The second to fifth positions are repeated, but the left and right sides are reversed.

- Return to starting position. After the above positions are repeated, both hands are lifted to the sides of the chest, with the palms facing up and the eyes looking straight-ahead. The elbows are flexed, and the palms are turned in and pressed down to hang loosely at the sides. The eyes look straight-ahead.
- Key points: When the arms are stretched out laterally, keep them as comfortably wide as you can in order to expand the chest as much as possible. When they are moved medially and downward, the chest should be contracted from both sides as much as possible. The upper and lower limbs should be moved in coordination and simultaneously inhale when raising the hands and exhale when lowering them.
- Functions and effects: Combined with the breathing exercise, moving of the arms up and down may promote respiration and expand the capacity of the chest, produce a massaging effect on the heart and lungs, and improve the blood's oxygenation function. The upthrust of the thumb and index finger stimulates the lung meridian (starting at the upper abdomen, extending along the medial surface of the upper arms, and stopping at the tips of the thumb and index finger), promotes circulation of Qi through this meridian, and improves the functions of the heart and lungs.

Practice above 1–12 sections movements, 10 minutes each time, three times total 30 minutes a day.

In the recent 3–4 years, I have traveled to many European countries to teach Taiji Qigong, such as Switzerland, Germany, France, Poland, Ireland, Italy, Spain, and others. As most of the students are elderly, I also teach them above 12 sessions of Tai Chi Qigong to improve balance function and prevent falls, and this, in turn, will enhance people's lifestyle.

You can follow the Video to practice: https://youtu.be/MryH57IwNYM.

18 Integrated Management in Elderly

Liu Xiao Hang
Tung Shin Hospital

CONTENTS

Main Differences Between Chinese and Western Medicine 205
    Advantages of Integrated Management in Elderly 206
    Basic Principles and Strategies of Integrated Management 206
    Features of Integrated Management in Common Diseases of the Elderly 206
        Coronary Heart Disease 206
        Congestive Cardiac Failure 207
        Stroke 207
        Chronic Obstructive Pulmonary Disease and Idiopathic Pulmonary Fibrosis ... 207
        Arthritis, Osteoporosis 207
        Hypertension 207
        Diabetes 208
        Dyslipidemia 208
        Renal Failure 208

MAIN DIFFERENCES BETWEEN CHINESE AND WESTERN MEDICINE

Chinese and western medicines are completely two different medical systems which have different development histories and characteristics.

Chinese medicine has a long history of thousands of years. The development of Chinese medicine is unlike western medicine. The experience was gained through the clinical practice which is treating diseases using syndrome differentiation according to the predecessors' experience. This syndrome differentiation method is unique. Chinese medicine practitioners analyse a patient's syndrome as yin or yang, deficiency or excess, cold or heat, external or internal from observation, olfaction, inquiry and pulse taking (including palpation), and give relevant treatment after the analysis. Comparatively, Chinese medicine attaches great importance to the holistic study of the human body. Symptoms would be treated first if the condition is urgent; when symptoms are relieved, regulating the body constitution (or curing the root cause) would be of utmost importance. Chinese herbs are made up of natural ingredients. Although the therapeutic effects are relatively slow, they have fewer side effects.

On the other hand, western medicine has only a few hundred years of history. The accomplishment of applying new technologies, such as modern biology, chemistry,

DOI: 10.1201/9781003043270-18

206 Healthy Ageing in Asia

physics, etc. in the western medical sector causes the rapid development of western medicine. The strength of western medicine is not only diagnosis but the surgical treatment and emergency rescue too. However, western medicine contains mostly chemical substances which have more side effects compared to Chinese medicine.

ADVANTAGES OF INTEGRATED MANAGEMENT IN ELDERLY

The majority of elderly patients have weak body constitution. In terms of regulating body constitution (by strengthening the weakness), western medicine doctors have limited strategy (or treatment method) such as prescribing CoQ10 and multivitamins. However, the application of Chinese herbs can be customised according to the individual's symptoms by regulating the imbalance of qi, blood, yin and yang to strengthen the body constitution. It adopts a targeted approach towards the disease, showing a promising result. Chinese herbs can relieve patients' symptoms, strengthen immunity resulting in less susceptibility to bacterial and viral infection, improve the overall quality of life, etc. In short, all elderly patients with a weak physique are suitable for the notifying treatment by regulating the imbalance.

Another objective of the integration of the Chinese and western medications is also to cut down the polypharmacy and the dosage of the western medication, on the condition that the disease is stable, in order to reduce the side effects of the western medication.

BASIC PRINCIPLES AND STRATEGIES OF INTEGRATED MANAGEMENT

First, a clear diagnosis according to the patient's examination report is made by using western medicine. Next, the analysis is made followed by the treatment plan. For those with critical illnesses, they require treatment with western medicine. During the integration of western and Chinese medication treatment, the role and focus of the western and Chinese medications would be different in each disease. For example, diseases such as acute myocardial infarction and stroke, Chinese medicine does not play an effective role in acute management. It is preferable to take western medication until the patient's condition is stable; subsequently, Chinese medication will come into play for the remission of diseases.

The polypharmacy and dosage of western medications can be reduced, on the condition that the disease is stable while using the Chinese herbs as basic treatment. But MUST continue taking western medications that cannot be replaced by Chinese medicine.

FEATURES OF INTEGRATED MANAGEMENT IN COMMON DISEASES OF THE ELDERLY

Coronary Heart Disease

Stable angina and stable myocardial infarction are mainly treated using western medicine but the treatment can be combined with Chinese herbs to regulate the body. Despite the use of percutaneous coronary intervention and surgical and medical

Integrated Management in Elderly **207**

treatment, symptomatic unstable angina can be treated with Chinese herbs. Patients are not advocated to stop the antiplatelet medication no matter how effective are the Chinese herbs. There is a possibility to reduce the polypharmacy of western medication, but it depends on patients' condition.

Unstable angina and acute myocardial infarction are mainly treated using western medication. Integrated management of Chinese and western medications is encouraged after the condition has been stabilised. After a period of taking integrated medicines, polypharmacy and the dosage of western medicine can be minimised gradually. However, the usage of basic antiplatelet drugs cannot be removed. There is an exception, i.e. for patients with unstable conditions despite going through all western medicine treatment, Chinese medicine could play an important role in this situation.

Congestive Cardiac Failure

Herbal medicine can compliment the western medicine treatment regimes. Diuretics (as well as ACEI and beta blocker can be reduced when the Chinese medicine is therapeutic. For patients with early-stage congestive cardiac failure (CCF) (mild CCF), they can choose to use Chinese medications ONLY to prevent deterioration. Meanwhile, integrated medicine can give an unexpectedly good result for patients with severe or end-stage CCF.

Stroke

During an acute stage, patients are mainly treated with western medicine. During the convalescence period, patients can be treated with integrated medicines of western and Chinese, especially acupuncture and Chinese herbs which play a major role.

Chronic Obstructive Pulmonary Disease and Idiopathic Pulmonary Fibrosis

During an acute stage, such as an acute exacerbation of asthma or acute respiratory infection, patients are mainly treated using western medications assisted by Chinese medicines to improve symptoms. During the remission stage, Chinese medication is used to regulate the body, improve the body condition and strengthen immunity in order to reduce or achieve no acute attacks at all.

Arthritis, Osteoporosis

Except for those indicated for surgery, the combination of Chinese herbs with acupuncture and tuina (Chinese massage) can control the symptoms and reduce the need for analgesics.

Hypertension

For those with early-stage hypertension, mild hypertension, white coat hypertension or menopause hypertension, we can give Chinese herbs a try before resorting to western treatment. Moreover, those with severe hypertension or those with complications due to hypertension are advised to take integrated medications. Furthermore, patients who are over-taking antihypertensive drugs can stop the western medication after Chinese medicine treatment.

Diabetes

Mild diabetes or early-stage diabetes patients are initially treated with a Chinese medication while patients with severe diabetes or diabetes with complications are treated with integrated management. The purpose of the Chinese medication in this condition is to improve the quality of life and to treat the complications.

Dyslipidemia

No replacement of western medication by Chinese medication is advocated for those patients with severe cardiovascular disease and cerebrovascular disease. For patients with mild hyperlipidaemia, Chinese medications should be the primary treatment. For asymptomatic patients, they can take red yeast tablets to control; for those with symptoms, they can take herbal decoction tailored accordingly.

Renal Failure

The goals of treating renal failure patients with Chinese medicine are to stabilise the condition, enhance renal function and delay the onset of dialysis. Patients with mild conditions (i.e. creatinine level is less than 300 µmol/L) are recommended to take long-term Chinese medications to maintain the condition. There are some precautions for renal failure patients such as patients who are prohibited to take herbs with toxicity especially herbs that are rich in aristolochic acids that would give more harm to the kidneys. During both Chinese and western treatments, the practitioners and patients MUST keep track of the changes in creatinine for patient safety.

19 Mental Health and Healthy Aging – Prevention and Management

Gerard Bodeker
University of Oxford

CONTENTS

Introduction 209
Aging and Mental Health in Malaysia 210
COVID-19: Mental Health and the Elderly 211
A Life Span Approach to Understand Mental Health 213
    Wellness Pathways 213
    Nutrition 213
    Exercise 215
    Yoga 215
    Tai Chi 216
    Dance 216
The Arts 217
    Music 217
    Art & Art Therapy 217
Social Support 218
Nature and the Environment 218
Japan's Ikigai 219
Japan's One Hundred Year Life Program 219
Bibliography 220

INTRODUCTION

There is no health without mental health.

– World Health Organization

WHO has taken the position that mental health leads to mental and psychological well-being. At the same time as WHO was taking this strong position, the World Health Organization, Mental Health Atlas (2018) has reported that the level of public expenditure on mental health in low- and middle-income countries was meager,

DOI: 10.1201/9781003043270-19

and more than 80% of funds went to mental hospitals. The allocation for human resources for mental health services has an extreme variation between low- and high-income countries (1 per 100,000 in low-income countries to 72 per 100,000 in high-income countries), while globally the median number of mental health workers is 9 per 100,000 population (WHO 2018).

The Committee on Ethical Issues of the European Psychiatric Association has proposed a new definition of mental health which is:

> Mental health is a dynamic state of internal equilibrium which enables individuals to use their abilities in harmony with universal values of society. Basic cognitive and social skills; ability to recognize, express and modulate one's own emotions, as well as empathize with others; flexibility and ability to cope with adverse life events and function in social roles; and harmonious relationship between body and mind represent important components of mental health which contribute, to varying degrees, to the state of internal equilibrium.
>
> *Galderisi et al. (2015)*

With mental health given its due importance in the United Nations Sustainable Development Goals, for the first time, leaders of the world have acknowledged that mental health promotion and well-being and the prevention and treatment of substance abuse are likely to have a positive impact on communities and countries where millions of people require much-needed help. The focus on ensuring healthy lives and promoting well-being for everyone of all ages lies in Goal 3 of the 17 Sustainable Development Goals. Goal 3, Target 3.4 calls on countries to reduce the premature mortality from noncommunicable diseases (NCDs) by one-third through prevention, treatment, and mental health and well-being promotion. Target 3.5 calls on governments to reinforce and increase efforts in the prevention and treatment of substance abuse, including narcotic drug abuse and the use of alcohol at harmful levels.

The Lancet Commission on Global Mental Health and Sustainable Development (2018) reported that:

> Despite substantial research advances showing what can be done to prevent and treat mental disorders and to promote mental health, translation into real-world effects has been painfully slow. The global burden of disease attributable to mental disorders has risen in all countries in the context of major demographic, environmental, and socio-political transitions.
>
> *Patel et al. (2018, p. 1553)*

AGING AND MENTAL HEALTH IN MALAYSIA

Asian economies are aging, some quite rapidly. And, according to the WHO, Southeast Asia has the highest number of cases of depressive and anxiety disorders compared to other regions, accounting for 7.2% and 2.8% of all years lived with disability, respectively (World Health Organization, 2017). In addition, several national reports from Asia have demonstrated that hypertension, depression, and anxiety disorders occur predominantly in older adults (Ministry of Health and National Institute of Health Research and Development, 2018). Therefore, the elderly, especially in

Asia, are vulnerable to the burden of hypertension, other NCDs, and mental health problems.

Given that Asia has the largest population of any region in the world and also given the vast cultural diversity within and between nations, it is unsurprising that mental health problems vary significantly between countries in Asia. It has been noted that, compared with other regions, Asia seems to have more cultural barriers such as stigma and discrimination around mental illness, superstitious beliefs, poor health literacy, and structural barriers such as poor personal and financial resources, which prevent people from seeking help from mental health professionals (Lauber and Rössler, 2007; Chong et al., 2016; Byrow et al., 2020).

An analysis of epidemiological data on depressive disorders (major depression and dysthymia) from South Asia found that depressive disorders accounted for 9.8 million disability-adjusted life years (DALYs) per 100,000 population in 2016. Of these, major depressive disorders (MDD) accounted for 7.8 million DALYs (95% UI: 5.3–10.5 million). India generated the largest numbers of DALYs due to depressive disorders and MDD, followed by Bangladesh and Pakistan. DALYs due to depressive disorders were highest in females and older adults (75–79 years) across all countries (Ogbo et al., 2018).

Depression in the elderly, often referred to as late-life depression (LLD), is defined as any depressive episode occurring at age 65 or later, regardless of the age of onset (Aizenstein et al., 2016). The biological dimensions of LLD include cerebrovascular pathology, disorders of the endocrine system, presence of inflammatory processes, and nutritional status (Tiemeier, 2003).

Loneliness is also associated with an increased risk of developing coronary heart disease and stroke. People with poor social relationships have a 29% and 32% higher risk of developing coronary heart disease and stroke, respectively (Valtorta et al., 2018; Boden-Albala et al., 2005).

COVID-19: MENTAL HEALTH AND THE ELDERLY

Neurological complications have emerged as a significant cause of morbidity and mortality in the ongoing COVID-19 pandemic. Besides respiratory insufficiency, many hospitalized patients exhibit neurological manifestations ranging from headache and loss of smell to confusion and disabling strokes. COVID-19 is also anticipated to take a toll on the nervous system in the long term. https://doi.org/10.1016/j.cell.2020.08.028.

A recent study found that anxiety and cognitive impairment are manifested by 28%–56% of COVID-19 convalescent individuals with mild respiratory symptoms and are associated with an altered cerebral cortical thickness (Crunfli et al., 2021). This study also found that the coronavirus that causes COVID-19 can infiltrate astrocyte cells in the brain, setting off a chain reaction that may disable and even kill nearby neurons, according to a new study. This could explain some of the structural changes seen in patients' brains, as well as some of the "brain fog" and psychiatric issues that seem to accompany some cases of COVID-19, the authors wrote.

While there is evidence for a strong antiviral defense system in the brain vasculature which, in concert with the endothelium's ability to sense circulating interferon type I signals, would limit SARS-CoV-2 entry into the brain, research is now showing that COVID-19 is more correctly viewed as a vascular disease that attacks the endothelium, impairing its ability to limit SARS-CoV-2 entry into the brain (Lei et al., 2021). This has implications for the elderly, who are already disposed to vascular and neurological vulnerability. A Lancet report on how mental healthcare should change as a consequence of the COVID-19 pandemic has noted that elderly people are at especially high risk of severe COVID-19 illness and mental-health-related consequences because they might already have some cognitive decline (Moreno et al., 2020).

In a Danish nationwide cohort including 144,321 patients with COVID-19, a Danish research team found that a medical history of severe mental illness (i.e., schizophrenia spectrum disorders, bipolar disorder, or unipolar depression) or a psychiatric disorder requiring active medical treatment is associated with an unfavorable outcome in patients with COVID-19. This was not the case for other psychiatric disorders (Barcella et al., 2021).

A Japanese study examined the prevalence of psychological distress during the COVID-19 pandemic and determined that the population is most affected by risk factors, such as the pandemic, socioeconomic status (SES), and lifestyle-related factors causing psychological distress in the early phases of the pandemic in Japan. Binary logistic regression analyses found that pandemic-related factors such as medical history, inability to undergo clinical tests immediately, having trouble in daily life, unavailability of groceries, new work style, and vague anxiety; SES-related factors such as lesser income; and lifestyle-related factors such as insufficient rest, sleep, and nutritious meals were significantly related to the psychological distress (Nagasu, Muto, and Yamamoto, 2021).

In a study on *long-COVID* published in JAMA in 2021, researchers from the University of Washington followed 177 people with laboratory-confirmed SARS-CoV-2 infection for up to nine months. They found that 30% of respondents reported persistent symptoms. The most common were fatigue and loss of smell or taste. More than 30% of respondents reported worse quality of life compared to before getting sick. And 14 participants (8%)—including nine people who had not been hospitalized—reported having trouble performing at least one usual activity, such as daily chores (Logue et al., 2021).

Physical distancing in eldercare institutions can be challenging, either because the nature of patients' conditions makes it difficult to manage (e.g., people with learning disabilities) or because of overcrowding. Increased death rates in assisted living facilities have been reported worldwide, especially among older people and people with learning disabilities (Moreno et al., 2020).

Quarantine and lockdown might particularly affect people with preexisting mental health problems: increased symptoms of anxiety and depression and high rates of post-traumatic stress disorder and insomnia have been reported (Brooks et al., 2020).

Simultaneously, physical distancing has reduced the availability of many family, social, and psychiatric supports. People with serious mental illness and associated socioeconomic disadvantages are particularly at risk of both the direct and indirect effects of the pandemic. Confinement at home, disruption of daily routines, and

Mental Health and Healthy Aging

physical distancing can exacerbate all these conditions and represent a challenge for service users and caregivers (Moreno et al., 2020).

A LIFE SPAN APPROACH TO UNDERSTAND MENTAL HEALTH

WHO has taken a life span approach to understand the risk factors and influencers on mental health and noted that these vary significantly for an individual as they move through the life course.

WELLNESS PATHWAYS

Asian cultural traditions of health care have wellness at their core. Central to these traditions is an understanding that people have different metabolic styles and that understanding these is the basis for developing personalized preventive health and wellness routines. Also, of primary importance in Asian wellness theories and practices is an individualized and balanced approach to nutrition based on body type and cultural food traditions. Integrative exercise is given priority along with stress-reducing and integrative breathing and meditative practice. Regular connection with nature is seen as a balancing influence on overall well-being. The following pathways to mental well-being for the elderly, and across the life span, will all have local forms that are applicable within the specific cultural contexts of the country concerned.

NUTRITION

Reflecting on a life span perspective, the World Health Organization has noted that many of the diseases suffered by older persons are the result of dietary factors, some of which have been operating since infancy. These factors are compounded by changes that naturally occur with the aging process (World Health Organization, 2020b).

Dietary changes seem to affect risk factor levels throughout life and may have an even greater impact on older people. Relatively modest reductions in saturated fat and salt intake, which would reduce blood pressure and cholesterol concentrations, could have a substantial effect on reducing the burden of cardiovascular disease. Increasing the consumption of fruit and vegetables by one to two servings daily could cut the cardiovascular risk by 30%.

Older adults are at increased risk of malnutrition, for a variety of physiological and psychological reasons. In turn, this has implications for health, quality of life, independence, and economic circumstances. Improvements in nutrition are known to bring tangible benefits to older people, and many age-related diseases and conditions can be prevented, modulated, or ameliorated by good nutrition.

The link between good nutrition and good mental health is also important to the mental well-being of older people. In recent years, research has been focusing on understanding the pathways that mediate relationships between diet, nutrition, and mental health. Findings point to the immune system, oxidative biology, brain plasticity, and the microbiome-gut-brain axis as key targets for nutritional interventions.

Writing for *The Lancet Psychiatry*, Jerome Sarris and colleagues at the International Society for Nutritional Psychiatry Research report:

> A traditional whole-food diet, consisting of higher intakes of foods such as vegetables, fruits, seafood, whole grains, lean meat, nuts, and legumes, with avoidance of processed foods, is more likely to provide the nutrients that afford resiliency against the pathogenesis of mental disorders. The mechanisms by which nutrition might affect mental health are, at least superficially, quite obvious: the human brain operates at a very high metabolic rate, and uses a substantial proportion of total energy and nutrient intake; in both structure and function (including intracellular and intercellular communication), it is reliant on amino acids, fats, vitamins, and minerals or trace elements. Dietary habits modulate the functioning of the immune system, which also moderates the risk for depression. The antioxidant defence system, which is also implicated in mental disorders, operates with the support of nutrient cofactors and phytochemicals. Additionally, neurotrophic factors make essential contributions to neuronal plasticity and repair mechanisms throughout life, and these too are affected by nutritional factors
>
> *Sarris et al. (2015)*

In a study on cognitive functioning and brain aging, higher levels of B-family vitamins, as well as vitamins C, D, and E, were all associated with higher scores on cognitive tests. The same positive relationship was found for omega-3 fatty acids, which have previously been linked to better brain health. Those with higher levels of trans fats, found in a variety of junk foods, performed more poorly in thinking and memory tests. Their magnetic resonance imaging scans also revealed more brain shrinkage than in people who had lower trans fat levels. The study found that, overall, nutrition accounted for 37% of the variation in brain volume (Bowman et al., 2012).

A landmark study has found that inexpensive B vitamins stopped the shrinkage in the area of the brain that defines Alzheimer's disease, called the medial temporal lobe. The study, led by David Smith from the University of Oxford, gave a combination of vitamin B_6 (20 mg), B_{12} (500 µg), and folic acid (800 µg) or placebo pills to people with mild cognitive impairment, the stage before a diagnosis of dementia or Alzheimer's. In those with high homocysteine levels, the specific areas of the brain associated with Alzheimer's disease shrank eight times more slowly in those taking B vitamins than in those on the placebo. This is strongly indicative that B vitamins may be substantially slowing down, or even potentially arresting, the disease process in those with early-stage cognitive decline. This is the first treatment that has been shown to do this (Douaud et al., 2013).

The Mediterranean diet is promoted globally as the dietary solution to NCDs. While it is clearly a beneficial dietary pathway to reduce inflammation and promote healthy nutrition, it is also a Western diet, studied by Westerners on Westerners, and it is being recommended for 75% of the world's population that is not Western (Bodeker and Kronenberg, 2015).

In Asia, the Japanese diet is well studied, and there are commonalities with the Mediterranean diet. They share a high intake of unrefined carbohydrates, moderate intake of protein, healthy fat profile, and low glycemic load, less inflammation and

Mental Health and Healthy Aging

oxidative stress, and potential modulation of aging-related pathways. A point of difference is that Asian diets typically include pharmacologically potent ingredients, such as turmeric in South Asia and Southeast Asia; *umeboshi* plums and *reishi* mushrooms in Japan; *goji* berry, ginkgo, and licorice root in the People's Republic of China; ginseng in the Republic of Korea; and *Centella asiatica* in Thailand and Malaysia.

The Prospective Urban Rural Epidemiology study, published in *The Lancet* in August 2017, collected data on more than 135,000 individuals from 18 countries for 4–7 years. The study assessed the association of nutrients with cardiovascular disease and mortality in low- and middle-income populations. Findings showed that higher intakes of fats (including saturated fatty acids, monounsaturated fatty acids, and total polyunsaturated fatty acids) and animal protein were each associated with lower mortality. Carbohydrate intake was associated with increased mortality (Miller et al., 2017).

The risk of total and non-cardiovascular mortality was in the order of 22%–23% lower for people who consume at least three servings per day of fruits, vegetables, and legumes, compared with participants who consumed less than one serving per day of these foods (Miller et al., 2017).

EXERCISE

As noted by Professor Keith Hill in his chapter in this book, aging populations have the potential for rapid increases in the incidence of health problems associated with aging, such as falls, dementia, osteoporosis, and osteoarthritis. Hill notes that a change of focus is needed in the population aging—i.e., to support prevention-focused approaches. "Health promotion and prevention approaches are essential across the full spectrum of health of older populations. Exercise is one health promotion and prevention approach that has an excellent potential to help the aging populations to age well."

Overall, approximately 89% of all published peer-reviewed research report a positive, statistically significant relationship between exercise/physical activity and mental health (John W Brick Foundation, 2021).

YOGA

Researcher Tiffany Field, director of the Touch Research Institute at the University of Miami, has published a review and a book on clinical research on yoga. The following is a summary of her findings on the impact of yoga.

Psychological effects: Field notes that at least two studies have demonstrated a significant increase in mindfulness. Studies of yoga's effects on anxiety are common, with significant series and single-session effects on measures of stress, anxiety, fatigue and depression, well-being, and vigor.

Pain syndromes: Field notes findings of significant pain reduction and less analgesic and opiate use in yoga than control groups, and these findings hold regardless of gender or age differences among participants.

Cardiovascular conditions: Field describes several studies addressing coronary artery disease and hypertension. In each, yoga was found to improve cholesterol and serum low-density lipid levels significantly. Yoga groups also had fewer anginal episodes, improved exercise capacity, decreased body weight, and lowered triglyceride levels than control groups. Blood pressure and blood glucose were reduced, and self-reported well-being and quality of life were increased.

Immune conditions: Field notes that for immune (and autoimmune) conditions, such as asthma, diabetes, multiple sclerosis, lymphoma, and breast cancer, yoga has been associated with several beneficial effects.

Tai Chi

Tai chi, also called tai chi chuan, is described by the UK's NHS Choices as combining deep breathing and relaxation with flowing movements. Originally developed as a martial art in 13th-century China, tai chi is today practiced around the world as a health-promoting exercise and a means of developing self-awareness. (National Health Services, 2018).

Tai chi has been shown to result in improved strength, balance, function, balance confidence, and improvement in some cardiovascular measures, even in the presence of health problems such as lower limb osteoarthritis. However, some forms of tai chi are more challenging (e.g., from a balance or fitness perspective) and therefore are most suitable for more healthy older people (e.g., Yang style), while other forms of tai chi such as the Sun style, including tai chi for arthritis, are more suitable and safe for people with comorbidities, such as lower limb arthritis or reduced balance (Song, 2007; Huang and Liu, 2015).

Dance

Research across the age span has highlighted the differing benefits of dance for different age groups. Research on the benefits of dance, as summarized in a Global Wellness Institute white paper on mental wellness, has found benefits across the life span (Bodeker et al., 2018; Fasullo, Hernandez, and Bodeker, 2020).

Older-aged dance participants with Parkinson's disease have shown improvements in mobility, reduced tremors, and improved social outreach. Dance for Parkinson's disease is an international program that began in New York and has spread to many countries. It offers dance as a means of enhancing the quality of life and improving symptoms in people with Parkinson's disease.

A study published in the *New England Journal of Medicine* examined physical and cognitive activities associated with a reduced risk of developing Alzheimer's disease. Researchers found that cognitive activities such as reading, playing board games, and playing musical instruments were associated with a lower risk of dementia. However, of 11 physical activities, "dancing was the only physical activity associated with a lower risk of dementia" (Verghese et al., 2003).

A comprehensive review of the neurobiology of dance found that dancing triggers the release of reward-related neurotransmitters, including endorphins and opioids. Dance, like all physical exercise, enhances immunoreactivity and improves caloric equilibrium, coordination, muscle tone, and cardiovascular health (Minton and

Mental Health and Healthy Aging

Faber, 2016). In addition, dance practice provides strong psychobiological learning opportunities. In this regard, dance provides socioemotional coping skills to increase self-confidence and boost self-esteem.

THE ARTS

Music

Music therapy has been found to improve anxiety and depression and enhance cognition in Alzheimer's patients (de La Rubia Ortí et al., 2018). Music played while patients are in intensive care units has been found to abate the stress response, decrease anxiety during mechanical ventilation, and induce an overall relaxation response without the use of medication. Music may also improve sleep quality and reduce patients' pain with a subsequent decrease in sedative exposure, leading to an accelerated ventilator weaning process and a speedier recovery (Mofredj et al., 2016).

Findings from multiple studies that have been recently reviewed show that patients with severe mental illness, including difficulties in expression and communication, obtained benefits when they participated in music therapy programs.

Art & Art Therapy

In a systematic review of art therapy and mental health, Uttley et al. (2015) reported the following:

Depression: Among nine studies examining depression, art therapy resulted in a significant reduction in depression in six studies. In four of these six studies, art therapy was significantly more effective than the control.

Anxiety: Among seven studies examining anxiety, art therapy resulted in a significant reduction in anxiety in six studies. In these six studies, art therapy was significantly more effective than the control.

Mood: Among four studies examining mood or affect, art therapy resulted in significant positive improvements in mood in three studies. In these three studies, art therapy was significantly more effective than control.

Trauma: Among three studies examining trauma, art therapy resulted in a significant reduction in symptoms of trauma in all studies. While trauma improved from baseline, there was no significant difference between the art therapy and control groups in any of the three studies.

Distress: Among three studies examining distress, art therapy resulted in a significant reduction in distress in all studies. In two studies, art therapy was significantly more effective than the control group.

Quality of life: In four studies examining the quality of life, art therapy resulted in significant improvements to some but not all components of the quality-of-life measures in all studies. In all studies, art therapy was significantly more effective than control.

Coping: Among three studies examining coping, art therapy resulted in significant improvements to coping resources in all studies. In one study, art therapy was significantly more effective than control. In another study, there was no difference between groups. In the third study, significant differences between the art therapy and control groups were not reported.

Cognition: In one study examining cognition, the control group (simple calculations) exhibited significant improvements in cognitive function relative to the art therapy group.

Self-esteem: In one study examining self-esteem, art therapy resulted in significant improvements in self-esteem relative to the control group.

SOCIAL SUPPORT

Aging is associated with an increased reliance on health-related and support services. Old age often goes hand in hand with increasingly complex and often interrelated problems, encompassing physical, psychological, and social health.

A study comparing the elderly in two provinces in East Asia (Tainan in Taipei, China, and Fuzhou in the People's Republic of China) found that participants identified children as the most important source of objective and subjective support, followed by spouse and relatives (Dai et al., 2016).

Tainan's elderly received more daily life assistance and emotional support, showed stronger awareness of the need to seek help, and maintained a higher frequency of social interactions compared with the elderly in Fuzhou. The mean objective support, subjective support, and support utilization scores as well as the overall social support among Tainan's elderly were significantly high compared with the scores among Fuzhou's elderly. Correlation analysis showed that social support was significantly correlated with the city, age, living conditions, marital status, and self-rated health.

NATURE AND THE ENVIRONMENT

Exercise for older people in the outdoors, where vitamin D, fresh air, and the benefits of being in nature all contribute toward enhanced mental well-being, has not been well researched.

Being in nature as a means of restoring mental well-being is not new in Asia. The master of Chinese medicine, Sun Simiao, advised that fresh air, daily walks in natural landscapes, and food from a fresh and wholesome garden—cultivated in part by the owner—were the fundamentals of creating and maintaining good health. Sun Simiao was born around 581 CE and died in 682 CE after completing his 30-volume *Encyclopedia of Medicine*, the first few volumes of which were not dedicated to medicine at all but to lifestyle, diet, and exercise. The Chinese poet and scholar Tao Yuanming, later known as Tao Qian (365–427), resigned his post as a civil administrator and chose a life of poetry, farming, family, friendships, wine, and, above all, a connection with the deep pulse of life, which is known in Chinese tradition as the Tao. Both Sun Simiao and Tao Qian have become Chinese icons of an ideal life in nature.

The ancient Indian tradition of going to the Himalayas for cold water bathing and doing morning exercises with the rising sun also have their roots in the healing power of nature and in humans balancing their lives by connecting with nature.

Mental Health and Healthy Aging

In Japan, there is the tradition of *shinrin-yoku*, a term that means "taking in the forest atmosphere" or "forest bathing." The group Shinrin-Yoku.org lists the effects of *shinrin yoku* as:

(i) boosted immune system functioning, with an increase in the count of the body's natural killer cells; (ii) reduced blood pressure; (iii) reduced stress; (iv) improved mood; (v) increased ability to focus, even in children with attention deficit hyperactivity disorder; (vi) accelerated recovery from surgery or illness; (vii) increased energy levels; and (viii) improved sleep.

People tend to live longer when they have access to green space, and perceived neighborhood greenness is strongly associated with better mental and physical health. Those living in highly green areas are much more likely to have better physical and mental health than those living near open areas that are not highly green (Park et al., 2010).

JAPAN'S IKIGAI

In Japan, *ikigai* is written by combining the kanji characters that mean "life" with "to be worthwhile." *Ikigai* is a Japanese concept that means "reason for being." It is the heart of things, the motivation at the center of our existence: the source of value in a person's life or the things that make them put one foot in front of the other each day.

Two Western researchers, Héctor García and Francesc Miralles, identified the characteristics and principles of Japanese who live longer with happiness. Their book *Ikigai: The Japanese Secret to a Long and Happy Life* defines the rules of *ikigai.* The authors conducted a total of 100 interviews in Ogimi, Okinawa, to try to understand the longevity secrets of centenarians and supercentenarians. They write, "What do Japanese artisans, engineers, Zen philosophy, and cuisine have in common? Simplicity and attention to detail" (García and Miralles, 2016).

A deep connection with, and appreciation for, *ikigai* is one probable reason for the remarkable longevity of the Japanese, particularly those residing in Okinawa. Here, there are 24.55 people over the age of 100 for every 100,000 inhabitants, far more than the worldwide average. The authors speculate that there are many factors that might collude to explain Okinawa's disproportionate populace of centenarians: their uncommon sense of community; a nonexclusionary sense of oneness wherein even strangers are treated like brothers; access to lush hills and crystalline waters; Moringa tea; a light, nutritious diet; and moderate exercise, even after retirement (Water for Health, 2019).

JAPAN'S ONE HUNDRED YEAR LIFE PROGRAM

Tomonori Maruyama has pointed out in his chapter in this book that in Japan, there is a gap of about 10 years between "healthy life span" and "average life span." He notes that Japanese people spend most of their medical expenses in the 10-year period between healthy life span and average life span, placing a considerable and growing pressure on the health system and the national budget as life span increases for the Japanese population. Accordingly, Japan has introduced a One Hundred Year

Life Program to promote wellness and a healthy life across the life span, which is being addressed cross-sectorally in Japan. During the 100-year life, there is a need to continually reskill because having a single skill or ordinary skills will not help us traverse a long life. The new approach is to acquire new skills and knowledge as people progress through life.

While the Japanese model necessarily reflects social and economic specifics unique to Japan, the idea of a life span approach to wellness stands as a model for the rest of Asia to look into and draw from.

BIBLIOGRAPHY

Adulyadej, B. (1999a) 'The practice of the arts of healing act B.E. 2542', *The Royal Thai Gazette*, 116 Article(39a), pp. 1–6.

Adulyadej, B. (1999b) *The Protection and Promotion of Thai Traditional Medicine Wisdom Act B.E. 2542, Thai Royal Gazette*. Available at: https://thailawonline.com/fr/thai-laws/laws-of-thailand/301-protection-and-promotion-of-traditional-thai-medicine-wisdom-act-be-2542-1999-.html (Accessed: 10 September 2020).

Afshar, S. et al. (2015) 'Multi-morbidity and the inequalities of global ageing: A cross-sectional study of 28 countries using the World Health Surveys', *BMC Public Health*, 15(776). doi: 10.1186/s12889-015-2008-7.

Aizenstein, H. J. et al. (2016) 'Vascular depression consensus report - a critical update', *BMC Medicine*, 14(1), pp. 1–16. doi: 10.1186/s12916-016-0720-5.

Al-Hashel, J. Y. et al. (2018) 'Use of traditional medicine for primary headache disorders in Kuwait', *Journal of Headache and Pain*, 19(1), pp. 3–9. doi: 10.1186/s10194-018-0950-3.

Al-Kindi, R. et al. (2011) 'Complementary and Alternative Medicine use among adults with diabetes in Muscat region, Oman', *Sultan Qaboos University Medical Journal*, 11(1), p. 62.

Al-Rowais, N. et al. (2010) 'Traditional healers in riyadh region: Reasons and health problems for seeking their advice. A household survey', *Journal of Alternative and Complementary Medicine*, 16(2), pp. 199–204. doi: 10.1089/acm.2009.0283.

Al Thiab Al Kendi, A. (2014) *Health and Medicall Care in the First Hijri Century (1–101 AH/ 622–719 AD)*. National Center for Complementary and Alternative Medicine. Kuala Lumpur: DTP Enterprise Sdn. Bhd.

Ang, J. Y. et al. (2021) 'A Malaysian retrospective study of acupuncture-assisted anesthesia in breast lump excision', *Acupuncture in Medicine*, 39(1), pp. 64–68. doi: 10.1177/0964528420920307.

Antman, F. (2012) 'How does adult child migration affect the health of elderly parents left behind? Evidence from Mexico', *SSRN Electronic Journal*. doi: 10.2139/ssrn.1578465.

Ao, X., Jiang, D. and Zhao, Z. (2016) 'The impact of rural-urban migration on the health of the left-behind parents', *China Economic Review*, 37, pp. 126–139. doi: 10.1016/j.chieco.2015.09.007.

Awad, A. I., Al-Ajmi, S. and Waheedi, M. A. (2012) 'Knowledge, perceptions and attitudes toward complementary and alternative therapies among Kuwaiti medical and pharmacy students', *Medical Principles and Practice*, 21(4), pp. 350–354. doi: 10.1159/000336216.

Barcella, C. A. et al. (2021) 'Severe mental illness is associated with increased mortality and severe course of COVID-19', *Acta Psychiatrica Scandinavica*, (March), pp. 1–10. doi: 10.1111/acps.13309.

Bernama. (2020) *Malaysia's Population Estimates at 32.7 million in 2020, Astro Awani*. Available at: http://english.astroawani.com/malaysia-news/malaysias-population-estimates-32-7-million-2020-251323 (Accessed: 15 July 2020).

Bhandari, H. and Yasunobu, K. (2009) 'What is social capital? A comprehensive review of the concept', *Asian Journal of Social Science*, 37(3). doi: 10.1163/156853109X436847.

Bodeker, G. and Kronenberg, F. (2015) 'Tackling obesity: Challenges ahead', *The Lancet*, 386(9995), pp. 740–741. doi: 10.1016/S0140-6736(15)61539-2.

Bodeker, G. et al. (2018) *Mental Wellness: Pathways, Evidence, Horizons*. Edited by G. Bodeker. Miami, FL: Global Wellness Institute.

Boden-Albala, B., Litwak, E., Elkind, M.S., Rundek, T. and Sacco, R.L. (2005) 'Social isolation and outcomes post stroke', *Neurology*, 64(11), pp. 1888–1892. doi: 10.1212/01. WNL.0000163510.79351.AF. PMID: 15955939.

Böhme, M. H., Persian, R. and Stöhr, T. (2015) 'Alone but better off? Adult child migration and health of elderly parents in Moldova', *Journal of Health Economics*, 39, pp. 211–227. doi: 10.1016/j.jhealeco.2014.09.001.

Bowman, G. L. et al. (2012) 'Nutrient biomarker patterns, cognitive function, and MRI measures of brain aging', *Neurology*, 78(4), pp. 241–249. doi: 10.1212/WNL.0b013e3182436598.

Brooks, S. J. et al. (2020) 'The psychologial impact of quarantine and how to reduce it: Rapid review of the evidence', *The Lancet*, 295(10227), pp. 912–920.

Byrow, Y. et al. (2020) 'Perceptions of mental health and perceived barriers to mental health help-seeking amongst refugees: A systematic review', *Clinical Psychology Review*, 75(July 2018), p. 101812. doi: 10.1016/j.cpr.2019.101812.

Chan, J., To, H. P. and Chan, E. (2006) 'Reconsidering social cohesion: Developing a definition and analytical framework for empirical research', *Social Indicators Research*, 75(2), pp. 273–302. doi: 10.1007/s11205-005-2118-1.

Chang, F. et al. (2016) 'Adult child migration and elderly parental health in rural China', *China Agricultural Economic Review*, 8(4), pp. 677–697. doi: 10.1108/CAER-11-2015-0169.

Chen, M. et al. (2020) 'Prescribing antibiotics in rural China: The influence of capital on clinical realities', *Frontiers in Sociology*, 5(October), pp. 0–10. doi: 10.3389/fsoc.2020.00066.

Chokevivat, V. and Chuthaputti, A. (2005) 'The role of Thai traditional medicine in health promotion', in *Department for the Development of Thai Traditional and Alternative Medicine*, pp. 1–25. Available at: http://citeseerx.ist.psu.edu/viewdoc/download?doi=10.1.1.496.5656&rep=rep1&type=pdf.

Chong, S. A. et al. (2016) 'Recognition of mental disorders among a multiracial population in Southeast Asia', *BMC Psychiatry*, 16(1). doi: 10.1186/s12888-016-0837-2.

CIA. (2020) *The World Factobook*. Available at: https://www.cia.gov/library/publications/the-world-factbook/fields/223rank.html.

Coburn D (2000) 'Income inequality, social cohesion, and the health status of populations.', *Social Science and Medicine*, 51, pp. 135–146.

Crawford Shearer, N. B., Fleury, J. D. and Belyea, M. (2010) 'An innovative approach to recruiting homebound older adults', *Research in Gerontological Nursing*, 3(1), pp. 11–17. doi: 10.3928/19404921-20091029-01.

Crosette, B. (1986) Vietnamese revive ancient medical arts. *The New York Times*. Available at: https://www.nytimes.com/1986/08/12/science/vietnamese-revive-ancient-medical-arts.html (Accessed: 16 October 2020).

Crunfli, F. et al. (2021) 'SARS-CoV-2 infects brain astrocytes of COVID-19 patients and impairs neuronal viability', *medRxiv*, pp. 2020-10. doi: 10.1101/2020.10.09.20207464.

Dai, Y. et al. (2016) 'Social Support and self-rated health of older people: A comparative study in Tainan Taiwan and Fuzhou Fujian Province', *Medicine*, 95(24), p. 3881. doi: 10.1097/MD.0000000000003881.

De La Rubia Ortí, J. E. et al. (2018) 'Does Music Therapy Improve Anxiety and Depression in Alzheimer's Patients?', *Journal of Alternative and Complementary Medicine*, 24(1), pp. 33–36. doi: 10.1089/acm.2016.0346.

Department of AYUSH. (2012) *Ayurveda: The Science of Life*, in Ramesh Babu, Katoch, D.C. Padhi, M.M. (eds.) Department of AYUSH. New Delhi: Ministry of Health & Family Welfare, Government of India. ISBN: 971-81-906489-0-5. www.indianmedicine.nic.in

Department of Statistics. (2020) *Current Population Estimates, Malaysia, Online*. Available at: https://www.dosm.gov.my/v1/index.php?r=column/cthemeByCat&cat=155&bul_id=OVByWjg5YkQ3MWFZRTN5bDJiaEVhZz09&menu_id=L0pheU43NWJwRWVSZklWdzQ4TlhUUT09 (Accessed: 22 February 2021).

Douaud, G. et al. (2013) 'Preventing Alzheimer's disease-related gray matter atrophy by B-vitamin treatment', *Proceedings of the National Academy of Sciences of the United States of America*, 110(23), pp. 9523–9528. doi: 10.1073/pnas.1301816110.

Engelhardt, U. (2000) 'Longevity techniques and Chinese medicine', in Stephen, T., Martin, K., Timothy, B., and Paul, W. K. (Eds.) *Handbook of Oriental Studies. Section 4 China*. Leiden: Brill, pp. 74–108. https://doi.org/10.1163/9789004391840_005.

Fasullo, L., Hernandez, A. and Bodeker, G. (2020) 'The innate human potential of elevated and ecstatic states of consciousness: Examining freeform dance as a means of access', *Dance, Movement & Spiritualities*, 6(1–2), pp. 87–117. doi: 10.1386/dmas_00005_1.

Fields, G. and Song, Y. (2020) 'Modeling migration barriers in a two-sector framework: A welfare analysis of the hukou reform in China', *Economic Modelling*, 84(59), pp. 293–301. doi: 10.1016/j.econmod.2019.04.019.

Fotoukian, Z. et al. (2014) 'Concept analysis of empowerment in old people with chronic diseases using a hybrid model', *Asian Nursing Research*, 8(2), pp. 118–127. doi: 10.1016/j.anr.2014.04.002.

Fu, S., Huang, N. and Chou, Y.-J. (2014) 'Trends in the prevalence of multiple chronic conditions in Taiwan From 2000 to 2010: A population-based study'. doi: 10.5888/pcd11.140205.

Fujikawa, Y. (1904) *Nihon igakushi (History of Japanese Medicine)*. Tokyo: Shokabo, 1036 pp.

Galderisi, S. et al. (2015) 'Toward a new defition of mental health', *World Psychiatry*, 14(2), p. 231.

García, H. and Miralles, F. (2016) *IKIGAI. The Japanese Secret to a Long and Happy Life*. New York : Penguin Books.

Google. (2020) *Singapore Ethnic Composition in 2019, Online*. Available at: https://www.google.com.my/search?q=singapore+ethnic+composition+in+2019&tbm=isch&ved=2ahUKEwiy6OHQs5DsAhVJB3IKHWjwCukQ2-cCegQIABAA&oq=singapore+ethnic+composition+in+2019&gs_lcp=CgNpbWcQAzoECAAQGFDp2gFYg8kCYPzNAmgAcAB4AIABXIgBrgqSAQIyOJgBAKABAaoBC2d3cyl3a (Accessed: 30 September 2020).

Hansa Jayadeva, S. (2010) *Yoga Teacher's Manual for School Teachers*. New Delhi: Morarji Desai National Institute of Yoga, Ministry of AYUSH.

Hu, Y. and Shi, X. (2020) 'The impact of China's one-child policy on intergenerational and gender relations', *Contemporary Social Science*, 15(3), pp. 360–377. doi: 10.1080/21582041.2018.1448941.

Huang, B., Lian, Y. and Li, W. (2016) 'How far is Chinese left-behind parents' health left behind?', *China Economic Review*, 37(71002056), pp. 15–26. doi: 10.1016/j.chieco.2015.07.002.

Huang, C. and Li, Y. (2019) 'Understanding leisure satisfaction of Chinese seniors: human capital, family capital, and community capital', *Journal of Chinese Sociology*, 6(1). doi: 10.1186/s40711-019-0094-0.

Huang, Y. and Liu, X. (2015) 'Improvement of balance control ability and flexibility in the elderly Tai Chi Chuan (TCC) practitioners: A systematic review and meta-analysis', *Archives of Gerontology and Geriatrics*, 60(2), pp. 233–238. doi: 10.1016/j.archger.2014.10.016.

Mental Health and Healthy Aging

Ibrahim, I. et al. (2016) 'A qualitative insight on complementary and alternative medicines used by hypertensive patients', *Journal of Pharmacology and Bioallied Science*, 8(4), pp. 284–288.

Institute for Public Health. (2015) *National Health and Morbidity Survey 2015: Traditional and Complementary Medicine, Ministry of Health Malaysia*. Putrajaya: Ministry of Health.

Institute for Public Health. (2020) *National Health and Morbidity Survey 2019: Non-Communicable Diseases, Health Demand, and Health Literacy - Key Findings*. Available at: http://iku.gov.my/images/IKU/Document/REPORT/NHMS2019/Fact_Sheet_NHMS_2019-English.pdf.

Institute of Medicine (US) Committe on the Use of Complementary and Alternative Medicine by the American Public. (2005) *Complementary Alternative Medicine in the United States*. Washington, DC. Available at: https://www.ncbi.nlm.nih.gov/books/NBK83804/.

Jaiswal, Y. and Williams, L. (2017) 'A glimpse of Ayurveda – The forgotten history and principles of Indian traditional medicine', *Journal of Traditional and Complementary Medicine*, 7(1), pp. 50–53. doi: 10.1016/j.jtcme.2016.02.002.

John W Brick Foundation (2021) *Move You Mental Wellness*. Available at: www.johnwbrick-foundation.org/move-your-mental-health-report/ (Accessed: 24 June 2021).

Kadetz, P. (2018) 'Collective efficacy, social capital and resilience: An inquiry into the relationship between social infrastructure and resilience after Hurricane Katrina', in Michael, Z., Nancy, M., Paul, K. (eds.) *Creating Katrina, Rebuilding Resilience*, 1st Edition. Oxford: Butterworth-Heinemann, pp. 283–304. Paperback ISBN: 9780128095577, eBook ISBN: 9780128095621.

Kalil, A. (2020) 'Treating COVID-19 Off-label drug use, compassionate use, and randomized clinical trials during pandemics', *Journal of the American Medical Association*, 323(19), pp. 1897–8.

Kavadar, G. et al. (2019) 'Use of traditional and complementary medicine for musculoskeletal diseases', *Turkish Journal of Medical Sciences*, 49(3), pp. 809–814. doi: 10.3906/sag-1509-71.

Kawachi, I. et al. (2004) 'Commentary: Reconciling the three accounts of social capital', *International Journal of Epidemiology*, 33(4), pp. 682–690. doi: 10.1093/ije/dyh177.

Keshet, Y. and Popper-Giveon, A. (2013) 'Integrative health care in israel and traditional arab herbal medicine: When health care interfaces with culture and politics', *Medical Anthropology Quarterly*, 27(3), pp. 368–384. doi: 10.1111/maq.12049.

Khalaf, A. J. and Whitford, D. L. (2008) 'The use of complementary and alternative medicine by patients with osteoporosis', *Nature Clinical Practice Endocrinology and Metabolism*, 4(3), p. 120. doi: 10.1038/ncpendmet0732.

Kuhn, R., Everett, B. and Silvey, R. (2011) 'The effects of children's migration on Elderly Kin's health: A counterfactual approach', *Demography*, 48(1), pp. 183–209. doi: 10.1007/s13524-010-0002–3.

Lauber, C. and Rössler, W. (2007) 'Stigma towards people with mental illness in developing countries in Asia', *International Review of Psychiatry*, 19(2), pp. 157–178. doi: 10.1080/09540260701278903.

Lee, D. Y. W. et al. (2021) 'Traditional Chinese herbal medicine at the forefront battle against COVID-19: Clinical experience and scientific basis', *Phytomedicine*, 80(September 2020), p. 153337. doi: 10.1016/j.phymed.2020.153337.

Lei, X. et al. (2014) 'Depressive symptoms and SES among the mid-aged and elderly in China: Evidence from the China health and retirement longitudinal study national baseline', *Social Science and Medicine*, 120, pp. 224–232. doi: 10.1016/j.socscimed.2014.09.028.

Lei, Y. et al. (2021) 'SARS-CoV-2 Spike Protein impairs endothelial function via downregulation of ACE 2', *Circulation Research*, 128, pp. 1323–1326.

Lhamo, N. and Nebel, S. (2011) 'Perceptions and attitudes of Bhutanese people on Sowa Rigpa, traditional bhutanese medicine: A preliminary study from Thimphu', *Journal of Ethnobiology and Ethnomedicine*, 7(January), pp. 1–9. doi: 10.1186/1746-4269-7-3.

Li, C. et al. (2020) 'Discussion on TCM theory and modern pharmacological mechanism of Qinfei Paidu decoction in the treatment of COVID-19', *Journal of Traditional Chinese Medicine*, pp. 1–4.

Li, T. et al. (2020) 'What happens to the health of elderly parents when adult child migration splits households? Evidence from rural China', *International Journal of Environmental Research and Public Health*, 17(5). doi: 10.3390/ijerph17051609.

Li, X. et al. (2020) 'Quality of primary health care in China: challenges and recommendations', *The Lancet*, 395(10239), pp. 1802–1812. doi: 10.1016/S0140-6736(20)30122-7.

Lo, V. (2001) 'The influence of nurturing life culture on early Chinese medical theory', in Hsu, E. (ed.) *Innovation in Chinese medicine*. Cambridge: Cambridge University Press, pp. 19–50.

Logue, J. K. et al. (2021) 'Sequelae in Adults at 6 Months after COVID-19 Infection', *JAMA Network Open*, 4(2), pp. 8–11. doi: 10.1001/jamanetworkopen.2021.0830.

Luo, H. et al. (2020) 'Reflections on treatment of COVID-19 with traditional Chinese medicine', *Chinese Medicine (United Kingdom)*, 15(1), pp. 1–14. doi: 10.1186/s13020-020-00375-1.

Ma, Z. and Zhou, G. (2009) 'Isolated or compensated: The impact of temporary migration of adult children on the wellbeing of the elderly in rural China', *Geographical review of Japan series B*, 81(1), pp. 47–59. doi: 10.4157/geogrevjapanb.81.47.

Ma, X., He, Y. and Xu, J. (2020) 'Urban-rural disparity in prevalence of multimorbidity in China: A cross-sectional nationally representative study', *BMJ Open*, 10(11), pp. 1–9. doi: 10.1136/bmjopen–2020–038404.

Malaysian Government. (2016) *The Traditional and Complementary Medicine Act 2016*. Putrajaya: Ministry of Health, Government of Malaysia.

Mauss, M. (2002) *The Gift: The Form and Reason for Exchange in Archaic Societies*. London: Routledge.

Miller, V. et al. (2017) 'Prospective Urban Rural Epidemiology (PURE) study investigators. Fruit, vegetable, and legume intake, and cardiovascular disease and deaths in 18 countries: A prospective cohort study.', *The Lancet*, 390(10107), pp. 2037–2049.

Ministry of AYUSH. (2015) *Homeopathy: Science of Gentle Healing*. New Delhi: Ministry of AYUSH, Government of India.

Ministry of AYUSH. (2016) *Unani System of Medicine: The Science of Health and Healing*. New Delhi: Government of India.

Ministry of AYUSH. (2019) *Introduction to Sowa-Rigpa, About the Systems*.

Ministry of Health and National Institute of Health Research and Development. (2018) *National Report on Basic Health Research, Riskesdas, 2018*. Jakarta.

Ministry of Health Turkey. (2016) *Traditioal and Complementary Medicine Practices and Related Legislation*. Ankara: Government of Turkey.

Ministry of Health Turkey. (2020) *What is Traditiona and Complementary Medicine, Traditional, Complementary and Functional Medicine Practices, Department*.

Minton, S. and Faber, R. (2016) *Thinking with the Dancing Brain: Embodying Neuroscience*. Lanham, MD: Rowman and Littlefield.

Mofredj, A. et al. (2016) 'Music therapy, a review of the potential therapeutic benefits for the critically ill', *Journal of Critical Care*, 35, pp. 195–199. doi: 10.1016/j.jcrc.2016.05.021.

Mohanty, S., Sharma, P. and Sharma, G. (2020) 'Yoga for infirmity in geriatric population amidst COVID-19 pandemic: Comment on age and ageism in COVID-19: Elderly mental health-care vulnerabilities and needs', *Asian Journal of Psychiatry*, 53, p. 102199.

Moreno, C. et al. (2020) 'How mental health care should change as a consequence of the COVID-19 pandemic', *Lancet Psychiatry*, 7(9), pp. 813–824. doi: 10.1016/S2215-0366(20)30307-2.

Nadareishvili, I. et al. (2019) 'Georgia's healthcare system and integration of complementary medicine', *Complementary Therapies in Medicine*, 45, pp. 205–210. doi: 10.1016/j.ctim.2019.06.016. Epub 2019 Jul 2. PMID: 31331562.

National Institute on Aging. (2011) Global health and aging. doi: 10.1016/j.ctim.2019.06.016.

Nagasu, M., Muto, K. and Yamamoto, I. (2021) 'Impacts of anxiety and socioeconomic factors on mental health in the early phases of the COVID-19 pandemic in the general population in Japan: A web-based survey', *PLoS ONE*, 16(3 March), pp. 1–19. doi: 10.1371/journal.pone.0247705.

National Health Services. (2018) *A Guide to Tai Chi, NHS UK*. UK. Available at: http://www.nhs.uk/Livewell/fitness/Pages/taichi.aspx (Accessed: 24 June 2021).

Nutbeam, D. and Kickbusch, I. (1998) 'Health promotion glossary', *Health Promotion International*, 13(4), pp. 349–364. doi: 10.1093/heapro/13.4.349.

Ogbo, F. A. et al. (2018) 'The burden of depressive disorders in South Asia, 1990–2016: findings from the global burden of disease study', *BMC Psychiatry*, 18(1), pp. 1–11. doi: 10.1186/s12888-018-1918-1.

Ozer, O., Santaş, F. and Yildirim, H. H. (2012) 'An evaluation on levels of knowledge, attitude and behavior of people at 65 years and above about alternative medicine living in Ankara', *African Journal of Traditional, Complementary, and Alternative Medicines : AJTCAM / African Networks on Ethnomedicines*, 10(1), pp. 134–141. doi: 10.4314/ajtcam.v10i1.18.

Pang, W. et al. (2020) 'Chinese herbal medicine for coronavirus disease 2019: A systematic review and meta-analysis', *Integrative Medicine Research* 9, 160(March), p. 100477. doi: 10.1016/j.phrs.2020.105056.

Park, H. (2003) *North Korea Handbook*. Yonhap News Agency. Available at: https://books.google.com.my/books?id=JI1h9nNeadMC&pg=PA439&lpg=PA439&dq=KORYO+MEDICINE&source=bl&ots=gy-.

Park, B. J. et al. (2010) 'The physiological effects of Shinrin-yoku (taking in the forest atmosphere or forest bathing): Evidence from field experiments in 24 forests across Japan', *Environmental Health and Preventive Medicine*, 15(1), pp. 18–26. doi: 10.1007/s12199-009-0086-9.

Patel, V. et al. (2018) 'The Lancet Commission on global mental health and sustainable development', *The Lancet*, 392(10157), pp. 1553–1598. doi: 10.1016/S0140-6736(18)31612-X.

Pusan National University School of Korean Medicine. (2015) *Korean Medicine: Current Status and Future Prospects*. Pusan: Pusan National University School of Korean Medicine.

Putnam, R., Leonardi, R. and Nanetti, R. (1993) *What Makes Democracy Work: Civic Traditions in Modern Italy*, Princeton: Princeton University Press. ISBN 9780691037387.

Ravishankar, B. and Shukla, V. J. (2007) 'Indian systems of medicine: A brief review', *Arfrican Journal of Traditional, Complementary and Alternative Medicine*, 4(3), pp. 319–337.

Republic of Phillipines. (1997) *Traditional and Alternative Medicine Act of 1997*.

Reyburn, S. (2019) *Rosa Parks: In her own words*. Atlanta: University of Georgia Press.

Roca, C. P. and Helbing, D. (2011) 'Emergence of social cohesion in a model society of greedy, mobile individuals', *Proceedings of the National Academy of Sciences of the United States of America*, 108(28), pp. 11370–11374. doi: 10.1073/pnas.1101044108.

Sarris, J. et al. (2015) 'Nutritional medicine as mainstream in psychiatry', *The Lancet Psychiatry*, 2(3), pp. 271–274. doi: 10.1016/S2215-0366(14)00051-0.

Scheffel, J. and Zhang, Y. (2019) 'How does internal migration affect the emotional health of elderly parents left-behind?', *Journal of Population Economics*, 32(3), pp. 953–980. doi: 10.1007/s00148-018-0715-y.

Shengelia, R. (1999) 'Study of the history of medicine in Georgia', *Croatian Medical Journal*, 40(1), pp. 38–41.

Shi, N. et al. (2021) 'Efficacy and safety of Chinese herbal medicine versus Lopinavir-Ritonavir in adult patients with coronavirus disease 2019: A non-randomized controlled trial', *Phytomedicine*, 81(January). doi: 10.1016/j.phymed.2020.153367.

Shih, C. C. et al. (2015) 'Use of folk therapy in Taiwan: A nationwide cross-sectional survey of prevalence and associated factors', *Evidence-based Complementary and Alternative Medicine*, 2015. doi: 10.1155/2015/649265.

Shuval, J. T. and Averbuch, E. (2012) 'Complementary and alternative health care in Israel', *Israel Journal of Health Policy Research*, 1(1), pp. 1–12. doi: 10.1186/2045-4015-1-7.

Song, Y. (2014) 'Mental support or economic giving: migrating children's elderly care behaviour and health conditions of left-behind elderly in rural China', *Population and Developemtn*, 20(4), pp. 37–44.

Song, L. et al. (2007) 'Effects of a sun style Tai Chi exercise on arthritic symptoms, motivation and performance of health behaviours in women with osteoarthritis', *Taehan Kanho Hakhoe chi*, 37(2), pp. 249–256.

Stickley, A. et al. (2013) 'Prevalence and factors associated with the use of alternative (folk) medicine practitioners in 8 countries of the former Soviet Union', *BMC Complementary and Alternative Medicine*, 13(83). doi: 10.1186/1472-6882-13-83.

Subramanian, S. V., Kim, D. J. and Kawachi, I. (2002) 'Social trust and self-rated health in US communities: A multilevel analysis', *Journal of Urban Health*, 79(1), pp. 21–34. doi: 10.1093/jurban/79.suppl_1.s21.

Thas, J. J. (2008) 'Siddha Medicine-background and principles and the application for skin diseases', *Clinics in Dermatology*, 26(1), pp. 62–78. doi: 10.1016/j.clindermatol.2007. 11.010.

The Law Commission Revisions. (2015) *The Statutes of the Republic of Singapore - Copyright Act*. Singapore: Government of Singapore.

The State Council Information Office (2016) *Traditional Chinese Medicine in China*. Available at: http://english.www.gov.cn/archive/white_paper/2016/12/06/content_281 475509333700.htm.

Thompson, N. and Thompson, S. (2001) 'Empowering older people', *Journal of Social Work*, 1(1), pp. 61–76.

Tiemeier, H. (2003) 'Biological risk factors for late life depression', *European Journal of Epidemiology*, 18(8), pp. 745–750. Available at: http://ovidsp.ovid.com/ovidweb.cgi?T= JS&PAGE=reference&D=emed6&NEWS=N&AN=2003347329.

Traditional and Complementary Medicine. (2020) *Guidelines for Registration of Traditional and Complementary Medicine Practitioners in Brunei Darussalam, Ministry of Health Brunei*. Brunei: Government of Brunei.

Traditional and Complementary Medicine Division. (2007) *National Policy on Traditional/ Complementary Medicine, Malaysia*. 2nd edn. Putrajaya: Ministry of Health.

Tse, C. (2013) *Migration and Health Outcomes of Left-Behind Elderly in Rural China. Available at SSRN 2440403*.

United Nations. (2016) *ESCAP Population Data Sheet Population and Development Indicators for Asia and the Pacific, 2012*. Available at: https://www.unescap.org/sites/ default/d8files/knowledge-products/SPPS PS data sheet 2016 v15-2.pdf.

United Nations. (2020) *Policy Brief: The Impact of COVID-19 on Older Person, Online2*. Available at: https://www.un.org/development/desa/ageing/wp-content/uploads/ sites/24/2020/05/COVID-Older-persons.pdf (Accessed: 5 June 2021).

Uttley, L. et al. (2015) 'Systematic review and economic modelling of the clinical effectiveness and cost-effectiveness of art therapy among people with non-psychotic mental health disorders', *Health Technology Assessment*, 19(18). doi: 10.3310/hta19180.

Valtorta, N.K., Moore, D.C., Barron, L., Stow, D., Hanratty, B. (2018) 'Older Adults' Social Relationships and Health Care Utilization: A Systematic Review'. *American Journal of Public Health*, 108(4):e1–e10. doi: 10.2105/AJPH.2017.304256. Epub 2018 Feb 22. PMID: 29470115; PMCID: PMC5844393.

Verghese, J. et al. (2003) 'Leisure activities and the risk of dementia in the elderly', *The New England Journal of Medicine*, 348, pp. 2508–2516.

Wang, H. et al. (2009) 'The flip-side of social capital: The distinctive influences of trust and mistrust on health in rural China', *Social Science and Medicine*, 68(1), pp. 133–142. doi: 10.1016/j.socscimed.2008.09.038.

Watanabe, K. et al. (2011) 'Traditional Japanese Kampo medicine: Clinical research between modernity and traditional medicine - The state of research and methodological suggestions for the future', *Evidence-Based Complementary and Alternative Medicine*, 2011. doi: 10.1093/ecam/neq067.

Water for Health. (2019) *Ten Rules of Ikigai: A Blueprint for a Fuller, Healthier Life?* Online. Available at: Water for Health (Accessed: 24 June 2021).

Wen, M., Browning, C. R. and Cagney, K. A. (2003) 'Poverty, affluence, and income inequality: Neighborhood economic structure and its implications for health', *Social Science and Medicine*, 57(5), pp. 843–860. doi: 10.1016/S0277-9536(02)00457-4.

WHO. (2002a) *WHO Traditional Medicine Strategy 2002–2005*. Geneva, Switzerland: WHO.

WHO. (2002b) *Active Ageing: A Policy Framework*.

WHO. (2009) *WHO Guidelines on Hand Hygiene in Health Care*. Available at: https://www.ncbi.nlm.nih.gov/books/NBK144013/pdf/Bookshelf_NBK144013.pdf.

WHO. (2013) *WHO Traditional Medicine Strategy*. Geneva, Switzerland: WHO.

WHO. (2017) *Depression and Other Common Mental Disorders: Global Health Estimates*. Geneva, Switzerland. Available at: https://apps.who.int/iris/bitstream/handle/10665/254610/WHO-MSD-MER-2017.2-eng.pdf.

WHO. (2018a) *Mental Health Atlas 2017*. Geneva, Switzerland: WHO.

WHO. (2018b) *Traditional, Complementary and Integrative Medicine, WHO TM Strategy*. Available at: https://www.who.int/health-topics/traditional-complementary-and-integrative-medicine#tab=tab_1 (Accessed: 30 August 2020).

WHO. (2019) *WHO Global Report on Traditional and Complementary Medicine 2019*. Geneva, Switzerland: WHO.

WHO. (2020a) *COVID-19 Strategy Update, Online*. Geneva, Switzerland: WHO.

WHO. (2020b) *Nutrition for Older Persons, Online*. Available at: https://www.who.int/nutrition/topics/ageing/en/index1.html.

WHO. (2020c) *WHO Timeline COVID-19, Online*. Available at: https://www.who.int/news/item/27-04-2020-who-timeline---covid-19 (Accessed: 24 June 2021).

Wilms, S. (2010) 'Nurturing life in classical chinese medicine: Sun Simiao on healing without drugs, transforming bodies and cultivating life', *Journal of Chinese Medicine*, 93, pp. 5–13.

Xiang, A., Jiang, D. and Zhao, Z. (2016) 'The impact of rural-urban migration on the health of the left-behind parents', *China Economic Review*, 37, pp. 126–139. doi: 10.1016/j.chieco.2015.09.007.

Yamaoka, K. (2008) 'Social capital and health and well-being in East Asia: A population-based study', *Social Science and Medicine*, 66(4), pp. 885–899. doi: 10.1016/j.socscimed.2007.10.024.

Yang, D. (2006) *Dusk Without Sunset: Actively Aging in Traditional Chinese Medicine*. Doctoral Dissertation, University of Pittsburgh.

Yip, W. et al. (2007) 'Does social capital enhance health and well-being? Evidence from rural China', *Social Science and Medicine*, 64(1), pp. 35–49. doi: 10.1016/j.socscimed.2006.08.027.

Zhang, Y. (2020) 'A case of severe COVID19 cured by Qinfei Paide decoction combined with Western Medicine', *Tianjin Journal of Traditional Chinese Medicine*, pp. 1–4.

Zhao, K. et al. (2016) 'A systematic review and meta-analysis of music therapy for the older adults with depression', *International Journal of Geriatric Psychiatry*, 31(11), pp. 1188–1198. doi: 10.1002/gps.4494.

Zhong, Y. et al. (2017) 'Association between social capital and health-related quality of life among left behind and not left behind older people in rural China', *BMC Geriatrics*, 17(1), pp. 1–11. doi: 10.1186/s12877-017-0679.

20 Laughter Is the Best Therapy for Happiness and Healthy Life Expectancy

Tetsuya Ohira
Fukushima Medical University

Masahiko Ichiki
Tokyo Medical University

CONTENTS

Introduction 229
    The Associations between Psychological Stress and Diseases 230
    Sex and Age Differences in Laughter 230
    Laughter and Pain 231
    Associations of Laughter with Lifestyle-Related Diseases 232
    Associations of Laughter with Functional Disability and Mortality 234
    Effects of Laughter on Lifestyle and Physical and Psychological Health 235
    Factors Associated with Increased Laughter in Daily Life 237
Conclusion 238
References 239

INTRODUCTION

Several epidemiological studies have reported associations of psychosocial factors with cardiovascular and lifestyle-related diseases. Since psychological stress and negative emotions are generally hard to control, an intervention for psychosocial factors to prevent lifestyle-related diseases has not been well elucidated. Thus, in recent years, it has been proposed that we should leave negative stress behind and increase positive emotions and behaviors. Particularly, it has been known empirically that laughing has a positive effect on the mind and body, as the old saying goes, "Good fortune comes to those who laugh" and "Laughter is the best medicine."

Laughter is defined as a behavior that occurs after we perceive an event or communication with a person as hilarious. In other words, it is not yet laughter when we think it is funny, but laughter is an action comprising two behaviors: a characteristic

DOI: 10.1201/9781003043270-20   **229**

voice saying "hahahaha" and a change in facial expression, which is known as a laughing face. Additionally, many muscles such as facial, abdominal, pectoral, and limb muscles move when we laugh, which may have some element of exercise and affect our health. Moreover, laughing itself improves physical and psychological health and enriches sociality, which may help prevent lifestyle-related diseases. In this article, we report on the factors related to laughter and health at different stages of life, especially on the relationship between laughter and stress and lifestyle-related diseases, and discuss the possibility that laughter can contribute to health promotion, happiness, and healthy life expectancy.

THE ASSOCIATIONS BETWEEN PSYCHOLOGICAL STRESS AND DISEASES

Cardiovascular diseases, including ischemic heart disease and stroke, not only are the leading causes of death in Japan but also are closely related to healthy life expectancy. It has been reported that, besides physical risk factors, psychosocial risk factors, including psychological stress and depression, are associated with the incidence and mortality of cardiovascular diseases and lifestyle-related diseases. In Japan, prospective epidemiological studies have shown that depressive symptoms are associated with stroke in a community-based population (Ohira et al., 2001), subjective stress increases the risk of death from ischemic heart disease (Iso et al., 2002), and social support reduces the risk of stroke death in men (Ikehara et al., 2008). Additionally, psychological stress has been implicated in cardiovascular risk factors, such as depression being associated with the accelerated sympathetic nervous system and abnormalities in glucose metabolism and suppressed anger being associated with the development of hypertension (Ohira et al., 2013). Moreover, psychological stress is known to affect various diseases, such as peptic ulcers, bronchial asthma, chronic low back pain, atopic dermatitis, and dizziness. Hence, psychological stress must be coped with to reduce the risk of cardiovascular and lifestyle-related diseases and to prolong healthy life expectancy.

SEX AND AGE DIFFERENCES IN LAUGHTER

We investigated the relationship between the frequency of laughter and sex and age among 4,780 residents of Akita Prefecture and Osaka Prefecture, who underwent health examinations between 2007 and 2008 (1,786 males and 2,994 females; mean age 59 years) (Ohira, Hirosaki, and Imano, 2011). The frequency of laughter was rated on a scale of "almost every day," "one to five days a week," "one to three days a month," and "almost never" as the frequency of "laughing out loud" in daily life.

Figure 20.1 shows the frequency of laughter by sex; 53% of women laughed "almost every day," whereas only 40% of men laughed, and women laughed aloud more often in their daily lives (p <0.001). Then, looking at the frequency of laughter by age, 65% of women younger than 40 years laughed "almost every day," but the frequency decreased according to age, that is, 46% of women older than 70 years (Figure 20.2). Men similarly laughed less frequently with age, dropping to 35% of those older than 70 years (Figure 20.3). Therefore, the frequency of laughter decreased with age for both men and women and was considered an indicator of aging.

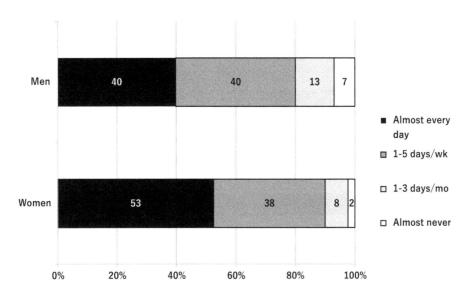

FIGURE 20.1 Frequency of laughter in daily life among 4,780 Japanese men and women.

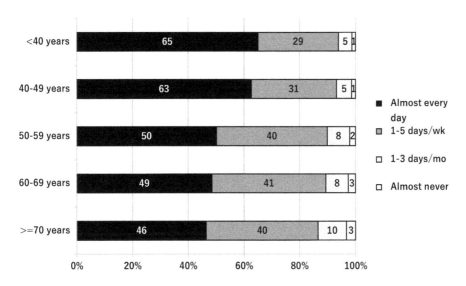

FIGURE 20.2 Frequency of laughter in daily life among women by age.

LAUGHTER AND PAIN

Reports on the effects of laughter on health did not come until after the 1960s, with one of the first reports of his own experience by Norman Cousins in the 1970s (Cousins, 1976). In 1964, at 49 years old, Cousins, editor-in-chief of the Saturday Review, was diagnosed with ankylosing spondylitis and was told by an attending physician that he had a 1-in-500 chance of recovering to his previous condition, as he could not walk because of the pain. Nonetheless, Cousins began treatment with

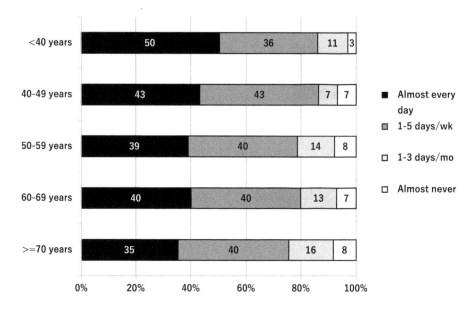

FIGURE 20.3 Frequency of laughter in daily life among men by age.

laughter and recovered to the point where he could return to his former job a few months later after conventional treatment failed to relieve his pain. Since that report on his progress, there has been some consideration of the effectiveness of laughter for pain. The Department of Rheumatology at Nihon Medical University studied how laughter changed pain in 26 rheumatoid arthritis patients and 31 control subjects (Yoshino, Fujimori, and Kohda, 1996). After watching a *rakugo*, a Japanese traditional sitting comedy, for about an hour, not only was subjective pain significantly reduced in the *rakugo* watching group, but interleukin-6, which is related to inflammation, and serum cortisol, a stress hormone, were also significantly reduced in the watching group. These changes were not observed in the control group, and thus, clearly, laughing reduced not only the subjective pain but also factors associated with the objective pain markers.

ASSOCIATIONS OF LAUGHTER WITH LIFESTYLE-RELATED DISEASES

In a study on laughter and diabetes, a research group at the University of Tsukuba conducted a 2-day study of 19 middle-aged diabetic patients (Hayashi et al., 2003). On the first day, the participants listened to a 40-minute lecture on diabetes after lunch, and on the second day, they watched a 40-minute comedy show after lunch and had a good laugh. On the day of the lecture, the blood glucose level elevated from 151 to 274 mg/dL, whereas on the day of the comedy show, the blood glucose level remained at 178–255 mg/dL, a difference of 46 mg/dL. Therefore, a good laugh was found to reduce the rise in blood glucose levels. We thus examined the association between the frequency of laughter in daily life and the prevalence of diabetes among 4,780 residents of Akita Prefecture and Osaka Prefecture (Ohira et al., 2013).

The results showed that those who laughed aloud 1–5 days a week were 1.26 (95% confidence interval [CI]: 0.97–1.65) times more likely to have diabetes than those who laughed aloud every day and those who laughed 1–3 days a month or rarely laughed were 1.51 times more likely to have diabetes (95% CI: 1.08–2.11) after adjustment for sex, age, body mass index, physical activity, smoking, alcohol intake, and depressive symptoms (Figure 20.4). Additionally, this population was followed for an average of 5.4 years to prospectively examine the association between the frequency of laughter and the incidence of diabetes, and a significant association was found between the frequency of laughter and the incidence of diabetes in both men and women, with those who laughed out loud almost daily having a 1.84-fold higher risk of developing multivariable-adjusted diabetes than those who laughed out loud less than once a week.

Additionally, the association of frequency of laughter with hypertension has been reported in a prospective cohort study of 1,441 men and women from the Ibaraki Prefecture community who participated in the Circulation Risk in Communities Study (CIRCS) (Ikeda et al., 2021). Blood pressure was followed for 4 years, and the results showed that among men who laughed aloud almost daily, systolic/diastolic blood pressure averaged 132.2/77.0 mmHg in 2010 and 133.0/76.6 mmHg in 2014, with little change. However, men who laughed less than once a week had a significant increase in both systolic and diastolic blood pressure over a 4-year period, averaging 130.7/75.9 mmHg in 2010 and 134.1/78.9 mmHg in 2014. In contrast, these associations were not observed in women.

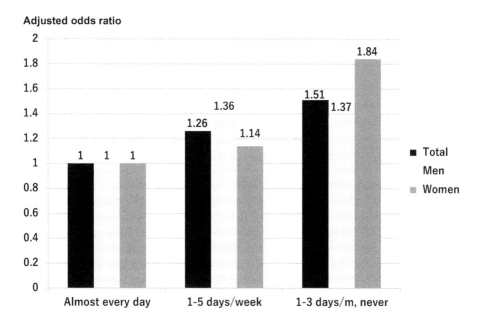

FIGURE 20.4 Association between the frequency of laughter and the prevalence of diabetes mellitus. Adjusted odds ratios for sex, age, body mass index, physical activity, smoking, alcohol consumption, and depressive symptoms for people who laugh almost every day.

234   Healthy Ageing in Asia

The association between laughter and cardiovascular diseases has been reported in a cross-sectional and prospective cohort study. In a cross-sectional study of 20,934 community-dwelling men and women aged 65 years or older who participated in the 2013 Japan Gerontological Evaluation Study (JAGES), the authors found that compared with those who laughed aloud almost every day, the multivariable-adjusted (adjusting for sex, age, body mass index, alcohol consumption, smoking, physical activity, and depression) prevalence ratios of heart diseases for the participants who laughed 1–5 days a week, 1–3 days a month, and almost never laughed were 1.13 (95% CI: 1.03–1.25), 1.18 (95% CI: 1.03–1.35), and 1.21 (95% CI: 1.04–1.41), respectively. Similarly, the multivariable-adjusted prevalence ratios of stroke were 1.12 (95% CI: 0.93–1.34), 1.28 (95% CI: 1.01–1.63), and 1.67 (95% CI: 1.30–2.15), respectively (Hayashi et al., 2016). Furthermore, the association between laughter and cardiovascular diseases (myocardial infarction and stroke) was examined in a prospective cohort study among 17,152 local residents in Yamagata Prefecture (Sakurada et al., 2020). Compared with those who laughed aloud more than once a week, the participants who laughed 1–3 days a month had a 1.63-fold greater sex- and age-adjusted risk of developing cardiovascular diseases (95% CI: 1.08–2.39), and the adjusted risk is 1.35 (95% CI: 0.52–2.85) for those who rarely laugh (less than once a month). The results suggest that cardiovascular diseases are more likely to occur in people who laughed less frequently.

We also conducted a questionnaire survey of 88,175 Japanese community residents aged 40–69 years to identify the effects of the perceived level of life enjoyment on cardiovascular disease incidence and mortality in the Japan Public Health Center–Based Study Cohort and found that, over the next 12 years, the multivariable hazard ratios of cardiovascular disease incidence for men in the high versus low perceived levels of life enjoyment group were 1.22 (95% CI: 1.01–1.47) for stroke and 1.23 (95% CI: 1.05–1.44) for total cardiovascular disease (Shirai et al., 2009). Moreover, men with a low perceived level of life enjoyment showed an increased risk of mortality from stroke and coronary heart disease: hazard ratios of 1.75 (95% CI: 1.28–2.38) and 1.91 (95% CI: 1.30–2.81), respectively. Therefore, laughter and life enjoyment may have a preventive role in the development of cardiovascular diseases by improving blood sugar and blood pressure control.

ASSOCIATIONS OF LAUGHTER WITH FUNCTIONAL DISABILITY AND MORTALITY

In a study of professional baseball players in the United States, the relationship between a player's photographic smile and longevity has been examined. Mugshots of 230 active professional baseball players in 1952 were analyzed, and the degree of smile was rated on a three-point scale and then related to later life expectancy (Abel and Kruger, 2010). One hundred eighty-four deaths in a follow-up study through 2009 and an analysis of the association with smiling showed that the average life expectancy of players who did not smile at all was 72.9 years versus 79.9 years for those who showed their teeth and wore a big smile, a difference of 7 years. However, in a subsequent reanalysis of similar U.S. professional baseball players, no association was found between smiles and life expectancy (Dufner et al., 2018).

Conversely, there have been few studies, including those in Europe and the United States, that have looked at the relationship between laughter and life expectancy

Laughter is the Best Therapy

(mortality), but a recent epidemiological study in Japan examined the relationship between laughter and all-cause mortality. In a study of 17,152 men and women aged 40 years or older living in seven cities in Yamagata Prefecture, the frequency of laughing out loud in daily life was evaluated in baseline health examinations and followed for up to 8 years (median 5.4 years). Compared with the participants who laughed once a week or more, the sex- and age-adjusted relative risk of all-cause mortality was 1.93 (95% CI: 1.15–3.06) for those who rarely laugh (Sakurada et al., 2020). A similar association between laughter frequency and mortality, besides sex and age, was found after adjusting for hypertension, diabetes, smoking, and alcohol consumption at baseline, suggesting that laughter frequency may be associated with reduced death independently of these factors.

Moreover, another study reported that laughter may affect not only death but also functional disability. Laughing out loud in daily life among 14,233 community-dwelling men and women aged 65 years and older living in 23 municipalities in nine prefectures who participated in a 2013 survey by the JAGES and who were not certified as needing long-term care (Tamada et al., 2021). The frequency of laughing out loud was evaluated with a questionnaire, and then, we looked at the association of laughter with all-cause mortality and new certification for the requirement of long-term care insurance over a period of more than 3 years (median 3.3 years) (Tamada et al., 2021). Compared with those who laugh aloud almost every day, the sex- and age-adjusted mortality rates for those who laugh 1–5 days a week, 1–3 days a month, and rarely (less than once a month) were 1.10 (95% CI: 0.92–1.32), 1.35 (95% CI: 1.07–1.70), and 1.52 (95% CI: 1.18–1.96). Similarly, the sex- and age-adjusted functional disability rates were 1.13 (95% CI: 0.94–1.37), 1.22 (95% CI: 0.94–1.59), and 2.14 (95% CI: 1.68–2.74), respectively. Besides sex, age, hypertension, diabetes, smoking and alcohol consumption, adjustments for family structure, social participation, depressive symptoms, cognitive functioning, daily functioning, educational history, and income showed no statistically significant differences in the association with mortality, but the association with a functional disability was 1.42 times greater in those who rarely laugh (95% CI: 1.10–1.85) even after adjustment for confounding factors.

An essential point from these two studies is that when the same laughter questionnaire was used to analyze the association with all-cause mortality in different geographical areas and age groups, similar trends were found between these two studies. These results were likely to apply to all Japanese (maybe Asians), with middle-aged and older adults, who rarely laughed aloud in their daily lives, being almost as likely to die 3–5 years later (for whatever reason) as those who laughed almost every day. Additionally, people older than 65 years who laugh very infrequently are also more likely to be functionally disabled within 3 years, revealing that laughing in daily life is associated with healthy life expectancy as well as future life expectancy.

EFFECTS OF LAUGHTER ON LIFESTYLE AND PHYSICAL AND PSYCHOLOGICAL HEALTH

We conducted a randomized interventional study to investigate the effect of the laughter program on blood glucose levels. Twenty-seven community residents aged 60 years or older were randomly divided into an intervention group and a control group, and the intervention group received 120 minutes of laughter therapy (a program that combines watching *rakugo*, comedy, etc., with mild exercise) for 10 weeks. The results showed that hemoglobin A1c, an indicator of diabetes control, improved significantly in the intervention group compared with that in the control group (Hirosaki et al., 2013). There was also an improvement in bone density and subjective health perception. Hence, it was suggested that laughter may improve the control of diabetes in the long term. Conversely, a study of 17 healthy subjects on the possibility that laughter may improve vascular endothelial function, an indicator of early atherosclerosis, reported a significant improvement in vascular endothelial function after viewing a comedy video for 60 minutes compared with viewing a documentary video (Sugawara, Tarumi and Tanaka, 2010). However, few studies, including this one, have been conducted on the long-term effects of other lifestyle diseases, such as hypertension, dyslipidemia, and atherosclerosis, and therefore, future reports are expected.

The effects of laughter on physical health have been mainly examined in terms of stress-related indices and effects on the autonomic nervous system. In 15 young healthy subjects, chromogranin A levels, as a measure of the sympathetic nervous system, were lower after viewing a video of laughter than after viewing a video without laughter (Toda and Ichikawa, 2012). Further, in a study that evaluated the autonomic nervous system function using heart rate variability, in 72 healthy subjects, after 6 minutes of fake laughter (in which participants were asked to engage in the behavior of laughing even if it was not funny) and after spontaneous laughter through humor video viewing, both increased the parasympathetic nervous system function, which is useful for mental and physical relaxation, after the intervention. Moreover, in a study of 90 college students, listening to laughter for 5 minutes after a stress load increased the parasympathetic function (Fujiwara and Okamura, 2018). Therefore, regarding the mental and physical relaxation effects of laughter, the act of laughing is more essential than the reason for laughing, and even if we are not laughing, just listening to the sound of laughter may affect us.

A study of the effects of laughter yoga on 38 healthy students reported improvements in overall well-being, particularly in physical symptoms, anxiety/insomnia, and depression, after participating in laughter yoga twice a week for 1 month compared with those on a control group (Yazdani et al., 2014). Similarly, the effects of laughter on depressive symptoms, anxiety, and sleep quality have been reported in community-dwelling older adults (Ko and Youn, 2011; Shahidi et al., 2011; Ghodsbin et al., 2015). Additionally, meta-analyses of the effects of laughter on depressive symptoms, anxiety, and sleep quality have been conducted, all of which reveal the usefulness of laughter in improving symptoms (van der Wal and Kok, 2019; Zhao et al., 2019; Demir Doğan, 2020). Furthermore, notably, the results of the meta-analysis showed that laughter without humor (e.g., laughter yoga) was more effective in improving depressive symptoms than laughter with humor (van der Wal and Kok, 2019). Although people with depressive symptoms are often unable to laugh with humor, they can still engage in the behavior of laughter. Thus, the behavior of laughing, not feeling funny, is essential for improving depressive symptoms.

Laughter is the Best Therapy

FACTORS ASSOCIATED WITH INCREASED LAUGHTER IN DAILY LIFE

In a study of 20,006 community residents aged 65 years and older who participated in the JAGES, the group with the highest equivalent household income laughed aloud almost every day of their daily lives more often than the group with the lowest equivalent household income, at an age-adjusted rate of 1.43 (95% CI: 1.33–1.54) for men and 1.30 (95% CI: 1.23–1.38) for women (Imai et al., 2018). Seeing friends more than twice a week and participating in more social activities were also factors that increased laughter. Furthermore, the family structure was also related to the frequency of laughter, with men laughing even more if they lived with their wives, but the association was weaker for women. In other words, even if both men and women were financially fortunate, living alone did not increase laughter much, but even if they were financially deprived, living with someone else may increase laughter in daily life. Additionally, if they did not have a family member, seeing friends more often and participating in social activities were regarded to be possible ways to increase laughter.

We surveyed 4,780 community residents aged 30 years and older in Akita and Osaka prefectures who participated in the CIRCS study to determine what the so-called "sources of laughter" were (Figure 20.5). Among women, the most common response was "Talking with family and friends," at around 82%, followed by "Watching TV or videos" and "Communicating with children or grandchildren."

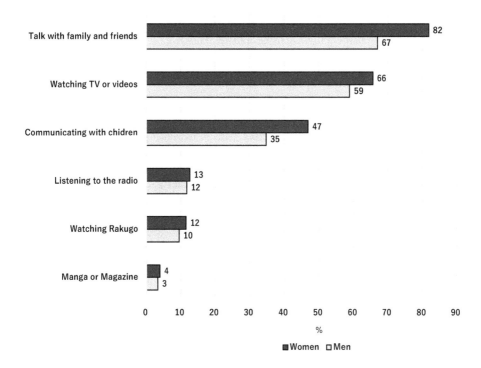

FIGURE 20.5 Sources of laughter in daily life by sex (multiple responses).

Similarly, men also chose "Talking with family and friends," "Watching TV or videos," and "Communicating with children or grandchildren," in that order but less frequently than women (Ohira, 2019). Therefore, laughter occurred most often while talking with people for both men and women, suggesting that increasing opportunities to talk with people is important. In other words, family structure and participation in social activities may lead to increased laughter by increasing opportunities to talk with people. Furthermore, among those who work, those who have a healthy lifestyle and support from their colleagues laugh more often almost daily (Inaba, 2015; Inaba and Hioki, 2019), suggesting that good lifestyle habits and relationships may influence the frequency of laughter as well as community members.

Conversely, it is possible that there are many people who live alone or who are not good at or unable to participate in social activities. In this case, the results of the aforementioned meta-analysis suggest that humorless laughter, such as laughter yoga, which involves laughing even when it is not funny, may be helpful. Laughter yoga is a health practice created by Dr. Madan Katarina, an Indian physician, in 1995 (Shahidi et al., 2011). Laughter yoga was from the idea that laughter, whether as a gymnastics exercise or when one feels funny and really laughs, has almost the same health benefits to the body (indeed, research has shown that this is true). In laughter yoga, there is no need for humor, jokes, or comedy, just laughter for no reason. At first, we laugh as a gymnastics exercise, but as we laugh together, the contagious power of laughter kicks in, and we gradually become funny and can laugh without difficulty (this is consistent with reports that stress is reduced simply by listening to the sound of laughter). By combining gymnastics and breathing exercises, laughter yoga is expected to have both aerobic and relaxation effects and be useful from a mechanistic standpoint as well.

CONCLUSION

The number of reports on the effects of laughter on lifestyle diseases and physical diseases such as those requiring nursing care is increasing, and prospective studies have shown that laughing may reduce death and nursing care and may prevent lifestyle diseases. Conversely, interventional studies on physical diseases are still scarce, and it is hoped that more studies using physical diseases and physical factors as outcomes will be conducted in the future.

The number of studies on laughter and health has increased dramatically over the past few decades, and more evidence is expected in the future. Laughter and smiles are increasing through people, and the effects of laughter have the potential to greatly expand beyond the individual and into society. Laughter has already been reported by several studies to be effective in maintaining immunity to new types of coronavirus-2019 (COVID-19) infections, so it may work as a preventive measure against COVID-19 infections. Conversely, communication with people has a significant impact on laughter, but the way we communicate with people may change to prevent infection, which may affect the frequency of laughter. Additionally, in terms of communication, systems for remote conversations using social network services have become more extensive and diversified. The challenge for the future is how to increase laughter and smiles in our recent limited lives.

Laughter can be increased in daily life without much cost, and it is very cost-effective as a health method for disease prevention and health promotion. Furthermore, laughter has the potential to improve the health of people of all ages, from children to the elderly, and if research on laughter and health is advanced, it can significantly contribute to greater happiness and extend healthy life expectancy.

REFERENCES

Abel, E. L. and Kruger, M. L. (2010) 'Smile intensity in photographs predicts longevity', *Psychological Science*, 21(4), pp. 542–544. Doi: 10.1177/0956797610363775.

Cousins, N. (1976) 'Anatomy of an illness (as perceived by the patient)', *New England Journal of Medicine*, 295, pp. 1458–1463. Doi: 1410.1056/NEJM197612232952605.

Demir Doğan, M. (2020) 'The effect of laughter therapy on anxiety: A meta-analysis', *Holistic Nursing Practice*, 34(1), pp. 35–39.

Dufner, M. et al. (2018) 'Does smile intensity in photographs really predict longevity? A replication and extension of Abel and Kruger (2010)', *Psychological Science*, 29(1), pp. 147–153. doi: 10.1177/0956797617734315.

Fujiwara, Y. and Okamura, H. (2018) 'Hearing laughter improves the recovery process of the autonomic nervous system after a stress-loading task: A randomized controlled trial', *BioPsychoSocial Medicine*, 12(1), pp. 1–9. doi: 10.1186/s13030-018-0141-0.

Ghodsbin, F. et al. (2015) 'The effects of laughter therapy on general health of elderly people referring to Jahandidegan community centre in Shiraz, Iran, 2014: A randomized controlled trial', *International Journal of Community Based Nursing and Midwifery*, 3(1), pp. 31–38.

Hayashi, K. et al. (2003) 'Laughter lowered the increase in postprandial blood glucose', *Diabetes Care*, 26(5), pp. 1651–1652. doi: 10.1331/154434503322452238.

Hayashi, K. et al. (2016) 'Laughter is the best medicine? A cross-sectional study of cardiovascular disease among older Japanese adults', *Journal of Epidemiology*, 26(10), pp. 546–552. doi: 10.2188/jea.JE20150196.

Hirosaki, M. et al. (2013) 'Effects of a laughter and exercise program on physiological and psychological health among community-dwelling elderly in Japan: Randomized controlled trial', *Geriatrics and Gerontology International*, 13(1), pp. 152–160. doi: 10.1111/j.1447-0594.2012.00877.x.

Ikeda, S. et al. (2021) 'Longitudinal trends in blood pressure associated with the frequency of laughter: Longitudinal study of Japanese general population: The circulatory risk in communities study (CIRCS)', *Journal of Epidemiology*, pp. 1–7.

Ikehara, S. et al. (2008) 'Alcohol consumption and mortality from stroke and coronary heart disease among Japanese men and women: The Japan collaborative cohort study', *Stroke*, 39(11), pp. 2936–2942. doi: 10.1161/STROKEAHA.108.520288.

Imai, Y. et al. (2018) 'Impact of social relationships on income-laughter relationships among older people: The JAGES cross-sectional study', *BMJ Open*, 8(7), pp. 1–10. doi: 10.1136/bmjopen-2017-019104.

Inaba, R. (2015) 'Study on the relationships between mirthful laughter and working condition, lifestyle and work-related stress among female nurses', *Japanese Journal of Occupational Medicine and Traumatology*, 63, pp. 81–87.

Inaba, R. and Hioki, A. (2019) 'Study on the relationships between mirthful laughter and working condition, lifestyle and work-related stress among female nurses', *Japanese Journal of Occupational Medicine and Traumatology*, 69, pp. 8–14.

Iso, H. et al. (2002) 'Perceived mental stress and mortality from cardiovascular disease among Japanese men and women: The Japan Collaborative cohort study for evaluation of cancer risk sponsored by Monbusho (JACC Study)', *Circulation*, 106(10), pp. 1229–1236. doi: 10.1161/01.CIR.0000028145.58654.41.

Ko, H. J. and Youn, C. H. (2011) 'Effects of laughter therapy on depression, cognition and sleep among the community-dwelling elderly', *Geriatrics and Gerontology International*, 11(3), pp. 267–274. doi: 10.1111/j.1447-0594.2010.00680.x.

Ohira, T. (2019) 'Life course and health - the associations of laughter with stress and lifestyle-related', *Comprehensive Medicine*, 17, pp. 20–27.

Ohira, T., Hirosaki, M. and Imano, H. et al. (2011) 'Prevention and improvement of dementia by laughter and humour therapy', *Geriatric Psychiatry*, 22, pp. 32–38.

Ohira, T. et al. (2001) 'Prospective study of depressive symptoms and risk of stroke among Japanese', *Stroke*, 32(4), pp. 903–907. doi: 10.1161/01.str.32.4.903.

Ohira, T. et al. (2013) *Epidemiological Study on the Effects of Positive Psychological Interventions such as Laughter on Prevention of Lifestyle-Related Diseases*. Available at: https://www.fmu.ac.jp/home/epi/report/index.html.

Sakurada, K. et al. (2020) 'Associations of frequency of laughter with risk of all-cause mortality and cardiovascular disease incidence in a general population: Findings from the yamagata study', *Journal of Epidemiology*, 30(4), pp. 188–193. doi: 10.2188/jea. JE20180249.

Shahidi, M. et al. (2011) 'Laughter yoga versus group exercise program in elderly depressed women: A randomized controlled trial', *International Journal of Geriatric Psychiatry*, 26(3), pp. 322–327. doi: 10.1002/gps.2545.

Shirai, K. et al. (2009) 'Perceived level of life enjoyment and risks of cardiovascular disease incidence and mortality. The Japan public health centre-based study', *Circulation*, 120(11), pp. 956–963. doi: 10.1161/CIRCULATIONAHA.108.834176.

Sugawara, J., Tarumi, T. and Tanaka, H. (2010) 'Effect of mirthful laughter on vascular function', *American Journal of Cardiology*, 106(6), pp. 856–859. doi: 10.1016/j. amjcard.2010.05.011.

Tamada, Y. et al. (2021) 'Does laughter predict onset of functional disability', *The Journal of Epidemiology*, 31(5), pp. 301–307.

Toda, M. and Ichikawa, H. (2012) 'Effect of laughter on salivary flow rates and levels of chromogranin A in young adults and elderly people', *Environmental Health and Preventive Medicine*, 17(6), pp. 494–499. doi: 10.1007/s12199-012-0279-5.

van der Wal, C. N. and Kok, R. N. (2019) 'Laughter-inducing therapies: Systematic review and meta-analysis', *Social Science and Medicine*, 232(January), pp. 473–488. doi: 10.1016/j. socscimed.2019.02.018.

Yazdani, M. et al. (2014) 'The effect of laughter of Yoga on general health among nursing students', *Iranian Journal of Nursing and Midwifery Research*, 19(1), p. 36.

Yoshino, S., Fujimori, J. and Kohda, M. (1996) 'Effects of mirthful laughter on neuroendocrine and immune systems in patients in rheumatoid arthritis', *The Journal of Rheumatology*, 23(4), pp. 793–794.

Zhao, J. et al. (2019) 'A meta-analysis of randomized controlled trials of laughter and humour interventions on depression, anxiety and sleep quality in adults', *Journal of Advanced Nursing*, 75(11), pp. 2435–2448. doi: 10.1111/jan.14000.

21 Impact of Music Therapy on Complicated Grief Reactions in Elderly Persons

Ranka Radulovic
Clinic for Psychiatry – Clinical Centre of Serbia
Hatorum – Centre for Education and
Counselling in Music Therapy

CONTENTS

Introduction 241
    Dimension of Problem 242
        Terminology Issues 242
        Prevalence 242
        Consequences and Comorbidity 244
        Treatment and Ethical Issues 244
        Aim 244
        Methodology 245
        Results 246
    Individual Case 248
    Discussion 250
Conclusion 250
References 250

INTRODUCTION

Music therapy (MT) represents a set of different techniques and methods applied by an educated music therapist who uses a sound which can be or doesn't have to be music. MT could be adapted to the cognitive, verbal, motoric and musical abilities of a client and applied in diagnostics, therapy, prevention, rehabilitation and stimulation of physical, mental and spiritual health. By providing a supportive environment, MT facilitates communication and maximises learning and makes a connection to the premorbid personality and previous coping styles of a client.

In the Oxford Handbook of Music Therapy, O'Callaghan and Michael (2016) listed some of the MT techniques applied in mourning: receptive music-based counselling, lyrical analysis, lyric substitution in familiar songs or instrumental music, music-based

DOI: 10.1201/9781003043270-21

life review, audio, visual and /contextual recording of one's reminiscences and significant reflections, playlists of significant musical milestones, songwriting; music improvisations, relaxation and/or guide imagery inductions with music, Bonny method of guide imagery and music; and song compositions, music-based audiovisual recordings.

MT techniques have ethnopsychology and ethnomusicology roots (Radulovic & Pejovic, 1997).

O'Callaghan et al. (2013) writes that MT was often still used to improve mood and sometimes used to confront grief. Specific music, however, was sometimes avoided to minimise sadness. Continuing bonds theory's focus on connecting with the deceased through memory and imagery engagement may expand to encompass musical memories, rework the meaning of familiar music, and discover new music related to the deceased. Pre-loss music involvement, including MT, between dying patients and families, can help in bereavement.

DiMaio and Economos (2017) discovered the unique roles of music in grief were as a pattern emerged that reflected the Dual Process Model of Grief (Stroebe & Schut, 1999).

Most of them are supportive and have a focus on creating a sense of connection with the deceased person ex. singing an imaginal dialogue with a deceased (Iliya, 2014) although in some cases the persisting connection with a deceased can result in enduring physical, psychological and psychosomatic difficulties in bereaved (Spillane et al., 2018).

Dimension of Problem

The issues of complicated grief reactions (CGR) are not resolved in psychiatry until today. There is no evidence that complicated grief (CG) criteria accurately identify individuals with a distinct mental disorder.

Terminology Issues

CGR which is also called prolonged grief disorder (PGD) represents intense grief after the death of a loved one that lasts longer than expected according to social norms and causes impairment in daily functioning (Shear, 2015).

Yale Bereavement Study (Maciejewski et al., 2016) showed that PGD and prolonged complex bereavement disorder (PCBD) (recently included in DSM-5 and ICD-11) but not CG are one and the same diagnostic entity. CG has a moderate agreement with PGD and PCBD in DSM-5 (Maciejewski et al., 2016; Prigerson & Maciejewski, 2017).

Significant modification is needed to improve case identification by DSM-5 persistent complex bereavement disorder diagnostic criteria (Cozza et al., 2016) and only systematic and well-designed empirical research can assess the validity and utility of this new grief disorder (Eisma, 2018).

Range issue: CGR research instruments usually consider the death of an important person. So, CGR in other kinds of loss are underestimated and untreated.

Prevalence

CG affects about 2%–3% of the population worldwide and is more likely (prevalence of approximately 10%–20%) after the loss of a child or a life partner and after a sudden death by violent means, suicide, homicide or accident (Shear, 2015).

Impact of Music Therapy on CGR in Elderly Persons

Meta-analysis made (Pan & Lui, 2019) focussed on the Chinese population revealed a pooled estimate of CG of 22.0%. The studies identified in this review were of methodological heterogeneousness and focussed on the population at high risk of CG.

In the study of Newson et al. (2011), a higher prevalence of CG in the age range of 75–85 years, suggesting that the very elderly have more difficulty in coping with a loss, was found. In a population study amongst the elderly, those between the ages of 75 and 84 years had a greater risk of developing CG compared with a younger age group.

The prevalence of CG is highest amongst women who are older than 60 years of age (Kersting, 2011).

Phenomenology of CGR in old age (Shear, 2015) writes that the hallmark of CG is represented by persistent, intense yearning, longing, and sadness; these symptoms are usually accompanied by insistent thoughts or images of the deceased and a sense of disbelief or an inability to accept the painful reality of the person's death. Rumination is common and is often focussed on angry or guilty recrimination related to the circumstances of death. Avoidance of situations that serve as reminders of the loss is also common, as is the urge to hold onto the deceased person by constantly reminiscing or by viewing, touching or smelling the deceased person's belongings. People with CG often feel shocked, stunned or emotionally numb, and they may become estranged from others because of the belief that happiness is inextricably tied to the person who died. They may have a diminished sense of self or discomfort with a changed social role and are often confused by their seemingly endless grief. Friends and relatives are often frustrated that they cannot help, and they may become critical or stop contacting the bereaved person, increasing his or her feelings of isolation.

Bereavement and grief in people with dementia (PWD) are represented by the usual phenomenology in the early stage of illness. But, sometimes in PWD, awareness of the loss may not always be possible. According to that, they stay stuck at an early stage (the first stage) of grief. So, denial of death may be protective. Some PWD are unable to retrieve the memory of someone's death, or they could have a constant delusion that the deceased person is still alive.

CGR in PWD are hard to detect because they could be characterised by somatic symptoms (headache, chest pain or palpitations); searching behaviour, denial of loss with depressive and anxiety states. On the other hand, some elderly patients going through bereavement may have no reactions to grief or they may displace hostility towards those still living. (Hashim, 2013).

Grieving people tend to find it difficult to ask for help. In most cases, old people don't want to burden their children or other family members. There is also a tendency for family members to dismiss these psychological symptoms and underestimate the severity of the distress or they could be occupied by their own grief.

Defence mechanisms often used by PWD are confusion of current loss for earlier losses and decline in cognitive functioning which may have eased their pain and suffering. The phenomenon of 'metaphone' is present when the metaphorical loss changes from being the loss of the son to the loss of an object; it could be expected an alienation of the PWD from the family's grief (Ling, 2016). Their attending to their own needs and their responses which are less predictable may sometimes be hurtful to family members. This 'self-threat' was described to reflect the PWD's perception of a threat to the 'self' with a shift of focus from the loss of the loved one to a more personal loss. They are unable to be a model of grief for their children (Howard et al., 2012).

Consequences and Comorbidity

CG is associated with other health problems, such as sleep disturbance (Milic, 2019), substance abuse in 32.4% (Masferrer, 2017), suicidal thinking and behaviour (Maple, 2016; Molina et al., 2019), connection between pain and CGR in Japanese older adults (Ghesquiere et al., 2020, abnormalities in immune function and increased risks of cardiovascular disease and cancer (Shear, 2015, O'Connor 2019).

The adverse psychological impact of bereavement on the elderly population cannot be underestimated, particularly in those with a pre-existing cognitive impairment. Neurobiological studies and neuropsychological studies suggest an alteration in the functioning of the reward system (in response to reminders of the deceased person) and abnormalities in autobiographical memory, as well as neural systems involved in emotional regulation and neurocognitive functioning (Saavedra Pérez et al., 2015; Fernández-Alcántara, 2016; O'Connor, 2018) including disrupted prefrontal activity during emotional processing in CG proved on an fMRI study (Arizmendi et al., 2016).

Schiele et al. (2018) for the first time suggests a gene–environment interaction effect of an oxytocin receptor gene variant with behavioural inhibition and possibly also symptoms of adult separation anxiety in the moderation of vulnerability for CG.

Treatment and Ethical Issues

Untreated CGR will result in somatic and psychiatric complications and disorders in the future. PDW have the right to grieve and mourn. The experience of acute grief and distress multiple times with 're-traumatisation' when the truth is revealed each time may be considered cruel and insensitive. It may be understandable that why some family members and care staff try to shield PWD from reality. There may be questions as to whether or not to tell, how to tell and how the revelation will impact their psychological well-being as well as their caregivers (Ling, 2016).

The study of Howard et al. (2012) was shown that in the grieving process, the ability of the bereaved to form new attachments and social connections is crucial. This will be an apparent challenge for many PWD. Difficulties communicating their distress may preclude PWD from participating in bereavement support groups. Interventions for the bereaved PWD will be aimed at facilitating and maximising learning and providing a supportive environment (Woods, 1982).

Aim

The aim of this paper is to consider the capacity of MUSICAL CHOICE METHOD THERAPEUTIC SINGING (MCM-TS) (Radulovic, R.) as a tool for the detection and treatment of CG reactions on the group level as well as on the individual level in a big group of elderly people in a nursing home.

Methodology

This pilot study represents a qualitative prospective analysis of 15 MT sessions in a big group of elderly persons.

Musical choice method-therapeutic singing (MCM-TS) was applied. It integrates the stage grief theory of Parkes (1998), dual-process model (Stroebe & Schut, 1999), 'ongoing' attachment theory (Hogan & DeSantis, 1992), 'continuing bonding' (Klass & Steffen, 2018) and the concept of 'disenfranchised grief' (Doka, 1989). The music therapist must be familiar with this.

The setting was a very important factor in spite of the fact that some group members' problem is with orientation. In the initial stage of the session, the therapist exchanged 'local' information with group members. In the singing phase, each member has been invited to sing a song according to their choice, as well as vocal, musical and cognitive capacities.

After performances, it was time for voting based on subjective preferences of each member and therapist's objective evaluation of results based on the performance, cognitive capacities, collaboration and level of initiative. The announcement of the winning song was at the end of the session.

MT sessions have a character of competition in memory. Grief was not mentioned as the focus of group meetings. The music therapist supports a collaboration between all group members without interpretations or judgement and actively collaborates with staff members after the sessions.

The method is based on the qualitative analysis of the song lyric in MCM-TS which defines the MCM forms: form of resistance, neutral songs, songs focussed on different stages of grief, separation anxiety, or phenomenon of psychopathology, social pathology or dependency (Table 21.1) and MCM – scale of cognitive performances represents the number of songs per session, number of strophes, level of participation, time and space orientation and musical skills.

The results of the scale of social skills (Radulovic, 2001) and qualitative analysis of the degree of client's projection are not presented in this paper.

During the therapeutic procedure, the therapist observes a move towards the basic aim – neutral song – and notices stagnation in other MCM forms which helps in the detection of CGR or elements of psychopathology or social pathology.

TABLE 21.1
Qualitative Analysis of the Song Lyrics in MCM

MCM Formes

MCM (−1)	Resistance song
MCM-0	Neutral song
MCM-1	Mourning song – stage 4
MCM-2	Mourning song – stage 3
MCM-3	Mourning song – stage 2
MCM-4	Mourning song – stage 1
MCM-5	Songs about fear, separation and anticipatory anxiety
MCM-6	Songs about psychopathological phenomena, addiction songs
MCM-7	Songs containing elements of structural problems and social pathology

Material is a qualitative analysis of the group therapy protocols during the 15 MT sessions which were made in a community MT setting, in the nursing home 'Stacionar Diljska' in Belgrade (Serbia), in the period 2014, September–December, in a setting, once a week, 90 minutes per session.

In MT sessions, participated seniors (≥65 years old) and younger were interested to come and participate in their initiative. The members had a mental and somatic illness, as well as disabilities and mental retardation, speech and language impairment. The members participated willingly and actively in sessions; they were invited to sing individually famous songs with lyrics, 3–5 minutes, by heart.

Results

The results are based on the qualitative analysis of the song lyric in MCM-TS in the group MT protocols. As examples, it would be presented in the group process and one individual case.

Descriptive analysis: 15 sessions were realised. Total number of participants varied between 21 and 7; average number per session was 12; range of age was between 47 and 89 (cc 68,7); there were 5 males and 16 females; most participants finished secondary school (11), elementary school 6, bachelor's 2, and special school 2; social level of group members was low.

Group was heterogeneous. Concerning mental disorders, there were eight patients with dementia F00-F09, two with alcoholism, one with paranoid schizophrenia (SCH), one with a residual type of SCH, nine had a depressive episode, and six members had general anxiety.

Dominant somatic problems were cardiovascular disorders in ten members, I10; I23, I63; diabetes mellitus in nine cases; cerebral palsy in two members, Guillain–Barre syndrome in one case. Five used a wheelchair and three patients had an amputation.

The group members preferred the Serbian folk songs and old town songs.

The lower number of participants in the last two sessions was due to the Christmas and New Year's holidays and departure of some members to visit their families.

Based on the Table 21.2, we can see that the dominant group's choice were songs about grief. Psychodynamic focus in grief was a loss of memory/body capacities and the cumulative effect of grief presented by regression from MCM-2 to MCM-4 (until 6 hours of session).

The winner in the 7th session was a Slovenian song in different languages, not understandable by most members (translated, this song also represents MCM-4, the first stage of grief for this group member). It was a group defence mechanism and represented a resistance MCM-1 form.

In the eighth session, the process started again and we had an MCM-3 form, but not for a long time.

In the next session, the group winner song is a confabulatory song – made from different parts of famous songs, and she composed a totally new song. The patient was absolutely sure that it was an original song, from her hometown. It can be the proof that confabulation, symptom of dementia, was the defence mechanism: denial

TABLE 21.2
The Analysis of Group Dynamic

Session	Number of Participants	Name of Winner	Song of the Winner / Serbian Translatio	MCM Form	Observation
1.	22	RJ	Moj, golube	MCM-2	
2.	17	J	O, Jelo, Jelena	MCM-2	
3.	11	R	O, moja ružo rumena	MCM-2	
4.	12	D	Ako ikad ozdravim	MCM-4	
5.	12	M	Ima dana	MCM-4	
6.	12	M	Kad bi ove ruže male	MCM-4	
7.	12	J	Solčence zahajalo (Slovenian song)	MCM-1/MCM-4	
8.	13	M	Za kim	MCM-3	
9.	11	R	New confabulatory song	MCM-6	
10.	11	s G with CP oR	Niška banja / New confabulatory song	MCM-0 / MCM-6	Compromise. Two votings: subjectively and objectively
11.	14	sM oMRS	Ima dana; Lepe li su nano; l Višnjičica rod rodila	MCM-4 MCM-0 MCM-2 / MCM-4	Two votings: based on subjective voting the winner is "Ima dana"; Three songs had a same number of points based on objective voting
12.	10	R	Confabulatory song	MCM-6	Other's confabulations. Splitting, Duel
13.	12	J	Tamo daleko	MCM-3	R. left group
14.	7	SB	Tekla reka Lepenica	MCM-0	
15.	7	Final session – new year wishes			

of the problem. Objectively, it is a clear symptom of psychopathology, negation of reality and lack of insight.

The group was faced with psychopathology. The winner didn't want to accept any kind of confrontation because she realised a huge number of rhymes (more than ten) and other group members were amazed by the "winner's memory".

For the next session, the therapist proposed a new rule for voting: subjective preferences of group members (signed "s" on the table) as before, and objective "o" – the points for rhymes; the number was limited to five, independently on the length of the song. The author of the confabulatory song was angry because of the decision. The result was splitting in the group: two winners with the same number of points. The winning song was a simple song proposed by a member with cerebral palsy form MCM-0 (the patient couldn't speak, but the group recognised the melody and participated with clapping in a common rhythm and gave support). Another winner was the same author of the confabulatory song.

The 11th session showed a deep group struggling for reality and motivation. We had four winners, only one MCM-0 form, all other songs about grief in the first and second stages.

In the 12th session, the group winner was again the confabulatory song but some group members made a strong confrontation. In spite of hard confrontation, the group voted for the confabulatory song, some members because of the lack of reality and some members because of the solidarity with the author of the confabulatory song.

The author of confabulatory songs left the group in the 13th session, and the winner was the MCM-3 form. During the second stage of grief, the group mourned because of the dropout of the author of a confabulatory song and some other members. But, for the 14th session, the winner was a neutral song, and we finished group sessions in reality.

INDIVIDUAL CASE

Case 1. Mrs. M., 70 years old, economist, mother of two in a good relationship with them.

Her main problems were somatic issues and illness, she was in a wheelchair due to double amputation as a consequence of diabetes and cardiovascular complications. She had mild cognitive deterioration. She lost her husband 15 years ago. The important loss was the separation of a younger lover who was discharged from the nursing home a year ago, due to bad behaviour (sexual nature in public) and alcoholism. She was isolated with reduced social interactions and worse somatic state after his departure. She accepted group music therapy but no individual music therapy treatment.

On Table 21.3, MCM-5 form dominates due to somatic problems which generate separation anxiety and fear of death. Neutral songs are connected to her husband and other people. Stage 2 is connected to the loss of a lover and loss of legs due to amputation, and MCM 7 is connected to her narcissistic traits sensitive to rejection. As her defence mechanism, she used sexualisation, self-idealisation and projection. She had a disfranchised grief, stocked at stage 2 till the end of therapy. She couldn't speak about the loss in front of the group because she couldn't get group support for inappropriate behaviours which resulted in the discharge of her lover.

TABLE 21.3
The Individual Therapeutics Protocol of the Mrs. M. During 15 Sessions

Session	The Song Name (Serbian Translasation)	Additional Songs/ Suggestions From Other Members	Verbalization Loss	Behavior	MCM Form
1.	Ti bi hteo pesmom da mi kažeš				Mourning MCM 3
2	Ajde Kato		Misssed app./love letters from the youth	Letter showed publicly, sexualisation	Anticipatory anxiety MCM 5
3.	Absent due to somatic health conditions				
4.	Ribar plete mrižu svoju		Death of husband 15 years ago	Stay in contact with common friends	Neutral song MCM 0
5.	Kad bi ove ruže male		Love separation, one years ago	Sexualisation	Mourning MCM 3
6.	Četri konja debela	U lepom, starom, gradu Višegradu	Dedicated to her husband Missed app. Italian	Sexualisation	Structural MCM 7
7.	Tiho noći		Dedicated to my dead aunt		Neutral MCM 0
8.	Za kim	Dunav, Dunav, tiho teče	Visited Japan Played accordion	Paranoid elaboration focussed on therapist	Mourning MCM 3
9.	No song, resistance			Paranoid elaboration focussed on therapist	MCM -1
10.	Ajd idemo Rado	U lepom, starom, gradu Višegradu			Anticipatory anxiety MCM 5
11.	Ima dana		Operation of blood vessels in plan	Aggressive towards other member becouse of confabulation	Mourning MCM 3
12.	Oj Moravo				Mourning MCM 3
13.	Gde si da si moj golube				Separation's anxiety MCM 5
14.	Sve ptičice				Mourning MCM 3
15.	Final session	New Year wish			

Her New Year's wish was to leave the institution, and she died in the next few months.

DISCUSSION

Grief is associated with various losses and all losses must be treated separately. The stages of grief are important for the strategy of treatment and prognosis. Nonverbal interventions are recommended in the first stage of grief.

Due to the cumulative effect of music, musical choices made by patients, his family or caregivers must be carefully considered. Listening to music or singing in the chorus could be beneficial but also in some cases can cause re-traumatisation.

CONCLUSION

MCM-TS in elderly people represents supportive techniques in the domain of active MT. By using this method as a diagnostic tool, we can monitor the stages of grief and detect CGR, psychopathological and sociopathology phenomena in individuals or in a group. A problem of disenfranchised grief can be also detected as well as psychodynamic connections between grief, other disorders and environmental problems.

As a therapeutic tool, this method can be used as a support during adaptation to the loss. It is a noninvasive and secure method to resolve personal and group stagnation in case of grief disorders and disorders connected to grief.

The method could be used in mild and severe forms of dementia, in a big heterogeneous group.

MCM-TS could open a new possibility in the treatment of PWD. For further MCM-TS researches, it needs to consider its application in different settings, with different selections of members with a focus on cognitive performance, behaviour in PWD, long-term effects and somatic effects during and after the therapy. Also, it needs to include family members and caregivers, check this method in intercultural research and compare the MCM and other MT techniques.

Family members and caregivers need to recognise and respond to the PWD's emotions about their illness, losses and death. They can participate in this kind of group activities and it could be beneficial for all participants.

REFERENCES

Arizmendi, B., Kaszniak, A. W., & O'Connor, M. F. (2016). Disrupted prefrontal activity during emotion processing in complicated grief—An fMRI investigation. *NeuroImage*, 124(Part A), 968–976. Doi: 10.1016/j.neuroimage.2015.09.054.

Cozza, S. J., Fisher, J. E., Mauro, C., Zhou, J., Ortiz, C. D., Skritskaya, N., Fullerton, C. S., Ursanom, R. J., & Shear, M. K. (2016). Performance of DSM-5 persistent complex bereavement disorder criteria in a community sample of bereaved military family members. *The American Journal of Psychiatry* 173(9), 919–929.

DiMaio, L. P. & Economos, A. (2017). Exploring the role of music in grief. *Bereavement Care* 36(2), 65–74. Doi: 10.1080/02682621.2017.1348585.

Doka, K. J. (1989). *Disenfranchised Grief—Recognizing Hidden Sorrow*. Lexington Books/D. C. Heath, Lexington, Massachusetts.

Eisma, M. C. & Lenferink, L. I. M. (2018). Response to—Prolonged grief disorder for ICD-11—the primacy of clinical utility and international applicability. *European Journal of Psychotraumatology* 9(1), 1512249. Doi: 10.1080/20008198.2018.1512249.

Fernández-Alcántara M., Pérez-García M., Pérez-Marfi M. N., Catena-Martínez A., HuesoMontoro C., & Cruz-Quintana F. (2016). Assessment of different components of executive function in grief. *Psicothema* 28(3), 260–265. Doi: 10.7334/psicothema 2015.257.

Ghesquiere A., Bagaajav A., Ito M., Sakaguchi Y. & Miyashita M. (2020). Investigating associations between pain and complicated grief symptoms in bereaved Japanese older adults. *Aging & Mental Health* 24(9), 1472–1478. Doi: 10.1080/13607863.2019.1594166.

Hashim, S. M., Eng, T. C., Tohit, N., & Wahab, S. (2013). Bereavement in the elderly—the role of primary care. *Mental Health in Family Medicine* 10(3), 159–162.

Hogan, N. & DeSantis, L. (1992). Adolescent sibling bereavement—an ongoing attachment. *Qualitative Health Research*, 2(2), 159–177. Doi: 10.1177/104973239200200204.

Howard, G., James, W. E., & Nicole, B. (2012). Identifiable grief responses in persons with Alzheimer's disease. *Journal of Social Work in End-of-Life & Palliative Care* 8, 151–164.

Iliya, Y. A. (2014). *Singing an Imaginal Dialogue—A Study of a Bereavement-Specific Music Therapy Intervention Expressive* Therapies Dissertations. 14. https://digitalcommons.lesley.edu/expressive_dissertations/14.

Kersting, A., Brähler, E., Glaesmer, H., & Wagner, B. (2011). Prevalence of complicated grief in a representative population-based sample. *Journal of Affective Disorders* 131, 339–43 and Com.

Klass, D., & Steffen, E. M. (2018). Introduction: Continuing bonds—20 years on. In Klass D & Steffen E. M. (eds) *Continuing bonds in bereavement: New directions for research and practice* (pp. 1–14). Routledge/Taylor & Francis Group, Oxfordshire.

Ling, T. L. (2016). Challenging aspects of bereavement and grief in older adults with dementia—a case series and clinical considerations. *Journal of Gerontology & Geriatric Research* 5, 276. Doi:10.4172/2167-7182.100027613.

Maciejewski, P.K., Maercker, A., Boelen, P.A., & Prigerson, H.G. (2016). "Prolonged grief disorder" and "persistent complex bereavement disorder", but not "complicated grief", are one and the same diagnostic entity—an analysis of data from the Yale Bereavement Study. *World Psychiatry*, 15(3), 266–275. Doi: 10.1002/wps.20348.

Maple, M., Cerel, J., Sanford, R., Pearce, T., & Jordan, J. (2016). Is exposure to suicide beyond kin associated with risk for suicidal behavior? A systematic review of the evidence. *Suicide & Life-Threatening Behavior*, 47(4), 461–474.

Masferrer, L., Garre-Olmo, J., & Caparrós, B. (2017). Is complicated grief a risk factor for substance use? A comparison of substance-users and normative grievers. *Addiction Research & Theory*, 25(5), 361–367. Doi: 10.1080/16066359.2017.1285912.

Milic, J., Perez, H.S., Zuurbier, L.A., Boelen, P.A., Rietjens, J., Hofman, A., & Tiemeier, H. (2019). The longitudinal and cross-sectional associations of grief and complicated grief with sleep quality in older adults. *Behavioral Sleep Medicine* 17(1), 31–40. Doi: 10.1080/15402002.2016.1276016.

Molina, N., Viola, M., Rogers, M., Ouyang, D., Gang, J., Derry, H., & Prigerson, HG. (2019). Suicidal ideation in bereavement—a systematic review. *Behavioural Sciences* 9(5), 53.

Newson, R.S., Boelen, P.A., Hek, K., et al. (2011). The prevalence and characteristics of complicated grief in older adults. *Journal of Affective Disorders* 132(2), 231–238. Doi: m10.1016/j.jad.2011.02.021

O'Callaghan C. & Michael N. (2016). Music therapy in grief and mourning. in *The Oxford Handbook of Music Therapy*. Doi: 10.1093/oxfordhb/9780199639755.013.42.

O'Callaghan, C.C., McDermott, F., Hudson, P., & Zalcberg, J.R. (2013). Sound continuing bonds with the deceased—the relevance of music, including preloss music therapy, for eight bereaved caregivers. *Death Studies* 37(2), 101–125. Doi :10.1080/07481187.2011.617488.

O'Connor, M.F. (2019). Grief—a brief history of research on how body, mind, and brain adapt. *Psychosomatic Medicine*, 81(8), 731–738. Doi: 10.1097/PSY.0000000000000717.

O'Connor, M.F. & McConnell, M.H. (2018). Grief reactions—a neurobiological approach. In Bui E. (eds) *Clinical Handbook of Bereavement and Grief Reactions. Current Clinical Psychiatry.* Humana Press, Cham.

Pan, H. & Liu F. (2019). The prevalence of complicated grief among Chinese people at high risk—A systematic review and meta-analysis. *Death Studies.* Doi: 10.1080/07481187. 2019.1648342.

Parkes, C.M. (1998). *Bereavement—Studies of Grief in Adult Life.* 3rd ed. International Universities Press, Madison, CT.

Prigerson, H.G. & Maciejewski, P.K. (2017). Rebuilding consensus on valid criteria for disordered grief. *JAMA Psychiatry* 74(5), 435–436. Doi: 10.1001/jamapsychiatry.2017.0293.

Radulovic, R. & Pejovic, M. (1997). *Muzika i depresija, Savremena administracija, Beograd.*

Radulovic, R. (2003). *Integrativna muzikoterapija i cerebralna paraliza,* Jugoslovensko udruženje za muzikoterapiju, Beograd.

Saavedra Pérez, H.C., Ikram, M.A., Direk, N., & Prigerson, H.G. (2015). Cognition, structural brain changes and complicated grief. A population-based study. *Psychological Medicine* 45(7), 1389–1399. Doi: 10.1017/S0033291714002499.

Schiele, M.A., Costa, B., Abelli, M., Martini, C., Baldwin, D.S., Domschke, K., & Pini, S. (2018). Oxytocin receptor gene variation, behavioural inhibition, and adult separation anxiety—Role in complicated grief. *The World Journal of Biological Psychiatry* 19(6), 471–479. Doi: the cognitive, verbal, motoric and musical abilities of a client.

Shear, K. M. (2015). Complicated grief. *The New England Journal of Medicine* 372, 153–160. Doi: 10.1056/NEJMcp1315618.

Spillane, A., Matvienko-Sikar, K., Larkin, C., et al (2018). What are the physical and psychological health effects of suicide bereavement on family members? An observational and interview mixed-methods study in Ireland. *The BMJ* 8, e019472. Doi: 10.1136/bmjopen-2017-019472.

Stroebe, M. & Schut, H. (1999). The dual process model of coping with bereavement rationale and description. *Death Studies* 23(3), 197–224. Doi: 10.1080/074811899201046.

Woods, R. (1982). *The Psychology of Aging—Assessment of Defects and Their Management, The Psychiatry of Late Life.* Blackwell Scientific Publications, Oxford.

22 Empowering the Community in Healthy Ageing

Goh Cheng Beh
Hospital Tuanku Ja'afar Seremban

Aaron K.T. Ang
Putra Polyclinic

CONTENTS

Introduction 253
    Definition of Empowerment 254
    Model of Empowerment 255
        Linear Empowerment Process Model 256
        Contextual Behavioral Empowerment Model 257
        The Social Work Model for Empowerment Oriented Practice 257
        The Iterative Empowerment Process Model 258
Empowerment in Malaysia 258
    Economic Dimension (Productive Ageing) 259
    Environment Dimension (Supportive Ageing) 259
    Health Dimension (Healthy Ageing) 260
    Social Dimension (Active Ageing) 260
    Spiritual Dimension (Positive Ageing) 261
Challenges in Empowerment 262
    Physical Accessibility Barrier 262
    Economic Barrier 262
    Social Barriers 262
    Unfriendly Nature of Healthcare Environment Barriers 262
Conclusion 263
References 263

INTRODUCTION

Globally, there were 703 million older persons aged 65 or over in 2019 (World Health Organization, 2002). The number of people aged 65 or older is projected to grow to nearly 1.5 billion in 2050, with most of the increase in developing countries (National Institute on Aging, 2011).

DOI: 10.1201/9781003043270-22

Malaysia, our focus in this chapter, has a large population of rapidly ageing people. According to the demographic statistics report, among Malaysia's population of 32.78 million in 2021, there has been an increase of 0.4% of ageing people as compared to the general population in 2020. Elders aged 60 and above are around 2.34 million in 2021 and were 2.24 million in 2019 (Department of Statistics, 2020). The worldwide report has indicated that in 2021, Hong Kong has the most elderly people with a longer life expectancy of 85.29 years old and is followed by Japan (85.03 years old) whereas Malaysia is ranked 74th (76.65 years old) and Singapore is ranked 5th (84.07 years old).

Morbidity and mortality can be secondary to communicable diseases and non-communicable (chronic) diseases with injuries. Non-communicable diseases including Alzheimer's disease and other dementias accounted for 74% of deaths worldwide in 2019. The rate of morbidity and mortality of females is 15% lower than males (Afshar et al., 2015). Hence, women would live longer with disability and with a poorer quality of life as compared to men.

An increasing ageing population has lots of challenges on ageism, mental and physical disabilities, socioeconomic/financial insecurity (poverty), legal issues, environmental issues (poor housing), inadequate and/or discriminatory healthcare services and social services accessibility. Consequently, a system is needed to be in place to enable the achievement of healthy ageing. Ultimately, the ageing population should thrive in a safe, friendly and happy environment with great dignity.

In January 2020, coronavirus disease-2019 (COVID-19) struck the world and a pandemic was announced by the World Health Organization (WHO) (World Health Organization, 2020). This pandemic has a negative impact on the health of people and socioeconomic standing of every country. COVID-19 began in December 2019 in Wuhan, China. It affects the most vulnerable elderly population most seriously and increases their morbidity and mortality, especially for those with other comorbidities.

Under this emergency period, elders face increased challenges while every government implements the 'new normal'. It is important for elders to have and continue a sustainable mental and emotional stability and healthy body. This is why the elders need to be empowered so as to reduce their morbidity, mortality and healthcare costs.

Definition of Empowerment

Application of the concept of empowerment is popular in healthcare service provision. The popularity of empowerment was brought to attention when societies encountered health cost enhancement and the government worked to reduce these costs through the transition from hospital to home care for patients and vulnerable people (Fotoukian et al., 2014). The elderly population is most likely to have suffered from a chronic illness or comorbidity and disability. Improvement of their health, quality of life and cost-effective hospitalization or health care will be possible with the community-based health empowerment intervention (Crawford Shearer, Fleury and Belyea, 2010). Consequently, empowerment is a process that provides mutual participation between old people and the society in order to achieve greater control on health, self-care acceptance, self-efficacy and the promotion of life quality. It is fundamental to the self-management of any chronic disease in the elderly.

Empowering the Community in Healthy Ageing

Different methods of empowerment have been promoted and implemented for elders in different countries globally. Empowerment was defined by the WHO as 'a process through which people gain greater control over decisions and actions affecting their health and should be seen as both an individual and a community process' (Nutbeam and Kickbusch, 1998). There could be 'individual' and 'community' empowerment. Individual empowerment refers primarily to one self's capability to make an informed choice and have control over one's personal life. Community empowerment involves many individuals acting mutually in order to produce greater influence and control over the determinants of health and the quality of life in their community. Both 'individual' and 'community' empowerment helps enhance the older population's self-confidence and self-esteem to acquire new skills. Subsequently, there will be an increase in elderly participation in community activities and a further improvement in their coping skills and self-care.

On the other hand, based on patient participation, knowledge and skills (self-efficacy and health literacy) and the presence of a facilitating environment, empowerment could be interpreted as 'a process in which patients understand their role, given the knowledge and skills by their healthcare provider to perform a task in an environment that recognises community and cultural differences and encourages patient participation' (World Health Organization, 2009). Through this empowerment, the elders participate in managing their health after obtaining accurate and proper information from the healthcare professionals. This helps decrease the morbidity and mortality of elders by early detection and management of their chronic disease or disability and improving their socioeconomic and environmental status which ultimately enhances their health further and promotes healthy ageing.

After appraising the view of Shearer and the WHO on empowerment, 'empowerment' could be interpreted as a means of processing the dignity of life through understanding the provided health status, knowledge and skills, followed by bearing their responsibility, particularly in making an informed choice and taking appropriate action for the betterment of their health in a facilitated environment with the participation from a recognized community.

MODEL OF EMPOWERMENT

Empowerment was developed as a three-level concept by Neil Thompson, based on 'personal, cultural and structural' (PCS) levels (Thompson and Thompson, 2001). The PCS approach doesn't offer formulae to generate empowerment but, rather, acts as a conceptual framework to help in understanding, exploring and addressing the complexities and challenges of ageing.

Empowerment training is about providing the necessary tools which will enable vulnerable elders to work constructively together to challenge oppression secondary to ageing. This, in turn, will bring about change in a society characterised by inequalities and discrimination. It is about personal development; it is about the social reconstruction of societal norms; and it is about promoting institutional change.

For further elaboration, the 'personal' level is related to the individual's ability to influence other people and the conditions he or she faces with self-confidence and self-esteem, which in turn impacts them having greater control over their lives. Moreover, good communication skills, interpersonal skills, charisma and strength of personality are required too.

At the 'cultural' level, it is important to have consciousness on shared meanings of the dominant culture, such as sets of assumptions, compartmentalisation, language and imagination during a discussion. This is because older people are often portrayed very negatively – for example, frail, dependent, a burden, disrespectful, undignified and being neglected in the community. If one wishes to promote empowerment from a cultural perspective, it is better to portray ageing positively.

There are structured patterns of inequality and differential social locations associated with ageing. This is most likely due to the fact that age, race or gender can operate as a form of social variance. Elders could be assigned to certain social positions with significant implications in different parts of the life of which can have differential awarding of life changes, status and social resources, hence, the need for policy development, constructive criticism of institutions and engagement in dialogue at the 'structural' level.

Let's explore models and strategies for developing empowering forms of social work practice in people with disabilities, older adults, women and others who lack power after understanding the concept of 'PCS'.

Linear Empowerment Process Model

Conger and Kanungo developed this model in 1988.[1] It focused on the process and action of empowering subordinates in the organization management context. It divided empowerment into five stages, namely psychological state of empowering experience, the managerial strategies and techniques used, self-efficacy information provision to subordinates, empowering experience of subordinates, and its behavioural consequences. This empowerment process focuses on diagnosis, intervention, and results.

The first stage is the diagnosis of conditions within the organisation that are responsible for feelings of powerlessness among subordinates. This leads to the use of empowerment strategies including goal setting, feedback system, and rewards by managers in Stage 2. The employment of these strategies is aimed not only at removing the external conditions responsible for powerlessness, but also (and more importantly) at providing subordinates with self-efficiency information to enact attainment and uplift emotion in Stage 3. As a result of receiving such information, subordinates feel empowered and have self-efficiency to perform tasks up to expectation in Stage 4, and the behavioural effects of empowerment are noticed in Stage 5.

The Linear Empowerment Process Model emphasised on the diagnosis of conditions or weaknesses before interventions. These interventions include directions, good settings, and rewards giving as well as personal development after obtaining information and support or encouragement. It does not touch on 'cultural' and 'structural' levels.

---

[1] Conger, J. A. and Kanungo, R. N. 'The Empowerment Process: Integrating Theory and Practice,' *Academy of Management Review* 13(3) (1988), pp. 471–482. See https://www.jstor.org/stable/pdf/258093.pdf?refreqid=excelsior%3Ab242cfc296e5073d451fdcab6fab2f7a (accessed June 28, 2021).

Contextual Behavioral Empowerment Model

Fawcett and colleagues developed this model of empowerment in 1994.[2] It focused on three components, namely the person or group, the environment, and the level of empowerment. There is an assumption that the level of empowerment is an outcome of the interaction between personal and environmental factors. Whereas the personal factor is mainly converting the degree of personal or a group's strength from vulnerable to strong. The outcome is that the people with physical disability, less knowledge or experience may become more empowered. Next is the factor of environment involving opportunity, discrimination, and accessibility of information may facilitate or restrict the outcome and status of empowerment. This empowerment model portrays the interrelation and combination of personal and environmental factors and formulates four main strategies. The strategies include (i) enhancing experience and competence; (ii) enhancing group structure and capability; (iii) removal of social and environmental barriers; and (iv) enhancing environmental support and resources. The empowerment strategy was used to improve agendas from the perspective of people with disabilities, enable access to homes through housing modifications or innovations, develop skills for personal self-advocacy, and promote self-directed behavioural change with personal and health concerns.

The Contextual Behavioral Empowerment Model portrays the interrelation of personal and environmental factors to empower people with physical disability, lack of knowledge or experiences via augmenting their competency and capability through resources and environmental support. This model encompasses 'personal' and 'structural' levels, but not 'cultural' level.

The Social Work Model for Empowerment Oriented Practice

This model was developed in 1994 by Cox and Parsons and was introduced in Japan in 1997.[3] This model was based on a theoretical and practical framework. The empowerment practice composes of a four-dimensional conceptualisation of problems and focus of interventions from micro to macro aspects.

The practical framework empathises on understanding the personal, interpersonal, and political aspects of at-risk populations and their situation, and developing interpersonal support networks. It stresses the identification and recognition of personal individual difficulties and needs, personal strengths and weaknesses, subsequently addresses them through training for skills development, providing or developing social support, and formulating relevant policies. The most important part is to encourage elders' active participation and a partnership in action.

Similar to the first model, the Social Work Model for Empowerment Oriented Practice involves establishing the conditions and weaknesses of the particular or specific individual or population and identifying the individual needs, personal training,

---

[2] Fawcett, S. B. et al., 'A Contextual-Behavioral Model of Empowerment: Case Studies Involving People with Physical Disabilities,' *American Journal of Community Psychology* 22(4) (1994), pp. 471–196. See https://www.researchgate.net/publication/15444191_A_contextual-behavioral_model_of_empowerment_Case_studies_involving_people_with_physical_disabilities (accessed June 28, 2021).

[3] Cox, E. O. and Parsons, R. J. *Empowerment Oriented Social Work Practice with Elderly* (Books/Cole Pub. Co., Pacific Grove, 1994).

258   Healthy Ageing in Asia

social and appropriate policy support. This model has reflected only the 'personal' and 'structural' stances and overlooked the 'cultural' aspects.

The Iterative Empowerment Process Model

Development of the Iterative Empowerment Process Model was based on "an iterative process, identifying core elements of that process, and defining the process in a way that is practically useful to both researchers and practitioners with terms that are easily communicated and applied."[4] The model comprises six main components, namely (i) personally meaningful and power-oriented goals; (ii) self-efficacy; (iii) knowledge; (iv) competence; (v) action; and (vi) impact.

Individuals move through the process with respect to a particular goal. Then, actions will be taken toward that goal and finally, there is observation and reflection on the impact of this action after drawing on the person's evolving self-efficacy, knowledge, and competence related to the goal. This model points out the importance of social context influencing all six components and their connection. Through this model, empowerment is attained through their own efforts.

The Iterative Empowerment Process Model mainly focuses on 'personal' facets. Following the goal direction, the people will be categorised based on their self-efficiency, knowledge, and confidence. Subsequently, they will be made aware of their weaknesses and attempt to achieve empowerment through their own efforts. This more independent approach without much support is mainly for professional groups of people or elders.

There are different categories of people with a lack of power such as people with dementia. The above four models are designed based on the different targeted populations. These models may not have complete "PCS" levels especially pertaining to the 'cultural' component. However, through adopting and adapting the different models which complement each other, one could ultimately design a holistic and inclusive model for older adults especially those who are helpless, isolated, and have low self-confidence.

EMPOWERMENT IN MALAYSIA

According to WHO, its Member States have their own empowerment model or program for the elders. As one of the Member States in the Western Pacific Region (WPR) of WHO, Hong Kong established the Hong Kong Society for Aged (SAGE) in 1997. SAGE is a non-governmental organisation that caters to the welfare needs of senior citizens. The Government of Hong Kong has provided senior citizens an accessible healthcare system pertaining to community care and socioeconomic support such as funds or homes for the lonely or disabled older people. The concept of an age-friendly city for its community of elders has been developed and implemented by the authorities. Similarly, Singapore has used its vast technology setting up a system

---

[4] Cattaneo, L. B. and Chapman, A. 'The Process of Empowerment A Model for Use in Research and Practice,' *American Psychologist* 65(7) (2010), pp. 646–659. See https://www.researchgate.net/publication/46576624_The_Process_of_Empowerment_A_Model_for_Use_in_Research_and_Practice (accessed June 28, 2021).

on health checks, physical or mental activity and employment, building up friendly and accessible environments for senior citizens.

Malaysia is one of the WHO Member States located in the WPR. Its implementation of empowerment varies based on the elders' sociodemographic characteristics including age group, gender, geographical area (rural vs urban), and level of education. In particular, approximately 30% of the older population live in rural areas and the majority of them are not well-educated – only 7.3% have received tertiary education. Therefore, their commonest social activities are gathering, conversation at leisure, watching television, listening to music, group Tai Chi and Yoga, as well as grocery shopping.

In Malaysia, the National Health Policy for Older Persons 2008 promotes "healthy, active and productive ageing by empowering the older persons, family and community with knowledge, skills, and enabling environments, and the provision of optimal healthcare services at all levels and by all sectors."[5] Subsequently, five wellbeing dimensions for the elderly were proposed by the Government in attempting to optimise the wellbeing of the older population, namely, (i) economy, (ii) environment, (iii) health, (iv) social, and (v) spiritual dimension.[6] Moreover, the four elements of socio-demographics, namely age group, gender, geographical area, and level of education play a role as a promoter for these five dimensions. Empowerment allows the creation of an appropriate approach for elders with regards to retirement, employment, social activity, and healthcare services.

Economic Dimension (Productive Ageing)

Malaysia's National Policy for Older Persons (2011) defines productive ageing as the participation of elders in either paid or unpaid activities that give meaning and satisfaction to them.[7] The aims were to encourage the elders to be more productive and independent and continue to participate in community or societal activities in paid or unpaid jobs. This is under the influence of factors such as socioeconomic background, religion, and education. Moreover, the retirement and pension scheme/employees provident fund (EPF) could help retired elders if other options are not available.

Environment Dimension (Supportive Ageing)

The National Policy for Older Persons (2011) has defined supportive ageing as the internal and external friendly environments that allow the older population to

---

[5] Ministry of Health, National Health Policy for Older Persons 2008 (Ministry of Health Malaysia, 2008), 11. See https://www.kpwkm.gov.my/kpwkm/uploads/files/Dokumen/Dasar/Dasar%20Kesihatan%20Warga%20Emas%20Negara.pdf (accessed June 29, 2021).

[6] Ramely, A. et al., 'Understanding Socio-demographic Patterns and Wellbeing Dimensions of the Elderly in Malaysia: The Way Forward in Reaching an Age Nation by 2030,' *Journal of Administrative Science* 15(1) (2018). See https://ir.uitm.edu.my/id/eprint/42493/1/42493.pdf (accessed June 29, 2021).

[7] Ministry of Women, Family and Community Development. *The National Policy for Older Person Malaysia* (2011). See http://www.kpwkm. gov.my/kpwkm/uploads/files/converted/6803/DasarWargaEmas1.pdf (accessed June 29, 2021).

function effectively and independently. Particularly, family members, friends, and colleagues can gather to learn or share amongst each other on the knowledge relating to the advancement of information technology applications (WhatsApp, video call), health services, transport, or environmental facilities (lift, disabled car park/road). A friendly and easy accessible environment can help the older population to function more effectively or independently.

HEALTH DIMENSION (HEALTHY AGEING)

Healthy ageing in the National Policy for Older Persons Malaysia (2011) has been interpreted as the fortitude in promoting a healthy lifestyle, the development of a better health system, and the existence of a healthy environment and local community that surrounds the elderly, for example, local community clinic (NCS medical clinic),[8] elderly activity program (Program Komuniti Sihat Pembina Negara/KOSPEN),[9] the financial support (Skim Peduli Keshatan for the B40 group known as PeKa B40),[10] and COVID-19 vaccination program for the elderly.

The severity of COVID-19 infection in the elderly could not be underestimated. Globally, elderly people are more likely to get very sick from COVID-19 infection needing hospitalisation, intensive care, or ventilator support. The risk increases with increasing age and with underlying medical conditions. Therefore, other than frequent hand washing, wearing a mask, and avoiding crowded places, vaccination is another strategy to prevent and to reduce the risk of getting severe infection. Adults 65 years old and older who were fully vaccinated with an mRNA COVID-19 vaccine (Pfizer-BioNTech or Moderna) had a 94% reduction in risk of COVID-19 hospitalizations and vaccination was 64% effective among those who were partially vaccinated (Pfizer-BioNTech or Moderna).[11] However, many elderly people chose not to be vaccinated for the fear of vaccine-induced side effects. In Malaysia, with proper educational tools and counselling, we have managed to encourage a good percentage (66% until 4 July 2021) of older population to come forth for vaccination which is not mandatory.[12]

SOCIAL DIMENSION (ACTIVE AGEING)

National Policy for Older Persons Malaysia (2011) has defined active ageing as the optimisation process of the involvement of the elderly person's family and community in empowering the wellbeing of the elderly. The re-enforcement of social activity

---

[8] https://www.healthhub.sg/directory/14/61189/ncs-medical-clinic (accessed June 29, 2021).

[9] http://iku.moh.gov.my/images/IKU/Document/REPORT/KOSPEN2016/KospenTechReport.pdf (accessed June 29, 2021).

[10] https://www.pekab40.com.my/eng/soalan-lazim (accessed June 29, 2021).

[11] https://www.cdc.gov/mmwr/volumes/70/wr/mm7018e1.htm (accessed June 28, 2021).

[12] https://www.google.com/search?q=National+Immunisation+program+for+elders&tbm=isch&ved=2a hUKEwjYz-DTzM3xAhUFGysKHbT3BBoQ2-cCegQIABAA&oq=National+Immunisation+progra m+for+elders&gs_lcp=CgNpbWcQAzoCCAA6BAgAEEM6BggAEAUQHjoECAAQGFCdZliPd2D1 eGgAcAB4AIABfIgBjgWSAQQxMC4xmAEAoAEBqgELZ3dzLXdpcei1pbWfAAQE&sclient=img& ei=39rjYJjkC4W2rAG075PQAQ&bih=657&biw=1366#imgrc=iyllM0On8MxccM (accessed July 6, 2021).

Empowering the Community in Healthy Ageing 261

amongst elders helps to increase their interest and participation. For example, during Chinese New Year or Hari Raya (Eid) or Deepavali festivals, the older people gather to do all the preparations (decoration, cooking, baking), and enjoy the joyful moment, as well as having information or skills sharing session. On other hand, if social or interactive activity has been reduced, it can lead to loss of confidence in the elderly, feelings of being socially isolated, and ultimately affecting their physical health status.

The social activities are to meet the needs of elders holistically through social, spiritual, physical, cognitive, and emotional perspectives. To further strengthen the social dimension, physical and social enablers and disablers will be touched upon to indicate how the elders' needs be addressed accordingly and holistically.[13] Re-ablement is to encourage, promote and assist older people continue to be socially, physically, and recreationally active. This allows the reduction or removal of the need for long-term ongoing or premature support, allowing them to remain as independent as possible.

Next, advocacy support is required for a person with care needs to address barriers or disablers, and enables them to remain active in the community. The advocate can be a family member, friend, and neighbor. The advocacy support could facilitate the access of social and recreational networks and maintain positive and respective relationships. Moreover, the advocates can play a role in listening to older people, helping them to solve problems, and upholding or protecting their rights. Religion and family background can influence the view and values of older people. Advocates need to have an open or broad mind to accept the fact that older people may have a different view, and should not attempt to change them. They are advised to place themselves in olders' shoes to listen, understand, and analyse to support their needs.

SPIRITUAL DIMENSION (POSITIVE AGEING)

Elderly must possess an optimistic spiritual mindset so as not to undermine their self-value and self-esteem even at old age. The elderly are encouraged to preserve a positive mindset and generate a good aura for society to perceive goodness in themselves. The National Policy for Older Persons Malaysia (2011) defines positive 'ageing' as the belief and positive value that become their life root and self-identity as well as possessing positive attributes and decent views on ageing. Elderly can age positively if they possess high self-esteem towards themselves and feel treasured by their family and society.

In optimising the wellbeing of the elderly in the context of the spiritual dimension, the application of four socio-demographic elements (age group, gender, geographical area, and level of education) in stimulating positive ageing is vital. For instance, while encouraging the elderly to feel cherished by their family and society, the consideration on their level of education is likewise apt. As most elders in Malaysia are poorly educated and underprivileged, they may feel inadequate in their later life.

---

[13] https://aspire-solidus-production.s3-ap-southeast-2.amazonaws.com/assets/CXAGE001/samples/CXAGE001.pdf (accessed June 29, 2021).

CHALLENGES IN EMPOWERMENT

When executing the empowerment of the community in healthy ageing, different resources or methodologies are used to improve and sustain a happy and comfortable environment for the elderly besides the attainment of good and quality health. It must be elaborated that there are many barriers that must be crossed to achieve this empowerment.

PHYSICAL ACCESSIBILITY BARRIER

In executing the empowerment of the community in healthy ageing, one of the most common barriers would be the high cost of transportation. As most elderly have lost their ability to travel independently, special arrangements have to be made for them. These include having disabled-friendly facilities at public transport systems, designated places or compartments for the elderly, and discounted fares. Besides that, roads system must be upgraded regularly to provide good and user-friendly roads. Public buildings and facilities must be elderly-friendly with ramps and lifts. All these features would require a huge allocation of the nation's budget each year.

ECONOMIC BARRIER

Most elderly have low income surviving only on a pension or Government's incentives. As not many establishments in Malaysia will hire them to work at this age, they have to live with the limited resources available. Their conditions are made worse by the high cost of living especially in the metropolitan areas. Some have had to rely on recycling wastes just to gain a few more dollars to sustain their life. To make matters worse, in rural areas, their healthcare facilities and services are not comprehensive enough. This leads to the elderly receiving substandard healthcare.

SOCIAL BARRIERS

Many elderly have poor communication and language skills. This could pose a great challenge for them to sustain their daily activities. Most of them also have poor family support which contributes to their low self-esteem.

UNFRIENDLY NATURE OF HEALTHCARE ENVIRONMENT BARRIERS

Due to their poor communication and language skills, they are ostracised by many people especially the younger generation. The poor attitude of healthcare providers can result in a lot of harm done to the elderly. Many elderly refuse to seek medical attention because of the rude and unbecoming behaviour of the health providers.

If we can address the above barriers, we could have a smooth connotation in the empowerment of the community in the healthy ageing of the elderly.

CONCLUSION

Empowerment is a holistic approach that encompasses the physical, psychological, emotional, health, and social issue of older population. Consequently, the ability to empower the community in healthy ageing will bring forth an improvement in the wellbeing of the elderly.

In conclusion, to obtain a successful, dignified well-meant ageing, we need to create or reinforce a holistic empowerment method that can cater for all elderly besides applying all kinds of measures to resolve the issue in the elderly. As the elderly are senior citizens who have directly and indirectly contributed to the growth, culture, and economy of the country in the past, it should be the duty of the present generation to look after them. Their physical and mental conditions, socioeconomic and cultural background, personality, coping skills, capability or strength, disability or weakness, psychological or emotional needs, attention to environment (sound judgement), good energy, urgency, commitment, concern of people or others should be properly addressed. Therefore, empowerment needs to focus strongly on the need to create or look for suitable jobs and to train the elderly to develop skills or technological knowledge and to avoid ageism or discrimination as well as to provide a suitable environment for them to live. All these could be realised if all government agencies can work in partnership with other non-governmental organisations (NGOs).

The stakeholders need to review, revise, reinforce the policies, and services, etc.; so that we can discover the pitfalls and perform countermeasures to improve the empowerment model which not only benefits the public but also the country. On the contrary, we need to share, updating own self and other regarding new information, facilities, resource, etc. so as that everyone can fully use these in a purposeful and meaningful way.

Finally, at the end of day, we aim for all in the elderly population to be able to maximise their engagement or participation in society or community activities or others which could increase independence and self-esteem indirectly reducing healthcare costs. They could become a valuable, meaningful person to their family and society at the end of the day. However, empowerment alone still has a long way to go, to prevent all ageism, inequities, etc. Therefore, we need to share and educate others, especially the younger generation because they will one day become old and all this can happen to them too.

REFERENCES

Afshar, S. et al. (2015) 'Multi-morbidity and the inequalities of global ageing: A cross-sectional study of 28 countries using the World Health Surveys', *BMC Public Health*, 15(776). doi: 10.1186/s12889-015-2008-7.

Crawford Shearer, N. B., Fleury, J. D. and Belyea, M. (2010) 'An innovative approach to recruiting homebound older adults', *Research in Gerontological Nursing*, 3(1), pp. 11–17. doi: 10.3928/19404921-20091029-01.

Department of Statistics. (2020) *Current Population Estimates, Malaysia, Online*. Available at: https://www.dosm.gov.my/v1/index.php?r=column/cthemeByCat&cat=155&bul_id= OVByWjg5YkQ3MWFZRTN5bDJiaEVhZz09&menu_id=L0pheU43NWJwRWVSZ klWdzQ4TlhUUT09 (Accessed: 22 February 2021).

Fotoukian, Z. et al. (2014) 'Concept analysis of empowerment in old people with chronic diseases using a hybrid model', *Asian Nursing Research*, 8(2), pp. 118–127. doi: 10.1016/j.anr.2014.04.002.

National Institute on Aging. National Institutes of Health, U.S. Department of Health & Human Services (2011) *Global Health and Aging.* Available at: https://www.who.int/ageing/publications/global_health.pdf

Nutbeam, D. and Kickbusch, I. (1998) 'Health promotion glossary', *Health Promotion International*, 13(4), pp. 349–364. doi: 10.1093/heapro/13.4.349.

Thompson, N. and Thompson, S. (2001) 'Empowering Older People', *Journal of Social Work*, 1(1), pp. 61–76.

World Health Organization. (2002) *Active Ageing: A Policy Framework.* Available at: https://apps.who.int/iris/handle/10665/67215

World Health Organization. (2009) *WHO Guidelines on Hand Hygiene in Health Care.* Available at: https://www.ncbi.nlm.nih.gov/books/NBK144013/pdf/Bookshelf_NBK144013.pdf.

World Health Organization. (2020) *WHO Timeline COVID-19, Online.* Available at: https://www.who.int/news/item/27-04-2020-who-timeline---covid-19 (Accessed: 24 June 2021).

23 Aging in Place
Beyond the Home

Jean Woo
Chinese University of Hong Kong

CONTENTS

Aging Successfully: Key to Aging in Place 265
Safe and Enabling Homes...266
Age-Friendly Environments Outside the Home..267
Pitfalls of the Digital Age 268
Conclusion 268
References..268

AGING SUCCESSFULLY: KEY TO AGING IN PLACE

Aging in place refers to the ability to remain living in the same environment without the need to relocate as a consequence of aging and accompanying physical or cognitive functional changes, if any. As the latter changes are common, it has been argued that successful aging describes those who have overcome any functional age-related changes and chronic diseases and limited disability to continue to lead productive lives, in line with the World Health Organization's concept of healthy aging that encompasses physical, cognitive, psychological, and social well-being. Other than lifelong learning and healthy lifestyles, a healthy environment (physical, social, and economic) plays an important role (Morley, 2015). A prerequisite for aging in place is a mechanism to detect unmet needs. Many healthcare systems do not include systematic screening for such needs, in particular early identification of common geriatric syndromes, such as frailty, sarcopenia, anorexia, mild cognitive impairment, and depression. These conditions may predispose to a functional decline, hence the call for rapid geriatric assessments in the community. A recent survey among 2,400 older persons aged 60 years and over attending community centers in Hong Kong showed a high prevalence of unmet needs, with memory problems, chewing difficulties, and pre-frailty and frailty being the most common problems (74%, 63%, and 38% respectively), while approximately 20% reported low subjective well-being and had problems with instrumental activities of daily living as well as insufficient income (Cheung et al., 2018).

It follows that aging in place is only desirable if conditions are met to optimize function to enable coping with common chronic disabling diseases, such as arthritis, stroke, as well as age-related syndromes, such as sensory impairment, chewing

DOI: 10.1201/9781003043270-23

difficulties, cognitive impairments (such as deficits in the domains of memory; processing speed; and executive function), impairments in instrumental activities of daily living, physical function, and psychosocial needs. Desirable goals with respect to aging in place include optimizing function by manipulating home design, furniture and aids, and reduction in isolation with the help of social network/support as well as technology. For the majority of people, aging in place will be synonymous with home-living; however, this may not be possible, and moving to a more enabling environment may be indicated to achieve active aging in spite of declining physical and cognitive function.

SAFE AND ENABLING HOMES

Ways to create a safe and enabling home include aids for bathing, dining, fall prevention, visual obstacle detection, transfer/lifting, cooking, emergency link, and ramp. Availability of personal care, communication external to home, and disease management are needed. Personal care may be provided by family members and/or formal carers. Both may require training in caring techniques, especially for those with dementia. A communication channel needs to be in place to allow rapid contact between the older person and carers in emergency situations (provided by alarm systems linked to mobile phones or dedicated services). In some countries, medical consultations may be provided with the primary care physician via telemedicine. From the point of view of maintaining social contacts to maintain a social network, technological advances have major contributions with smart TVs and mobile devices and related software such as FaceTime. In terms of disease management, technology has also provided various monitoring devices that can identify deviations in the usual pattern of movements and aid in physical training, medication management, as well as promotion of healthy diets.

There are some examples of promoting and building smart homes for aging in place in Hong Kong. The Hong Kong Science and Technology Park runs a demo showcase on smart living–aging in place that has a thematic focus on the role of technology on health monitoring, home safety, daily living, and rehabilitation [https://www.hkstp.org/en]. The Housing Society provides the first private senior housing in Hong Kong with monitoring and sensing equipment at the Tanner Hill development [http://www.thetannerhill.hkhs.com]. Some countries such as the United Kingdom have websites managed by nongovernment organizations listing aids and equipment for different aspects of home living that are available and may be purchased online for home delivery. Computer programs used for ongoing rehabilitation may also be installed at home to allow earlier return home from hospitals, such as the upper limb movement-based computer training program using "able X" (Lam et al., 2018). Computer-assisted interventions using touch screen video game technology have also been used in older Chinese adults with mild-to-moderate dementia to improve cognitive function and behavioral symptoms (Yu et al., 2015). The development of robots to aid in home tasks as well as providing social interaction has been spearheaded by Japan, particularly for use in eldercare. The use of the baby-seal PARO is well known and used in many countries including Denmark, Canada, Italy, and the United States since 2003, particularly for dementia care. In 2009, it was certified by the Food and Drug Administration as a therapeutic device. Efficacy has been documented in various clinical trials in eliciting positive responses, improved moods, reduced depressive symptoms, and caregiver burden (Robinson et al., 2016; Mervin et al., 2018).

Aging in place requires an understanding of needs from an older person's perspective and must be personalized. A common response to home adaptations for older people is an "universal design" [https://www.bd.gov.hk/english/documents/code/BFA2008_e.pdf]. However, this concept is not tailored for the specific needs of elders but follows general principles of a barrier-free environment for all ages and disabilities. There is a conflicting interest between end users and between design and practicality.

AGE-FRIENDLY ENVIRONMENTS OUTSIDE THE HOME

Age-friendly environments outside the home should also be considered, which includes the immediate surroundings as well as the spaced and urban characteristics at a further distance from the home, such as walkability, supportive neighborhoods that build a sense of community, and green spaces—designs of healing environments for hospitals. The design of immediate environment for homes and hospitals that have health benefits (healing environments) has been championed by some architects, emphasizing close proximity to nature (Goto et al., 2013; Visvanathan, 2018), and exemplified by the design of the geriatric unit of the Queen Elizabeth Hospital in Adelaide, Australia (Visvanathan, 2018).

The overall principles of age-friendly environments are summarized by the World Health Organization's concept of Age-Friendly Cities (AFC), covering age-friendly transport; housing; respect and social inclusion; civic participation and employment; health and community services; information and communication; social participation; outdoor spaces and buildings (Wong et al., 2017; Woo et al., 2017). Since many older people live in urban cities, attention to these principles may make a difference in promoting healthy aging instead of being obstacles. For example, a large cohort study of older people in Hong Kong aged 65 years and over showed that neighborhood green space is associated with a lower risk of all-cause mortality, in particular those caused by circulatory diseases, as well as frailty progression (Wang et al., 2017; Yu et al., 2018). There is also a variation in psychological health within a city, depending on urban characteristics, such as building height and density interacting with socioeconomic characteristics (Ho et al., 2017). A key mediator in the relationship between the physical environment and well-being is walkability. It is the predominant factor associated with health-related quality of life and social support, which is rated higher than leisure and social facilities in the older age-group aged 65 years and over compared with younger people (Chau et al., 2010; Woo, 2011). A study on community living of older people aged 65 years and over showed that walkability, walking time, well-being, and loneliness are linked (Yu et al., 2017). Social experiments are currently being carried out to redesign age-friendly communities in Kashiwa and Fukui in Japan, which incorporates all the AFC domains (Akiyama, 2010).

PITFALLS OF THE DIGITAL AGE

The use of information technology has transformed how populations lived in the past two decades. It has the power to facilitate healthy aging and aging in place. Yet, aging often leads to limitations in taking up new concepts and skills required for the use of new technology and may lead to societal exclusion through increasing adoption of technology by service providers (Bujnowska-Fedak and Grata-Borkowska, 2015). For example, many older people find it difficult just to get services due to the widespread use of automated voice recordings with various choices, without talking to an actual person. This caveat has been described as "information without wisdom: innovation working in the interest of medical–industrial complex versus the individual." 'Despite all its cleverness, big data and biometric sensors cannot access the lonely subjective experience of the fearful and distressed individual in the face of the threat of disease and death (Heath, 2017).

CONCLUSION

To conclude, aging in place requires an understanding of needs from an older person's perspective and must be personalized. The home environment needs to have suitable adaptations, and age-friendly environments outside the home should also be considered.

REFERENCES

Akiyama H (2010). Aging well: an update. *Nutr Rev* 78(S3):3–9.

Bujnowska-Fedak MM, Grata-Borkowska U (2015). Use of telemedicine-based care for the aging and elderly: Promises and pitfalls. *Smart Homecare Techn.* 3:91–105.

Chau PH, Chan KC, Cheung SH, Chan CMY, Woo J (2010, October 8–9). Neighbourhood and health outcomes. Age-Friendly World Cities Environment, Hong Kong.

Cheung JTK, Yu R, Wu Z, Wong SYS, Woo J. Geriatric syndromes, multimorbidity, and disability overlap and increase healthcare use among older Chinese. *BMC Geriatr.* 2018;18(1):147.

Goto S, Park BJ, Tsunetsugu Y, Herrup K, Miyazaki Y (2013). The effect of garden designs on mood and heart output in older adults residing in an assisted living facility. *HERD* 6(2):27–42.

Ho HC, Lau KK, Yu R, Wang D, Woo J, Kwok TCY, et al (2017). Spatial variability of geriatric depression risk in a high-density city: A data-driven socio-environmental vulnerability mapping approach. *Int J Environ Res Public Health* 14(9).

Heath I (2017). Information without wisdom. *BMJ.* 358(j3203). doi: 10.1136/bmj.j3203.

Lam S, Ng SSM, Lai C, Woo J (2018). Effectiveness of bilateral movement-based computer training program to improve the motor function of upper limb in sub-acute stroke patients - a randomized controlled trial. In *Speed and Poster Presentations in HA Convention*. HA Convention; May 7–8, Hong Kong.

Mervin MC, Moyle W, Jones C, Murfield J, Draper B, Beattie E, et al (2018). The cost-effectiveness of using PARO, a therapeutic robotic seal, to reduce agitation and medication use in dementia: Findings from a cluster-randomized controlled *Trial J Am Med Dir Assoc* 19(7):619–22 e1.

Morley JE (2015). Aging successfully: The key to aging in place. *J Am Med Dir Assoc* 16(12):1005–7.

Robinson H, Broadbent E, MacDonald B (2016). Group sessions with Paro in a nursing home: Structure, observations and interviews. *Australas J Ageing* 35(2):106–12.

Wang D, Lau KK, Yu R, Wong SYS, Kwok TTY, Woo J (2017). Neighbouring green space and mortality in community-dwelling elderly Hong Kong Chinese: a cohort study. *BMJ Open* 7(7):e015794.

Woo J (2011, November 16–17). Neighbourhood matters: Exploring spatial patterns in older people's health in Hong Kong. Cities Health and Well-being Urban Age Hong Kong, Hong Kong.

Wong M, Yu R, Woo J (2017). Effects of perceived neighbourhood environments on self-rated health among community-dwelling older Chinese. *Int J Environ Res Public Health* 14(6): 614. doi:10.3390/ijerph14060614.

Woo J, Yu R, Leung J, Wong M, Lau K, Ho HC, et al (2017). Urban characteristics influencing health of older people: What matters. *Int J Innovative Res Med Sci* 2(12):1561–8.

Yu R, Cheung O, Lau K, Woo J (2017). Associations between perceived neighborhood walkability and walking time, wellbeing, and loneliness in community-dwelling older Chinese People in Hong Kong. *Int J Environ Res Public Health* 14(10):1199. doi:10.3390/ijerph14101199.

Yu R, Poon D, Ng A, Sit K, Lee J, Ma B, et al. (2015). Computer-assisted Intervention using Touch-screen Video Game Technology on Cognitive Function and Behavioural Symptoms for Community-dwelling Older Chinese Adults with Mild-to-Moderate Dementia - Preliminary Results of a Randomized Controlled Trial. In *Proceedings of the 1st International Conference on Information and Communication Technologies for Ageing Well and e-Health* 297–302. doi: 10.5220/0005490402970302.

Yu RB, Wang D, Leung J, Lau K, Kwok T, Woo J (2018). Is neighborhood green space associated with less frailty? Evidence from the Mr. and Ms. Os (Hong Kong) study. *J Am Med Dir Assoc* 19(6):528–34.

Visvanathan R (2018). Implementing geriatric programmes of excellence in Adelaide, Australia. *Asian J Gerontol Geriatr* 13(1):31–5.

24 Mapping Healthy Ageing Start-ups

The Role of Accelerators and Incubators in Supporting Innovation for Prevention and Wellness in Southeast Asia

Kishan Kariippanon
University of Wollongong

CONTENTS

Introduction 272
  Technology for Health 272
  What is a Start-up? 274
  A Snapshot of Asian Start-ups Tackling Healthy Ageing Challenges 274
  Accelerators and Incubators 276
  A Snapshot of Accelerators/Incubators in Asia 277
  Knowledge Translation in Health Prevention and Wellness 277
    Problematization 278
    Interessement 278
    Enrolment 278
    Mobilization 279
  Dementia-Friendly Design: The Desert Rose House and
  iAccelerate – A Case Study 279
  Methodology 282
  Critical and Collective Reflexivity 283
  Privacy 284
  Master Bedroom 285
  Bathroom 285
  Kitchen 285
Conclusion 286
References 287

DOI: 10.1201/9781003043270-24

271

INTRODUCTION

There is little doubt that the global health crises in the world, brought by the COVID-19 pandemic, were exacerbated by a significant increase in the global burden of non-communicable diseases (NCDs) in the last three decades. The number of years lived with disability (YLD) has increased between 1990 and 2017 by 61.1% according to James et al. (2018) creating synergistic health problems that affect vulnerable populations under persistent socio-economic inequities. Mendenhall et al. (2017) argue in The Lancet that 'syndemic' is a term that captures the best approximation of health burdens of transitioning populations, particularly in low-to-middle-income countries (LMICs). A clear example of a syndemic is the interaction of people living with diabetes in the context of persistent poverty which may include added challenges such as 'forced migration, unemployment, gender inequality, racism and a lack of social capital' (Corburn and Hildebrand, 2015).

In the context of the 21st-century crisis in NCDs and low mental health support in LMICs, the importance of critical and creative thinking has never been more important in the history of public health. The need to expand student learning in interdisciplinary training outside their disciplinary concentration has become the norm for universities, especially the Mailman School of Public Health at Columbia University (Begg et al., 2014). To tackle complex problems facing public health administrators, interdisciplinary collaboration becomes a foundation for reflection and action (reflexivity is, therefore, reflection in action). The action begins at an organizational level through innovation in leadership (Hougaard and Carter, 2018; Mathias, Fargher, and Beynon, 2018). As LMICs bear nearly 90% of the global burden of diseases and have severe shortages of trained healthcare providers, innovative health and medical technologies become the next frontier for exploration. These innovative health and medical technologies are included in one of the six essential building blocks of the WHO Health System Framework and have the potential for a positive impact on LMICs (Olson et al., 2017) (Table 24.1).

TECHNOLOGY FOR HEALTH

Developments in health technology can be transformative. These technologies can afford to offset the limitation of the healthcare workforce by optimizing the efficiency, accuracy and effectiveness of providers, but the growth of health medical technology in Asia has only recently begun to gain momentum. Approximately 40%–70% of technologies developed in high-income countries (HICs) fail when implemented in LMICs (Olsen et al., 2017). There is a broad scope for partnerships, but locally driven innovation between LMICs and HICs ensures relevance, cultural effectiveness, feasibility and acceptability are attained in regard to developing new technologies. This could help reap the benefits of what Olson et al. (2017) refer to as relative 'value', otherwise defined as health outcomes over cost.

Mobile health or mHealth has seen an accelerated expansion in LMICs, becoming ubiquitous and more powerful. An estimated USD 4.3 billion was invested in digital health technologies in 2015 with a market share of more than 160,000 iOS- and Android-related healthcare applications or apps. It is certainly unrealistic to think that global health challenges along its social costs can be solved by technology

TABLE 24.1
Comparison of the Elderly Population across Regions between 2015 and 2030 (Asia Pacific Risk Center, 2018)

Geographical Region	2015	2030
North America	🚶🚶🚶🚶🚶	🚶🚶🚶🚶🚶🚶🚶
European Union	🚶🚶🚶🚶🚶🚶🚶🚶🚶 🚶	🚶🚶🚶🚶🚶🚶🚶🚶🚶🚶🚶 🚶🚶
Rest of the world	🚶🚶🚶🚶🚶🚶🚶🚶🚶 🚶🚶🚶🚶🚶🚶🚶	🚶🚶🚶🚶🚶🚶🚶🚶🚶🚶🚶 🚶🚶🚶🚶🚶🚶🚶🚶🚶🚶🚶 🚶🚶🚶🚶
East Asia, South Asia, South East Asia and Oceania (excl, Central Asia)	🚶🚶🚶🚶🚶🚶🚶🚶🚶 🚶🚶🚶🚶🚶🚶🚶🚶🚶 🚶🚶🚶🚶🚶🚶🚶🚶🚶 🚶🚶🚶	🚶🚶🚶🚶🚶🚶🚶🚶🚶🚶 🚶🚶🚶🚶🚶🚶🚶🚶🚶🚶 🚶🚶🚶🚶🚶🚶🚶🚶🚶🚶 🚶🚶🚶🚶🚶🚶🚶🚶🚶🚶 🚶🚶🚶🚶🚶🚶

or mobile apps. The low-hanging fruits of healthcare challenges are constantly addressed by high-tech innovations, but very few attempt to tackle systems-level factors contributing to poor health or managing chronic diseases. There is still a lack of mHealth app adoption across the population that has led to sustained improvements in health outcomes. A mHealth app will have the potential to succeed if it fits into a comprehensive, systemic solution from the bottom up (Angelidis et al., 2016).

A report from Galen Growth, a leading digital intelligence and analytics consultancy for investors, showed that in 2019, the total funding for health tech in Southeast Asia doubled to USD 266 million. With a 2.25 times growth, this rate represents growing maturity in the health technology ecosystem. Singapore and Indonesia comprised 93% of the total funding value in the region, while countries such as Myanmar, Malaysia and Vietnam expand their ecosystem and attractiveness for start-up health tech development. India made a significant increase in attracting investors to their health tech ecosystem with a total investment of USD 723 million. China remains at the top as the country with the most health tech investments at USD 3.4 billion in 2019. The country remains the top funder with mainland Chinese making up the bulk of investors of the top ten health tech investments across the Asia–Pacific region (https://indvstrvs.com/healthtech-in-south-east-asia-breaks-funding-records/).

In just over a decade, four in five people living in Southeast Asia had only limited Internet access. Today, there are more than 360 million Internet users in the region, with about 100 million added only in the last 4 years. Healthcare professionals (85% in Southeast Asia) are now more confident in using data or interacting with the patient via mobile apps, wearables and other forms of technology in their future practice. Governments such as Indonesia, Malaysia, the Philippines and Thailand are catching up and have introduced measures to include technology into their healthcare system (Huizingh, 2017).

Partnerships are a key variable in deciding where venture capital funding is funnelled to scale the innovation. Halodoc (https://www.halodoc.com/) is an online platform in Bahasa Indonesia that provides patients with a one-stop portal for medical consultation and treatments including an online pharmacy. Patients can even locate a hospital of their choice. Halodoc entered a partnership agreement with Prudential Life Assurance who has invested in Halodoc to provide services to over two million of its customers in Indonesia. MyDoc Pty Ltd (Singapore) and AXA Singapore created a partnership to enable employees and clients to conduct video and messaging consults with a qualified healthcare professional through their smartphone. Intudo Ventures, Monk's Hill Ventures, Wavemaker and Openspace Ventures are just some of the top venture capital firms investing in the health tech ecosystem in Southeast Asia.

What is a Start-up?

The industry that spurs technological innovation for social and technological change is made up of functional units called a start-up. A start-up is an organization or corporate entity that is designed to work in limited financial resources, a small number of founder innovators or staff with a sole purpose to work on a solution of a specifically identified problem which in this context is affecting the health of the population. Often the problem itself is identified by the start-up through various methods which potentially begins with a hunch (Perez-Breva, 2017; Tracey and Stott, 2017), and then includes qualitative interviewing of key stakeholders, observations and prototyping solutions to validate the problem (Perez-Breva, 2017; Langås-Larsen et al., 2018). A start-up becomes an expert in the problem they are trying to understand and solve with innovation by creating either a new product or service but under conditions of uncertainty (Frederiksen and Brem, 2017). A product or service by a start-up provides value to the customer experience. The word 'innovation' according to Frederiksen and Brem (2017) is to be understood broadly such that a new scientific discovery, a new use for old technologies and the identification of a new business model that taps into a hidden value are all efforts that create a product or service to meet new market demand. Start-ups are used to facing extreme uncertainty and are very different to duplicating a business model that competes via pricing, target customer or products (Frederiksen and Brem, 2017). Start-ups often face unlimited challenges in their journey to innovate, and very often they are housed and supported in organizations called an accelerator or incubator.

A Snapshot of Asian Start-ups Tackling Healthy Ageing Challenges

As Singapore's baby boomer generation (1946–1964) celebrated their 65th birthdays, they are not only living longer but thriving as healthy and active members of their community. An elderly care start-up called Homage announced its series B funding

Mapping Healthy Ageing Start-ups

that it plans to use for expansion into Asia. This start-up offers a digital platform that connects healthcare providers with elderly people and their loved ones or carers in need of home-based care. Homage has raised more than USD 15 million from investors such as Golden Gate Ventures, HealthXCapital, EV Growth, Alternate Ventures and KDV Capital. Homage paved the way for more digital health start-ups to offer 'active ageing' products and services that support the healthy ageing population to stay active and more importantly independent while still being connected (https://www.techinasia.com/singapore-seniors-startups-step-up).

The success of Homage can also be attributed to the Singaporean government's policy to become a global healthcare technology hub. The city state is already home to about 9% of Asia's health tech start-ups after India and China (https://www.techinasia.com/singapore-seniors-startups-step-up).

Biofourmis is a biotechnology company founded in Singapore that uses wearables and artificial intelligence (AI) to collect and analyse patients' health data to predict the possibility of adverse outcomes such as heart attacks. Having raised USD 40 million in equity financing, the start-up aims to partner with pharmaceutical companies to further develop products that are effective in managing heart disease.

In Japan, the manufacturing of e-skin wearable technology by a company called Xenoma (https://xenoma.com/news/article/200911.php) has the potential to significantly collect, analyse and improve the daily vitals of their elderly users. Their technology is smart apparel that creates a multi-modal sensor infrastructure. It is essentially a tight-fitting bodysuit with sensors built in to monitor sleep as well as a separate fitness training suit to measure the efficiency of the fitness training programme. This healthcare company is interested not only in e-skin technology but especially in the use of big data collected by their products to predict and prevent early signs of diseases.

mClinica is an example of a health tech start-up that may directly benefit the ageing population in Asia. Their digital platform enables patient adherence to pharmacological treatments. Using a data-driven program, patients are enabled to better afford and understand their medication while improving health outcomes for their clients (https://www.top10asia.org/main/rankings/top-10-asian-healthtech-startups/).

A health tech start-up based in China called iCarbonX combines genomics and health factors such as metabolites, bacteria and lifestyle behavioural data to create a digital repository. By combining data from new biological measures and millions of people around the world, the founder Jun Wang uses AI to search the data for signals about health, disease and ageing. iCarbonX is using AI to better classify conditions, refine diagnoses and create a targeted treatment for biologies in a specific way (https://www.top10asia.org/main/rankings/top-10-asian-healthtech-startups/).

Ping An Good Doctor is a one-stop healthcare ecosystem with more than 250 million users founded by Wang Tao in China. Ping An Good Doctors works by employing medical personnel in its in-house medical team and contracts renowned external doctors. Together with AI, a 24×7 online consultation service, Ping An Good Doctor also collaborates with over 3,000 hospitals to provide referrals, appointments and inpatient management (https://www.top10asia.org/main/rankings/top-10-asian-healthtech-startups/).

Medifi (https://www.medifi.com/) is an online medical platform that connects patients with doctors using a propriety video calling feature. Patients may choose from over 3,000 doctors available via an app, with no subscription fees, and pay only for each consultation. Patients may also receive digital prescriptions via the app, including lab requests and medical certificates. This HIPAA compliant app democratizes healthcare and allows healthcare to be personalized and home-based or wherever you are.

DocDoc (https://www.docdoc.com/patients) is a healthcare technology run by a group of professionals who have been patients using AI to connect patients, insurers and doctors with telemedicine and cashless services on one platform. The patients benefit from the optimization of health expenditure and enhance patient end-to-end health journey.

Alodokter (https://www.alodokter.com/) is an online platform in Bahasa Indonesia that provides medical information to patients and carers that is easy to understand, accurate and accessible to everyone. The platform is managed by a team of doctors and has the support of the Ministry of Health of the Republic of Indonesia.

The chairman and CEO of ROKIT Healthcare (https://rokithealthcare.com) claims that 'Aging is a Disease' and that as a company they endeavour to change the world with proprietary biofabrication technologies across all types of applicable diseases in the field of regenerative medicine.

ACCELERATORS AND INCUBATORS

Accelerators are also known as seed accelerators, start-up accelerators or business accelerators and are short programs that are time-limited, often lasting up to no more than 6 months, with a core business goal to coach and support start-up ventures to achieve their entrepreneurial potential and aspirations. Accelerators have a physical building where start-ups are provided with a co-working space with an Internet connection, small seed capital and a wide range of networking, educational and mentorship opportunities from the directors of the accelerator, external participants from successful businesses, venture capitalists and angel investors referred to as 'mentors' (Cohen et al., 2019). The most notable accelerator programs are Y Combinator, founded in 2005, and Techstars, founded in 2007. Both accelerators have helped launch over 2000 start-ups that have, in turn, collectively raised more than USD 16 billion in funding. The use of accelerators as a training and mentoring platform to guide the innovation and learning process of start-ups to bring a viable solution to a specific market is the new norm, where a third of all start-ups receiving venture capital in 2015 had been through an accelerator program (Cohen et al., 2019).

Start-up incubation continues from accelerators to provide a platform and support for commercialization research. The start-up ecosystem contributes to the economy by

generating employment, empowering the poor, regenerating and revitalising communities, encouraging and supporting innovation, creating export revenues, encouraging young graduates to create their businesses, developing new industry sectors (such as creative industries, alternative energy, rural livelihood, healthcare, and social services), and increasing the competitiveness of an existing sector.

Baskaran, Chandran, and Ng (2019 p. 388)

A Snapshot of Accelerators/Incubators in Asia

China is home to 159 accelerators and incubators. The Hong Kong Science and Technology Parks Corporation (HKSTP) is an incubator/accelerator with more than 890 companies and 9,000 researchers working towards innovation that enable technology transfer and commercialization. The HKSTP connects start-ups with their vast network of investors, assists in market adoption of technology solutions, expands and nurtures the talent pool in research and development and go-to-market support (https://www.hkstp.org/about-us/who-we-are/). Another example is Cyberport (https://www.cyberport.hk/en/about_cyberport/about_overview), which is committed to enabling a supportive tech ecosystem, promoting entrepreneurship among youth, integrating new and traditional economies by accelerating digital adoption in the private and public sectors.

BlueChilli is an Australian accelerator with a new base in Singapore (https://www.bluechilli.com/healthtech/). Their interest in Asia is to scout for bold ideas and domain experts and have partnered with Enterprise Singapore's Start-up SG Accelerator initiative to support health tech start-ups in the region. Together both BlueChilli and Startup SG provide funding and non-financial support for start-ups to develop new products and services, obtain business financing and improve market access (https://www.startupsg.gov.sg/programmes/4900/startup-sg-accelerator).

In Thailand, the National Innovation Agency was assigned by the Ministry of Science and Technology to spearhead the start-up development and promotion project. Two accelerators support health tech start-ups in Thailand: DEPA Accelerator Program (https://techsauce.co/depa-accelerator/) and SPRINT (https://sprintacceleratorthailand.com/).

Knowledge Translation in Health Prevention and Wellness

Public health interventions that focus on promoting healthy ageing are now joined by a new hybrid generation of researchers using a preventative framework and the use of digital technology, wearables and mobile technology. It is still uncommon for mainstream public health practice to venture into the area of design to integrate seamless prevention of lifestyle diseases (Lupton, 2018).

The practical application of design-led public health efforts in Asia would naturally incorporate the elements of tradition and culture without mimicking western practices of health promotion, for example promoting the consumption of salads as opposed to Malay 'ulam' in the local Malaysian diet. Lupton (2018) adopts an engineering-based innovation lens to look at public health challenges. For example, instead of an aetiological approach or assumptions of stakeholders as lacking in basic health information, the researcher or practitioner is encouraged to define the problem and engage with it from the standpoint of the stakeholder and their lived experiences. Researchers and practitioners who attempt to translate knowledge may also consider that the problematization of lifestyle-based diseases is challenging and requires multiple stakeholders. For example, it would only be practical if women who are now juggling career and household responsibilities in certain contexts, can be enabled to prepare a healthy meal instead of providing healthy meal plans to men who are most at risk of metabolic syndrome.

Translation of research requires empathy and understanding of the lived experiences of the population at risk and utilizing health technology through an iterative process that requires time and financial investment. The pain points for the disadvantaged population are also more often felt by the government and not for profits, as the normalization or acceptance of pathology has become rampant in LMICs.

There are four phases of knowledge translation according to Waerass and Nielsen (2016): Problematization, Interessement, Enrolment and Mobilization. This section is relevant to this chapter as it outlines a very clear picture of the co-design-led approach to knowledge translation.

Problematization

In this earliest phase of knowledge translation for prevention and wellness, a link to research on the context of the intervention is pertinent. The researcher or practitioner studies carefully the traditional and cultural, understanding systematic challenges or even entrenched practices that need decolonization. All the actors are identified, including the non-human actors. Non-human actors such as mobile phones, the Internet, wearables and other Bluetooth-friendly devices such as a glucometer or digital sphygmomanometer (for measuring blood pressure) have their capability for influence, or convenience, but more importantly of acceptance to both the culture and practice of the host context.

Interessement

In the next phase of knowledge translation, the researcher or practitioner calls upon 'other actors', different stakeholders that contribute to engaging with the innovation ecosystem. In this instance, healthy ageing healthcare providers and start-ups or organizations are invited to share different perspectives on the identification of the true problem. The topic for discussion and reflection is based on the results of phase 1, the 'problematization' based on the views and experiences of the previous set of actors. Through a series of research activities, one entity of actors is asked to define and stabilize the identity of another group of actors. This stage of reflection between a different set of actors is where many shortcuts are taken. Design requires a level of collective reflexivity which new start-ups cannot afford to don't miss an opportunity to design and implement programmes for prevention and wellness that (i) implement technology that is not needed, (ii) solve a problem that is not a pain for the user and (iii) the solution is cumbersome and does not take into consideration cultural context and sensitivities.

Enrolment

The role of collective reflexivity is positioned to align all the immediate stakeholders or actors with the other set of actors who are at arm's length but still have a role to play in implementing prevention and wellness interventions that are culturally sensitive and traditionally relevant. In this phase, the collective of actors or stakeholders understand their roles in the ecosystem of innovation and have come to an agreement on the 'problem' and what their efforts will be in addressing the issue.

Mobilization

In the final phase of knowledge translation mobilizing social change and, implementing innovation in using culture and traditional methods for prevention and wellness, requires strategies for sustainability. Leadership qualities in researchers and other vested entities are key to keeping focus and traversing the trial and error stages of innovation to find out how best knowledge can be translated to have an impact in the lives of the people.

In the next section, a case study is provided to show how knowledge translation between researchers and a university-based accelerator can support innovation and engagement with the local community using co-design principles and researcher reflexivity.

The Solar Decathlon is both an academic and industry-led design challenge started by the US government to tackle real-world housing challenges with solutions that use renewable energy, from sustainable material, and improve the well-being of the dwellers (https://www.solardecathlon.gov/event/challenges-design.html). Teams from various tertiary education institutions from around the world attend the Solar Decathlon and present their design and construction projects to a panel of industry jurors, learn from other teams, compare their solutions and engage with a variety of stakeholders on the career pathways as engineers in the design and energy industry.

In 2018, the University of Wollongong took part in the Solar Decathlon Middle East organized by the Government of Dubai. Fifteen teams took part in this challenge, and over 3 weeks, the team assembled their houses in the desert not far from Dubai to showcase how their innovation can meet the challenges of a hot climate with religious requirements. The University of Wollongong team decided to build a dementia-friendly home for the ageing population of Dubai and incorporate sustainable design and renewable energy and incorporate the aesthetics of the Middle East into their build. The next section elaborates further on the process that was used to design and build a dementia-friendly dwelling, which encourages ageing in place and is affordable to maintain.

DEMENTIA-FRIENDLY DESIGN: THE DESERT ROSE HOUSE AND IACCELERATE – A CASE STUDY

More than 50 million people are living with dementia, which costs the economy more than USD 1 trillion. These numbers are expected to rise with time, and in Asia, this will predominantly be driven by increasing life expectancy. Two goals were decided upon in 2013 where the G8 (now G7) nations held a dementia summit. The nations committed to develop a cure for dementia by 2025 or to significantly increase the amount of funding for dementia research through greater innovation to improve the quality of life for those living with dementia and their carers (Pickett and Brayne, 2019).

The Desert Rose House is an innovative residential construction that provides maximum comfort, elegance and privacy, backed by a design that compliments the needs of sustainable living and healthy ageing in the Middle East. The house enables ageing in place and was built based on the Dementia-Friendly Environmental Design

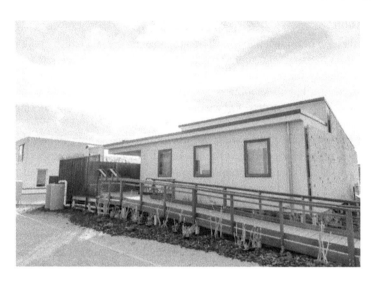

FIGURE 24.1 The Desert Rose House as constructed in Dubai for 2018. (Solar Decathlon Middle East.)

framework. The co-design process involved people living with dementia, carers, retirees, industry professionals, researchers and doctoral students (Figure 24.1).

The co-design process allowed counter-narratives to influence its design and construction. The use of ethnographic and autoethnographic methods from the social sciences provided a rich perspective from all stakeholders. The aim of the autoethnographic approach, which gave importance to the experiences of people living with dementia, was to disrupt norms of research practice and representation. Through a multidisciplinary team represented by faculty and students from engineering, the humanities and vocational institutions, these data were further analysed and reflected upon during the iterative co-design process until a consensus was reached. The Desert Rose House was shipped to Dubai in 2018 to participate in the Solar Decathlon Middle East competition with 14 other teams from around the world.

The Desert Rose House was designed and built not only to suit the climatic challenges of the Middle East but also to be culturally sensitive to religious norms and allow for social interactions in the house when entertaining guests. The Middle East takes pride in hospitality, and allowing for privacy in the household is important. Designing these elements for a dementia-friendly house was not an easy task. Through a 6-month training programme at iAccelerate, an accelerator/incubator based at the University of Wollongong, the construction and design team came together to map out the key driving principles that combine cultural sensitivities and dementia-friendly design.

The design process results could be distilled into four major areas:

1. Familiarity and emotions: The interior of the house needed to be built around old and strong memories, incorporated with meaningful items that

evoke understandable associations. Familiar music, pictures and colour comfort the occupants and lift them emotionally.
2. Minimize complexity and choice: The design eschewed any urge to automation which removes the agency of the occupants. Rather, the design focused on clarity and simplicity, making it easier for the occupants to choose and act without confusion. Too many buttons and options are often the cause of confusion that is detrimental to people living with dementia.
3. First impression and acceptance: The Desert Rose design team took great care in learning how to design without 'othering' the user or causing more stigma for those living with dementia. The interaction with the everyday appliances and the use of the bathroom and laundry facilities all evoke curiosity and are attractive but make acceptance quite easy. The technology is reliable and has a quick response time.
4. Positive and supportive feedback: The design elements on the Desert Rose House incorporated simple feedback mechanisms through vision, hearing and touch. For example, when turning on the tap, the user has the option of twisting the tap or simply pushing the tap. The usability of the tapware can be adjusted to suit the specific needs of the occupant (Figure 24.2).

The role of the accelerator in this case study was to provide a framework for leadership in design and construction that meets industry needs and challenge the current norms of designing retirement dwellings for the elderly. iAccelerate provided training in preparing a business model, customer engagement, creating a value proposition for multiple stakeholders and also how to pivot in the face of insurmountable challenges (Figure 24.3).

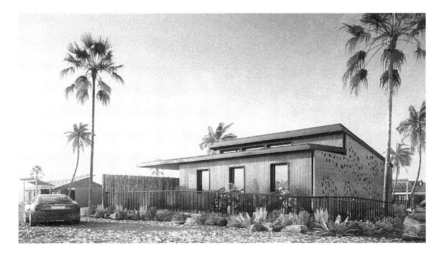

FIGURE 24.2 First rendering of the Desert Rose House.

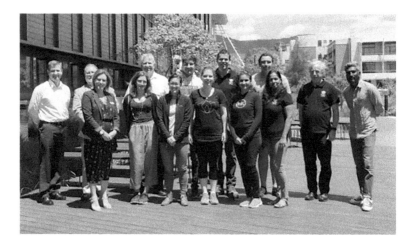

FIGURE 24.3 The multidisciplinary team of faculty and students working with people living with dementia in the design process (leadership team).

Methodology

The co-design process allowed counter-narratives to influence its design and construction. The use of ethnographic and autoethnographic methods from the social sciences gave importance to the experiences of people living with dementia and disrupted norms of design, research practice and representation. The data in the form of talks, narratives, video narratives and photo-voice including observations were analysed with the help of a multidisciplinary team represented by faculty and students from engineering, the humanities and vocational institutions (TAFE) (Figure 24.4).

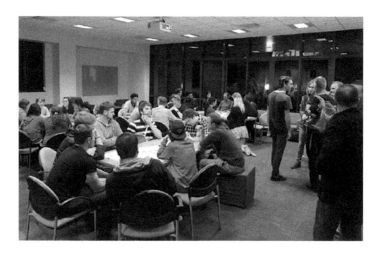

FIGURE 24.4 Workshops with a diverse student's representation from across the university.

Mapping Healthy Ageing Start-ups

CRITICAL AND COLLECTIVE REFLEXIVITY

The process of analysis required collective reflexivity to layer the different requirements and needs of the various stakeholders to create solutions and decisions that are comprehensible, meaningful and manageable (Lindström and Eriksson, 2006). Regular meetings with members of the community and people living with dementia were organized to provide consistent critique and feedback to the team. The co-design process acknowledged that there were assumptions that required validation and a paucity of design decisions that were meaningful to elderly people. The collected narratives transformed professional practice by providing insights into the lived experience of people who want to age in place. As a result of this reflexive co-design process, a shift from a clinical design to one that reduces the stigma of ageing and dementia was achieved. The house is relevant to all age groups but capable of allowing its residents to age in place (Figure 24.5).

The Desert Rose House was conceptualized to incorporate contemporary residential construction innovations that provide maximum comfort, elegance and privacy backed by a design that compliments the needs of sustainable living in the Middle East. The interior design adopts both Middle Eastern and European design concepts to produce a house that combines features sought by both mainstream Australian and traditional Muslim culture.

To accomplish this, the interior design team adopted a neutral design that allows aspects of both cultures to be seamlessly intertwined throughout the living spaces (Figure 24.6).

Strong weighting has been placed upon the colours chosen such as blues and greys have been chosen as they can make rooms appear larger – while the former has the added benefit of inducing feelings of calm, safety, protection and spirituality. This is an important feature as the home is known as a place of safety and family unity.

As the house has strict solar envelope requirements as well as an architectural footprint, clever use of colour and light was incorporated into the design to help maximize lighting and give the effect of greater open space. As the house was designed to grow with the ageing population, special considerations were incorporated into the design, which included the following:

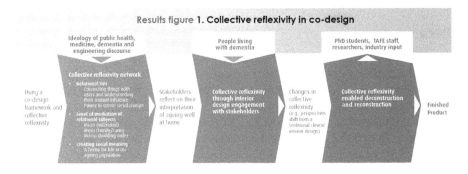

FIGURE 24.5 The process of collective reflexivity.

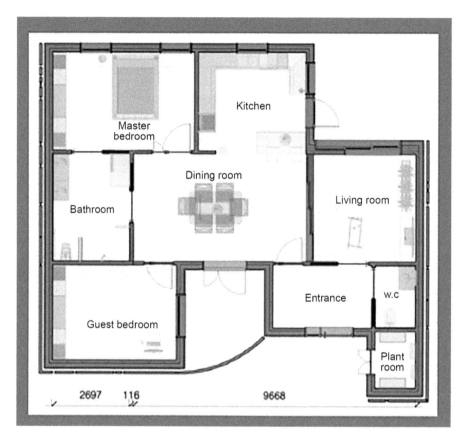

FIGURE 24.6 The interior layout of the Desert Rose House.

Light reflective values (LRVs) – a minimum of 30 LRV difference is required between different surfaces: wall and floor, furniture and wall. We have endeavoured to provide where possible LRV of up to 62. Keeping flooring colour consistent and reducing reflection throughout the house can improve the quality of life for elderly residents living with dementia (Figure 24.7).

Privacy

Many Islamic cultures emphasize modesty, privacy, personal space and hospitality within the confines of one's home. Given these cultural customs, special consideration had to be taken while developing the house layout. Firstly, regarding privacy, it was decided that a front door should be designed in such a way that it does not give immediate access to domestic quarters, but least to a vestibule, or a lobby, which will prevent the interior from being exposed to the outside world when the front door is opened. Taking into consideration the cultural sensitivities around gender and the interaction with men who are not close relatives by the female residents of the household inspired the design and construction of a partitioned living or multipurpose room.

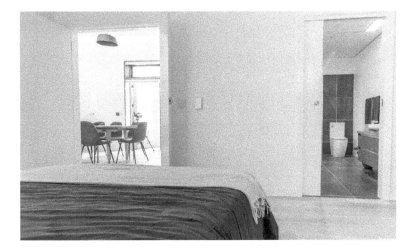

FIGURE 24.7 View from the master bedroom. The clear line of sight to the bathroom and dining area enables elderly people with dementia to navigate without confusion. Easy access at night to the bathroom with automatic lighting when movement is detected.

To provide privacy as well as hospitality characteristics in the design, the Desert Rose House facilitates an unobstructed movement of people. The layout of the dwelling allows for the 'awrah', or privacy and peace, dwelling to keep certain spaces of the house private while entertaining guests and being hospitable.

MASTER BEDROOM

The master bedroom is accessible from the dining area and is connected to the bathroom via an internal entrance. The bedroom is equipped with a bedside table and a queen-size bed built from recycled Australian timber. A series of built-in cupboards are installed to be wheelchair-friendly with shelves that can be accessed easily from a sitting position. The position of the bed has been taken into consideration relative to the direction of Mecca, the Holy City for Muslims (Figure 24.8).

BATHROOM

The bathroom has also been designed to be accessible by wheelchair and with anchor points for future installation of handrails and supporting points as the occupants of the house age. The taps in the bathroom are digital but simulate a normal twist motion that is easy to use. Elderly people with difficulty in turning taps due to arthritis will find it easy to use. The taps also turn off automatically if the user forgets.

KITCHEN

In the kitchen, designs have been implemented which are stylish and embedded with features that aid the use of residents who are bound by a lack of physical ability,

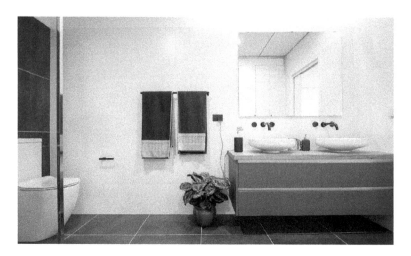

FIGURE 24.8 Digital taps in the bathroom.

for example a resident in a wheelchair. We have incorporated appliances that are user-friendly in a kitchen layout that makes it a safer place for aged/disabled occupants and those with dementia. Design features include cupboards with enough room underneath for wheelchair footplates, adjustable bench heights, and roomier areas underneath benches if the occupant prefers to sit while preparing food. All kitchen materials have been chosen to be shatter-proof and able to mitigate any possible risk of injury to disabled occupants, while non-slip tiles, the elimination of any sharp corners, cabinets and cabinet/cupboard doors are implemented as a further risk mitigation measure.

Standard features such as an induction cooktop and an oven are installed – with the oven designed with a slide-open door for ease of use for wheelchair-bound occupants; other nuanced features for convenience include wall-lift cabinets, crosshead taps and a pull-out shelf below the oven (Figure 24.9).

The Desert Rose House won the 2nd prize overall at the Solar Decathlon Middle East 2018. It took 2 years and 40 students from both the University of Wollongong and vocational educational institution TAFE NSW with the support of individuals living with dementia to achieve this incredible outcome. The Desert Rose House came first in interior design, comfort and innovation as separate categories. The house has been reconstructed in the new Sustainability Precinct on Innovation Campus, University of Wollongong, for public tours and for educational sessions for school STEM programmes and to promote the technology and furniture donated by the sponsors who believe in sustainability.

CONCLUSION

The multidisciplinary approach to health ageing has gained more support from the business and technology innovation sector. Researchers and potential academic spin-offs can reach out to their preferred or local accelerator and incubator to learn how

Mapping Healthy Ageing Start-ups

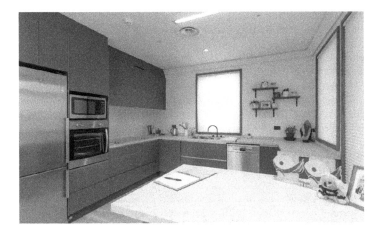

FIGURE 24.9 The kitchen is designed for use in a wheelchair, and accessible storage allows for decluttering. The cabinets are scratch resistant, and the benchtop is a synthetic material that dampens noise.

to commercialize their innovation and bring suitable, culturally relevant and usable products and technology to the ageing market in Asia.

This chapter's effort to map the healthcare innovation activity in the Asian regions was to enable the readers, researchers and small-to-medium enterprises to see that innovation and commercialization for healthy ageing is taking place in Asia at a rapid pace attracting multimillion-dollar series of funding. The challenges for the Asian context will be in finding solutions that are not only technologically savvy, but promote local practices and are culturally sensitive. Accelerators and incubators are potentially key stakeholders in the process of promoting healthy ageing and will be better poised to support technology start-ups if they are made aware of the traditional and complementary practices in the region before scaling to a wider audience. Understanding the Asian market is necessary, as a lack of adoption will increase attrition of users and force the start-up to abandon their ideas or pivot to another market.

REFERENCES

Angelidis, P. et al. (2016) 'The hackathon model to spur innovation around global mHealth', *Journal of Medical Engineering and Technology*, 40(7–8), pp. 392–399. doi: 10.1080/03091902.2016.1213903.

Baskaran, A., Chandran, V. G. R. and Ng, B. K. (2019) 'Inclusive entrepreneurship, innovation and sustainable growth: Role of business incubators, academia and social enterprises in Asia', *Science, Technology and Society*, 24(3), pp. 385–400. doi: 10.1177/0971721819873178.

Begg, M. D. et al. (2014) 'MPH education for the 21st century: Design of Columbia University's new public health curriculum', *American Journal of Public Health*, 104(1), pp. 30–36. doi: 10.2105/AJPH.2013.301518.

Cohen, S. et al. (2019) 'The design of startup accelerators', *Research Policy*, 48(7), pp. 1781–1797. doi: 10.1016/j.respol.2019.04.003.

Corburn, J. and Hildebrand, C. (2015) 'Slum sanitation and the social determinants of women's health in Nairobi, Kenya', *Journal of Environmental and Public Health*, 2015. doi: 10.1155/2015/209505.

Frederiksen, D. L. and Brem, A. (2017) 'How do entrepreneurs think they create value? A scientific reflection of Eric Ries' Lean Startup approach', *International Entrepreneurship and Management Journal*, 13(1), pp. 169–189. doi: 10.1007/s11365-016-0411-x.

Hougaard, R. and Carter, J. (2018) *The Mind of the Leader: How to Lead Yourself, Your People and Your Organization for Extraordinary Results*. Boston, MA: Harvard Business Press.

Huizingh, E. K. R. E. (2017) 'Moving the innovation horizon in Asia', *Technovation*, 60–61(February), pp. 43–44. doi: 10.1016/j.technovation.2017.01.005.

James, S. L. et al. (2018) 'Global, regional, and national incidence, prevalence, and years lived with disability for 354 Diseases and Injuries for 195 countries and territories, 1990–2017: A systematic analysis for the global burden of disease study 2017', *The Lancet*, pp. 1789–1858. doi: 10.1016/S0140–6736(18)32279-7.

Langås-Larsen, A. et al. (2018) '"We own the illness": a qualitative study of networks in two communities with mixed ethnicity in Northern Norway', *International Journal of Circumpolar Health*, 77(1), p. 1438572. doi: 10.1080/22423982.2018.1438572.

Lindström, B. and Eriksson, M. (2006) 'Contextualizing salutogenesis and Antonovsky in public health development', *Health Promotion International*, 21(3), pp. 238–244. doi: 10.1093/heapro/dal016.

Lupton, D. (2018) 'Towards design sociology', *Sociology Compass*, 12(1), pp. 1–11. doi: 10.1111/soc4.12546.

Mathias, M., Fargher, S. and Beynon, M. (2018) 'Exploring the link between integrated leadership in government and follower happiness: the case of Dubai', *International Review of Administrative Sciences*, 85(4), pp. 780–798.

Mendenhall, E. et al. (2017) 'Non-communicable disease syndemics: poverty, depression, and diabetes among low-income populations', *The Lancet*, 389(10072), pp. 951–963. doi: 10.1016/S0140-6736(17)30402-6.

Olson, K. R. et al. (2017) 'Health hackathons: theatre or substance? A survey assessment of outcomes from healthcare-focused hackathons in three countries', *BMJ Innovations*, 3(1), pp. 37–44. doi: 10.1136/bmjinnov-2016-000147.

Perez-Breva, L. (2017) *Innovating: A Doer's Manifesto for Starting from a Hunch, Prototyping Problems, Scaling Up, and Learning to be Productively Wrong*. Boston, MA: MIT Press.

Pickett, J. and Brayne, C. (2019) 'The scale and profile of global dementia research funding', *The Lancet*, 394(10212), pp. 1888–1889. doi: 10.1016/S0140-6736(19)32599-1.

Tracey, P. and Stott, N. (2017) 'Social innovation: a window on alternative ways of organizing and innovating', *Innovation: Management, Policy and Practice*, 19(1), pp. 51–60. doi: 10.1080/14479338.2016.1268924. https://www.un.org/development/desa/indigenouspeoples/publications/state-of-the-worlds-indigenous-peoples.html.

United Nations. (2017) *State of the World's Indigenous Peoples: Education*. Available at: https://www.un.org/development/desa/indigenouspeoples/wp-content/uploads/sites/19/2017/12/State-of-Worlds-Indigenous-Peoples_III_WEB2018.pdf.

Waerass, A. and Nielsen, J. A. (2016) 'Translation theory "Translated": Three perspectives on translation in organizational research', *International Journal of Management Reviews*, 18(3), pp. 236–70. doi: 10.1111/ijmr.12092.

25 Translational Research
A Novel Yam Protein with Tremendous Potential for Menopausal Syndrome

Stephen Cho Wing Sze
The Golden Meditech Centre for
NeuroRegeneration Sciences

CONTENTS

Introduction 290
    Hormone Replacement Therapy (HRT) for Menopausal Symptoms 290
    Population Aging in Mainland China, Hong Kong SAR,
    Asia, Europe, and the USA 291
    Estrogen, Healthy Aging, and Longevity 291
    Isolation of Estrogenic and Osteogenic Protein DOI from Yam
    (*Dioscorea opposita*) Rhizomes 292
    Characterization of DOI from Yam (*Dioscorea opposita*) Rhizomes 292
    Stimulatory Effect of DOI on Viability of Normal Cells (Rat Ovarian
    Granulosa Cells and Mouse Splenocytes) and Its Suppressive Effect
    on Cancer Cells (Ovarian Cancer OVCA-429 Cells and Breast Cancer
    MCF-7 Cells) 293
    Estradiol-Stimulating Effect of DOI *In Vitro* 293
    Estradiol-Stimulating Effect of DOI *In Vivo* 294
    Stimulatory Effect of DOI on Expression of FSHR and Aromatase *In Vivo* 294
    Stimulatory Effect of DOI on Bone Mineral Density and Microarchitecture ...294
    Stimulatory Effect of DOI on Expression of BDNF and Its Receptor
    TrkB gp145 in the Prefrontal Cortex of the Brain 295
    DOI-Like Proteins from Other Dioscorea Species 295
Discussion 296
Acknowledgments 296
References 296

DOI: 10.1201/9781003043270-25

INTRODUCTION

This intent of this chapter is to describe the discovery of a protein from yam which would benefit postmenopausal women who are afflicted by uncomfortable symptoms and facing health problems due to estrogen deficiency that accompanies their increasing age.

Hormone Replacement Therapy (HRT) for Menopausal Symptoms

Menopausal syndrome refers to the variety of symptoms manifested by women in menopause, encompassing difficulty going to sleep, nervousness, mood disorders, depression, night sweat, and hot flushes. There is an ensuing heightened risk of osteoporosis and cardiovascular disease due to the decline in estrogens. The total worldwide population of postmenopausal women is expected to be 350% of that in 1990 by 2030. The current approach for alleviating menopausal syndrome is HRT, which aims at compensating for the postmenopausal decline in estrogen. Systemic hormone estrogen therapy employing a higher dose is utilized to treat the common menopausal symptoms. Low-dose vaginal estrogen is used to deal with urinary and vaginal menopausal symptoms. Estrogen is often administered in conjunction with progesterone or progestin since estrogen alone enhances the risk of endometrial cancer. Long-term use of HRT may protect against cataract genesis. HRT reduces inflammation and elevates antioxidant levels in the blood of postmenopausal women (Jee et al., 2021). However, the estrogen–progestin pill heightens the risk of blood clots, breast cancer, cardiac disease, and cerebrovascular accidents. Patients who commence HRT in their sixties or older or more than 10 years from the onset of menopause are at greater risk of the above conditions. Family history, personal medical history, and risk of blood clots, heart disease, stroke, liver disease, and osteoporosis cancer are important factors. HRT is not recommended for treating postmenopausal symptoms in triple-negative breast cancer patients with lack of expression of the estrogen receptor (ER) and progesterone receptors (PRs), and without amplification of human epidermal growth factor receptor-2 (*HER2* or *ERBB2*) (Bauer et al., 2007, Horstman et al., 2012; van Barele et al., 2021). Hence, there is a pressing need for safe and effective therapeutic agents such as plants capable of inducing estrogen secretion to attenuate menopausal syndrome and prevent deterioration in memory and cognition (Echeverria et al., 2021). It is presented in this chapter that a 33.5-kDa protein designated as DOI isolated from rhizomes of the yam *Dioscorea opposita* has the attribute of augmenting estradiol secretion from ovarian granulosa cells, upregulating expression of ovarian aromatase and expression of brain-derived neurotrophic factor (BDNF) and its receptor TrkB gp145 in the prefrontal cortex of the brain, and in addition, fortifying the bone mineral density and microarchitecture. The yam protein is a promising therapeutic candidate for menopausal syndrome, especially in view of the fact that it exhibits antiproliferative activity toward breast cancer cells and ovarian cancer cells and proliferative activity toward spleen cells and ovarian granulosa cells.

Population Aging in Mainland China, Hong Kong SAR, Asia, Europe, and the USA

Mainland China has one of the world's largest populations as well as one of the most rapidly aging populations, caused by years of declining birth rate and escalating life expectancy. As the aging of the population has strong repercussions on the economy, it will become a major challenge for Chinese society in the decades to come. The increase in life expectancy is accompanied by deteriorating health, impaired cognitive function, and disabilities. The speedy economic development and urbanization in mainland China have led to a separation of the elderly from their children, raising the need for community-based health care. The situation is similar in Asia, Europe, and the USA, albeit to a less serious extent. This highlights the importance of a focus on healthy aging in order to improve the quality of life.

At present, population aging in Hong Kong SAR is a less serious problem compared to Japan and Italy, and about the same as that in the UK. However, the elderly population in Hong Kong will increase from 15% in 2013 to 30% in 2033, even more rapidly than the expected pace in Japan. The elderly population in South Korea and Taiwan is expected to double in 17 and 20 years, respectively. The elderly population in Europe and America will remain under 30% even 50 years later (Wong and Yeung, 2019).

Population aging is a global issue. The population aged above 65 is to double to 1.5 billion in 2050. Population aging has been fastest in Eastern and South-Eastern Asia (doubled during the period 1990–2019) and Latin America and the Caribbean (60% increase during the period 1990–2019). Between 2019 and 2050, the share of older persons is expected to double or increase more in Northern Africa and Western Asia, Central and Southern Asia, Latin America and the Caribbean, and Eastern and South-Eastern Asia. Life expectancy is expected to lengthen globally. Women currently live longer than men by about 5 years, but the difference is expected to narrow over the next 30 years (United Nations, 2019).

Estrogen, Healthy Aging, and Longevity

Aging is related to a decline of gonadal hormone in both sexes: andropause in men and menopause in women. In men, reductions in testosterone can initiate a fall in bone mass, muscle mass, and physical function. In women, the effect of estradiol on bones is well known, but there is only some evidence regarding whether decline of estradiol adversely impacts muscle mass and physical function. Nevertheless, the lack of anabolic hormones has been demonstrated to predict health status and longevity in people of an older age. Thus, whether targeted HRT may have an effect in treating age-associated sarcopenia, cancer cachexia, and acute or chronic illnesses merits attention. HRT in women may prevent and reverse fall in bone mass, muscle mass, and physical function and perhaps enhance healthy aging and longevity (Horstman et al., 2012).

Isolation of Estrogenic and Osteogenic Protein DOI from Yam (*Dioscorea opposita*) Rhizomes

In China, the *Dioscorea opposita* species of Chinese yam is the most commonly used of the genus 'group' of Dioscorea species for improving female health and regulating menstruation. Furthermore, the rhizome part of the stem of the species has been classified as a Chinese herbal medicine by the Chinese government. *Dioscorea opposita* rhizomes purchased from a market in Hong Kong were authenticated by an expert, peeled, and homogenized in 5% acetic acid–0.1% β-mercaptoethanol (1:2 w/v) for 3 hours at 4°C. The homogenate was centrifuged before precipitation of the proteins with 80% saturated ammonium sulfate. The precipitated proteins were collected by centrifugation, resuspended, dialyzed, and then ultra-centrifuged. The supernatant collected was subjected to anion exchange chromatography on a HiPrep 16/10 DEAE Fast Flow column using an AKTA Purifier FPLC system. Gradient elution of the column was employed (buffer A: 100 mM Tris, pH 8.0; buffer B: 1 M NaCl, with 100 mM Tris, pH 8.0; gradient: 0%–45% buffer B). The large unadsorbed fraction D1 and the first adsorbed fraction D2 lacked estrogen-stimulating activity. The most strongly adsorbed fraction D3 was the only fraction with estrogen-stimulating activity. After dialysis, fraction D3 was subjected to FPLC on a HiPrep 16/10 Phenyl Fast Flow (high sub) column using gradient elution (buffer A: Milli-Q H_2O; buffer B: 10 mM sodium phosphate, pH 7.0, with 1 M $(NH_4)_2SO_4$; gradient: 30%–0% buffer B). The first and largest fraction P1 with estrogen-stimulating activity was collected, dialyzed, and lyophilized before FPLC-gel filtration on a Superdex 75 10/300 GL column in 50 mM sodium phosphate buffer (pH 7.2) containing 150 mM NaCl. The bulk of the eluate present in the major peak fraction S1 containing the purified protein DOI with estrogen-stimulating activity was collected, dialyzed, and then lyophilized. The yield of DOI from *Dioscorea opposita* rhizomes was 0.36% of the total soluble proteins.

Characterization of DOI from Yam (*Dioscorea opposita*) Rhizomes

DOI displayed a molecular weight of 33.5 kDa as determined with mass spectrometry, and 32.5 kDa as determined by gel filtration on Superdex 75, 15% native PAGE, and 15% SDS-PAGE followed by silver staining. The N-terminal sequence GIGKITTYWGQYSDEPSLTE was determined by Edman degradation using a protein sequencer. The partial amino acid sequence was determined using mass spectrometry. DOI was dissolved in 50 mM NH_4HCO_3, treated with 300 ng trypsin/Lys-C mix at 37°C for 16 hours, and dried using a SpeedVac. Peptide analysis was performed using nanoLC-MS/MS. The mass spectrometer was operated in a data-dependent mode with a single MS full scan (m/z 350–1200), followed by top 20 MS/MS scan. The data were searched with MaxQuant using the UniProt/Swiss-Prot plant database.

BLAST analysis of the N-terminal sequence of DOI disclosed an elevated E-value exceeding 10^{-3}, showing its novelty. DOI belongs to the chitinase-like superfamily. BLAST analysis of the partial amino acid sequence of DOI revealed its pronounced

Translational Research

resemblance to the 27.9-kDa *Dioscorea japonica* chitinase (AAB23692.1) and the 31.4-kDa *Dioscorea oppositifolia* chitinase (BAC56863.1). Mass spectrometry analysis of DOI tryptic peptides revealed ten peptides that matched peptides in *Dioscorea japonica* acidic endochitinase. The identified peptides are highlighted in bold in the partial sequence of acidic endochitinase. The N-terminal sequence manifested dissimilarities from the 31.4-kDa *Dioscorea oppositifolia* chitinase (BAC56863.1). DOI did not exhibit any discernible chitinase activity toward different chitinase substrates, including 4-nitrophenyl N-acetyl-β-D-glucosaminide, 4-nitrophenyl N,N′-diacetyl-β-D-chitobioside, and 4-nitrophenyl β-D-N,N′,N″-triacetylchitotriose (N8638).

Hemagglutinating activity was indiscernible in DOI, indicating that it is not a lectin. DOI is also without chitinase activity, and DOI (1–10 nM) displayed estrogen-stimulating activity in rat ovarian granulosa cells. DOI (10 nM) showed acid stability as its estrogen-stimulating activity remained intact after treatment with HCl (0.01–1 M) and also showed thermostability at 80 °C, but it did not show alkali stability in NaOH (0.01–1 M).

STIMULATORY EFFECT OF DOI ON VIABILITY OF NORMAL CELLS (RAT OVARIAN GRANULOSA CELLS AND MOUSE SPLENOCYTES) AND ITS SUPPRESSIVE EFFECT ON CANCER CELLS (OVARIAN CANCER OVCA-429 CELLS AND BREAST CANCER MCF-7 CELLS)

In the MTT assay, DOI increased the viability of rat ovarian granulosa cells and mouse splenocytes in a dose-dependent manner. At 100 nM DOI, there was an approximately 40% and 60% increase, respectively. The viability of ovarian cancer OVCA-429 cells and breast cancer MCF-7 cells underwent a dose-dependent decline after exposure to DOI, and at 100 nM DOI, a circa 20% reduction was observed. Thus, DOI did not exert toxicity toward normal cells *in vitro* but curtailed the viability of cancer cells.

ESTRADIOL-STIMULATING EFFECT OF DOI *IN VITRO*

Rat ovarian granulosa cells were isolated as follows. Pregnant mare serum gonadotropin (80 IU) was injected into Sprague-Dawley rats (21–23 days old) to stimulate ovarian follicular development. The rats were sacrificed 48 hours later. Granulosa cells were isolated from the ovarian follicles by puncturing with a needle and then incubated with DOI for 12 hours. The cell culture medium was collected for determination of estradiol levels, and cellular proteins were extracted for Western blot analysis.

Rat ovarian granulosa cells exposed to DOI (10 nM) exhibited an 8% increase in estradiol biosynthesis, 100% increase in aromatase expression, and 1200% follicle-stimulating hormone receptor (FSHR) expression compared to the control. In the presence of protein kinase A inhibitor, 10 nM DOI-induced estradiol levels in the culture medium of granulosa cells were reduced.

ESTRADIOL-STIMULATING EFFECT OF DOI *IN VIVO*

In response to treatment of the rats with 2.5, 5, and 10 mg/kg DOI for 6 weeks, estradiol and progesterone attained zenith levels, with a 120%, 180%, and 180% rise in estradiol and 85%, 100%, and 100% increment in progesterone, respectively. Estradiol biosynthesis was also promoted by 12.4 mg/kg premarin. The lack of a change in body weights of the rats signifies that DOI is devoid of toxicity. The ratio of final ovarian weight to final total body weight remained steady after treatment with DOI (2.5 and 5 mg/kg). However, treatment with 10 mg/kg DOI and premarin increased the ovarian weight, with the ratio of final ovarian weight to final total body weight from 0.032% to 0.047% and 0.048% ($p < 0.05$), respectively.

STIMULATORY EFFECT OF DOI ON EXPRESSION OF FSHR AND AROMATASE *IN VIVO*

Following treatment with DOI, FSHR and CYP19 mRNA expression in the rat ovaries determined by real-time PCR was significantly enhanced, with the maximal effect produced by DOI observed at 2.5 mg/kg. Rat ovarian protein kinase A mRNA expression was significantly increased by 72% in response to treatment with 10 mg/kg DOI.

Western blotting analysis disclosed that the protein expression levels of ovarian aromatase were significantly upregulated by 77% as a result of treatment with DOI at 2.5 mg/kg and by 66% after treatment with DOI at 5 mg/kg. In contrast, the breast aromatase protein expression level was unaffected by DOI, *in vitro* as well as *in vivo*. The protein expression level of aromatase in MCF-7 breast cancer cells remained unaltered after treatment with DOI. DOI at the dosages of 2.5, 5, and 10 mg/kg significantly heightened the protein expression level of ovarian FSH receptor by 67%, 100%, and 56%, respectively. Following treatment with 10 mg/kg DOI, the protein expression level of protein kinase A was significantly enhanced.

The mechanism with which DOI promotes estradiol and progesterone formation awaits elucidation. DOI increases the ovarian expression of ovarian and ovarian aromatase. The pituitary hormone FSH binds to FSH-specific G protein-coupled receptors (FSH receptors) on granulosa cells. FSH activates the membrane-bound adenyl cyclase, increases intracellular cAMP formation, and activates protein kinase A. FSH stimulates the activity of 3β-hydroxysteroid dehydrogenase on the steroidogenic pathway and enhances the conversion of pregnenolone to progesterone in granulosa cells. FSH is the major inducer of aromatase which catalyzes the conversion of testosterone to estradiol (Stocco, 2008; Oktem et al., 2017; Casarini and Crépieux, 2019). DOI resembles the action of FSH in some ways. It remains to be seen how it produces its actions, for instance, by using ovariectomized rats to see whether the estrogen induced is of ovarian estrogen.

STIMULATORY EFFECT OF DOI ON BONE MINERAL DENSITY AND MICROARCHITECTURE

Regarding the action of DOI in osteogenesis, apparent trabecular bone mineral density and bone microarchitecture were assessed with the built-in program of an *in vivo*

Translational Research

MicroCT 40 computed tomography system using the model-independent direct 3D morphometry. All 18-month-old female SD rats that had received DOI in different doses for 6 weeks exhibited an apparent bone mineral density of the second lumbar vertebra (L2) higher than that of the control group. The apparent bone mineral density was significantly elevated due to treatment with DOI (87% increase in the 2.5 mg/kg group and 157% increase in the 5 mg/kg group). The bone volume fraction was augmented by 60% following treatment with DOI (2.5 mg/kg) compared with the control group. L2 trabecular thickness was raised by 10% and 20%, respectively, compared with the control rats after treatment with DOI (2.5 and 5 mg/kg). DOI at various dosages brought about a decline in the structure model index of vertebra L2 compared with the control, and the 30% reduction observed after treatment with 2.5 mg/kg DOI group reached statistical significance. There were no significant changes in trabecular separation of vertebra L2 after DOI treatment, except for the 23% decrease seen after treatment with 5 mg/kg DOI.

STIMULATORY EFFECT OF DOI ON EXPRESSION OF BDNF AND ITS RECEPTOR TRKB GP145 IN THE PREFRONTAL CORTEX OF THE BRAIN

In order to ascertain how DOI impacts cognitive function, BDNF protein levels in the rat hippocampus and prefrontal cortex were determined with ELISA and normalized using the total protein concentration of the individual samples. Regarding determination of receptor TrkB gp145, immunoblotting was carried out using antibody against TrkB receptor and using anti-GAPDH antibody as the internal standard. Chemiluminescence was measured using densitometry following incubation with horseradish peroxidase-conjugated secondary antibody. The results revealed that as a consequence of administration of 5 mg/kg DOI, a significant increase was observed in BDNF concentration in both the prefrontal cortex (34% increase) and the hippocampus (30% increase) and also in TrkB gp145 receptors (43% increase) in the prefrontal cortex.

DOI-LIKE PROTEINS FROM OTHER DIOSCOREA SPECIES

Microscopic authentication of four Dioscorea species (*D. alata* L., *D. zingiberensis* C.H. Wright, *D. collettii* var. hypoglauca (Palib.) S.J. Pei & C.T. Ting, and *D. oppositifolia* L.) was carried out using paraffin and powder sections of the rhizomes. Basic features typical of rhizomes of Dioscorea species comprising suberized cells, cortex, and starch granules and basic features of the powder of Dioscorea species including starch granules and vessels were examined. The methodologies are well established. Affinity-purified polyclonal antibodies were raised in New Zealand white rabbits against purified DOI protein. An affinity column with the aforementioned anti-DOI antibodies covalently attached using AminoLink® Plus Immobilization kit was employed to bind and purify DOI-like proteins from four Dioscorea species. The SDS-PAGE gel showed that different Dioscorea species possessed DOI-like proteins with different molecular weights, but a 32.5-kDa major band appeared after purification. The denatured protein extracts of *D. alata, D. collettii, D. oppositifolia* (synonymous with *D. opposita*), and *D. zingiberensis* displayed three major bands from

26 to 34 kDa, three major bands around 32.5 kDa, two bands at 32.5 and 34 kDa, and two major bands at 30 and 34 kDa, respectively. The different protein isoforms of DOI-like proteins from four Dioscorea species may possess regions with analogous structures/epitopes that bind the DOI antibodies. DOI (0.01 µM) significantly elevated estradiol secretion in ovarian granulosa cells and aromatase expression. The DOI-like proteins from three other Dioscorea species only exhibited a tendency to enhance aromatase expression.

Whereas DOI at 0.01 µM significantly enhanced steroidogenic acute regulatory protein (StAR) expression, DOI-like protein from D. alata at 0.01 µM, that from *D. zingiberensis* at 0.1 µM, that from *D. collettii* at 0.01 µM, and that from *D. collettii* at 0.1 µM slightly upregulated expression of StAR. DOI-like protein from *D. alata* at 0.01 µM, that from *D. zingiberensis* at 0.1 µM, and that from *D. oppositifolia* at 0.01 µM significantly increased the expression of Erβ (estrogen receptor agonist β). Our data demonstrate that the protein from *D. opposita* (*D. oppositifolia*) was the most active protein (Lu et al., 2016; Zhang et al., 2019).

DISCUSSION

It is revealed in the foregoing account that an estrogenic and osteogenic protein designated as DOI, with antiproliferative activity toward breast cancer and ovarian cancer cells and proliferative activity toward ovarian granulosa cells and rat splenocytes, can be isolated from yam (*Dioscorea opposita*) rhizomes. The counterparts of this protein in other *Dioscorea* species have much lower activity. DOI has good potential for development into the first protein drug in the future, which can be deployed for the alleviation of symptoms and health risks associated with menopause.

ACKNOWLEDGMENTS

This study (with findings reported in the papers Sze et al., 2018; Sze et al., 2016, and Wong et al., 2015) was partially supported by grants from the Innovation and Technology Fund (ITF) of the Innovation and Technology Commission, Government of Hong Kong SAR (HKSAR) (project no. ITS/262/09FP); General Research Funding, University Grants Committee, HKSAR (Ref: 12102919); and Start-Up Grant (Tier 1 and Tier 2), Hong Kong Baptist University, HKSAR (Ref: 18–19/0287).

REFERENCES

Bauer KR, Brown M, Cress RD, Parise CA, Caggiano V. Descriptive analysis of estrogen receptor (ER)-negative, progesterone receptor (PR)-negative, and HER2-negative invasive breast cancer, the so-called triple-negative phenotype. *Cancer.* 2007;109:1721–1728 doi: 10.1002/cncr.22618.

Casarini L, Crépieux P. Molecular mechanisms of action of FSH. *Front Endocrinol (Lausanne).* 2019;10:305. doi: 10.3389/fendo.2019.00305.

Echeverria V, Echeverria F, Barreto GE, Echeverría J, Mendoza C. Estrogenic plants: To prevent neurodegeneration and memory loss and other symptoms in women after menopause. *Front Pharmacol.* 2021;12:644103. doi: 10.3389/fphar.2021.644103.

Horstman AM, Dillon EL, Urban RJ, Sheffield-Moore M. The role of androgens and oestrogens on healthy aging and longevity. *J Gerontol A Biol Sci Med Sci*. 2012;67(11):1140–52. doi: 10.1093/gerona/gls068.

Jee D, Park SH, Hwang HS, Kim HS, Kim MS, Kim EC. Effects of hormone replacement therapy on lens opacity, serum inflammatory cytokines, and antioxidant levels. *Ann Med*. 2021;53(1):707–714. doi: 10.1080/07853890.2021.1928275.

Lu J, Wong RNS, Zhang L, Wong RYL, Ng TB, Lee KC, Zhang YB, Lao LX, Liu JY, *Sze SCW. Comparative analysis of proteins with stimulating ovarian estradiol biosynthesis from four different *Dioscorea* species in vitro: Implication for treating menopause. *App Biochem Biotech*, 180(1):79–93. doi: 10.1007/s12010-016-2084-x.

Oktem O, Akin N, Bildik G, Yakin K, Alper E, Balaban B, Urman B. FSH Stimulation promotes progesterone synthesis and output from human granulosa cells without luteinization. *Hum Reprod*. 2017;32(3):643–652. doi: 10.1093/humrep/dex010.

Stocco C. Aromatase expression in the ovary: Hormonal and molecular regulation. *Steroids*. 2008;73(5):473–87.

Sze SCW, Wong KL, Tong Y, Zhang YB, Cheung HP. Novel Bioactive Protein Isolated from Chinese Yam and uses thereof. US Patent and Trademark Office, U.S. Patent No.: US9273105B2. Patent Date: Mar. 1, 2016.

Sze SCW, Wong KL, Tong Y, Zhang YB, Cheung HP. Novel Bioactive Protein Isolated from Chinese Yam and uses thereof. European Patent Office, EU Patent Pub. No EP2750684B. Patent Date: Oct. 17, 2018.

United Nations, Department of Economic and Social Affairs, Population Division. (2019). *World Population Ageing 2019: Highlights* (ST/ESA/SER.A/430), United Nations, New York. https://www.un.org/en/development/desa/population/publications/pdf/ageing/WorldPopulationAgeing2019-Highlights.pdf

Van Barele M, Heemskerk-Gerritsen BAM, Louwers YV, Vastbinder MB, Martens JWM, Hooning MJ, Jager A. Estrogens and progestogens in triple negative breast cancer: Do they harm? *Cancers (Basel)*. 2021 May 21;13(11):2506. doi: 10.3390/cancers13112506.

Wong K, Yeung M. *Population Ageing Trend of Hong Kong. Economic Letter 2019/02. Office of the Government Economist the Government of the Hong Kong Special Administrative Region*. 2019, Office of the Government Economist, Hong Kong SAR. https://www.hkeconomy.gov.hk/en/pdf/el/el-2019-02.pdf

Wong KL, Lai YM, Li KW, Lee KF, Ng TB, Cheung HP, Zhang YB, Lao L, Wong RN, Shaw PC, Wong JH, Zhang ZJ, Lam JK, Ye WC, *Sze SCW (*Corresponding author). A novel, stable, estradiol-stimulating, osteogenic yam protein with potential for the treatment of menopausal syndrome. *Sci Rep*. 2015;5:10179. doi: 10.1038/srep10179.

Zhang L, Ng TB, Lam JKW, Wang SW, Lao L, Zhang KY, *Sze SCW (*Corresponding author). Research and development of proteins and peptides with therapeutic potential from yam tubers. *Curr Protein Pept Sci*. 2019;20(3):277–284. doi: 10.2174/1389203719666180622094356.

26 Conclusion – The Way Forward

Goh Cheng Soon
T&CM Division, MOH Malaysia

Gerard Bodeker
University of Oxford

Kishan Kariippanon
University of Wollongong

An ageing population is a huge challenge. Healthy ageing, however, is the biggest challenge. Many countries in Asia are rapidly moving towards an ageing population just like many developed countries in the West. People are living longer due to the current medical advancements and improved standards of living in the developed countries. However, the quality of life of the ageing population is still a cause for concern. This concern is not merely confined to the numbers involved; it is also regarding the future policies, health care, welfare and living arrangements of this group of people. This is the reason why promoting and advocating for healthy ageing has become a necessity.

The authors of the chapters in this book believe that the right resources (such as proper regulation), right organization, right incentives and right measurement are recipes to strengthen healthy ageing across the nation and globe. Universal Health Coverage (UHC) and Sustainable Development Goals (SDGs) cannot be achieved if institutions are not inclusive and held accountable for vulnerable groups being left behind.

Policy changes and/or policy innovations are required to support Asia's rapidly growing elderly population without jeopardizing economic growth and social development. Asian countries have the benefits of having stronger family ties since the majority of Asian elders are living with their families, stronger community support from neighbourhoods and accessibility to domestic helpers. In short, policy encourages healthy ageing by optimizing opportunities for health, participation and security in order to enhance quality of life as people age.

The strong connections among the different aspects of healthy ageing could be strengthened through an integrated approach centred on how older people live and to empower elders in taking control of their health. Taking the integrated approach means coordinating actions across different areas of healthy ageing policy and medical services so that they are mutually reinforcing. This joint action respects the

DOI: 10.1201/9781003043270-26

relationships among all perspectives of healthy ageing and allows accessibility by everyone at all times.

Furthermore, the collaboration of conventional and traditional and complementary medicine is allowed to thrive for the benefit of the public. Integrated medicine could improve the older population's health and enhance the quality of healthcare services in an affordable and sustainable manner. We certainly need to encourage and nurture these collaborations or integrations, break through the silos and embrace new ways of thinking in order to deal with challenges standing in the way of healthy ageing.

The groundbreaking levels of corporate funding in the Southeast Asian region, supporting researchers and spin-off academics in the field of healthy ageing are astounding. Many new start-ups are innovating be it in digital health technologies or services for ageing at home. This can be seen clearly as there are ample evidences that venture capital investment will spur more academic spin-offs along with collaborations between researchers and industry as well as policy level support for start-up. The evolution of the technology parks where accelerators and incubators are working hand in hand between government agencies and venture capital firms proves to us that a community of practice is engaged in high-level knowledge translation. As digital health technologies can be scaled and suited for context-specific consumers, an interdisciplinarity public health curriculum agenda will prepare postgraduate students to bridge the knowledge translation gap through the use of scalable technology and entrepreneurial thinking by creating services that are sustainable.

This has direct implications for public health and medical education in the future. Where health promotion concepts and frameworks have dominated public health curriculum for the past three decades, we anticipate a potential surge in social innovation, people-centred design and social entrepreneurship and leadership courses become part of the global public health agenda. Collaboration between disciplines and the partnership with industry are becoming more common. In the medical education field, physician training takes a turn into prioritizing local or regional approaches, and traditional practices that contribute to prevention and well-being. An evidence-based medical education on traditional and complementary practices will enable physicians to implement the sustainable prevention and treatment strategies using local resources and traditional knowledge.

The SDGs act as a policy and strategy-level guide for industry, government and research collaborations to integrate traditional and complementary approaches to prevention and well-being with the help of novel services and appropriate digital technologies.

In today's complex and rapidly changing world, this book would like to conclude with an emphasis on multisectoral policy and action, as integrated health services coupled with empowered people and communities are crucial to address the main causes and risks of poor health and well-being, on top of handling the emergency challenges that threaten health such as the COVID-19 pandemic. Only with the combination of policies with integrated health services and empowerment will the achievement of the health-related SDGs and UHC be possible.

Index of Countries

Note: **Bold** page numbers refer to tables and *italic* page numbers refer to figures.

Afghanistan
    traditional medicine in 118, **119**
Armenia **121**
Australia 8, 12, 33, 190, 267
Azerbaijan **121**

Bahrain 118
    traditional medicine in **119**
Bangladesh 211
    traditional medicine in **116**
Bhutan
    medicine practice in 115
    traditional medicine in **116**
Brazil 12, 189
Brunei
    traditional and complementary medicine in
        111, **112,** 114

Cambodia
    Khmer traditional medicine in 124
Canada
    baby-seal PARO in 266
China 123, 152, 273, 277, 292
    adult-child migrants 94–97
    agency role 98–100
    China Health and Nutrition Survey
        (CHNS) 92
    China Health and Retirement Longitudinal
        Study (CHARLS) 92
    coronavirus outbreak in 3, 254
    exercises in 154
    factors impacting 90–92
    healthcare technique in 158
    health preservation in 6
    health tech start-up 275
    The Hukou System 91–92
    left-behind elderly health 5, 89–101
    martial art in 216
    New Urbanization (2014–2020) 91
    One-child policy 92
    population aging in 291
    rural migration impacts 92–94
    social capital 98–100
    social cohesion 98–100
    social safety network 90
    TCM therapy in 111, 114
    traditional medicine in **112,** 115
    understand recuperation 98–100
Cyprus **119**

Denmark
    baby-seal PARO in 266

Fiji 33n2
France 12, 26–27, 189, 204

Georgia
    traditional medicine in **121,** 123
Germany 204

Hong Kong
    Hong Kong Science and Technology Parks
        Corporation (HKSTP) 266, 277
    Hong Kong Society for Aged (SAGE) 258
    smart homes for aging in 266

India
    AYUSH embracing Ayurveda 115
    classical system 4
    disability-adjusted life years 211
    health tech ecosystem 273, 275
    homoeopathy 115
    Indian traditional systems 111
    India's classical system 4
    nature and environment 218
    naturopathy 115
    population doubling in 12
    Siddha 115
    Sowa-Rigpa 115
    traditional Indian system, Yoga 171, 172, 181
    traditional medicine in 6, **116,** 117, 118, 124
    Unani 115
    yoga 115
Indonesia 189
    Alodokter 276
    health tech in 273, 274
    traditional medicine in **116**
Iran **119**
Iraq
    Complementary or alternative medicine
        118, **119**
Ireland 204
Israel
    traditional medicine in 110, 120, **121,** 122
Italy 204, 266, 291

Japan
    age-friendly communities in 267
    ageing population 5, 11, 190, 291

Index of Countries

Japan (*cont.*)
    COVID-19 pandemic in 212
    diet in 214–215
    e-skin wearable technology in 275
    government policies 64–65
    healthcare system 64
    healthy body and mind 65–67
    ICT and healthcare technologies in 55
    ikigai 65–67, 219
    Ikigai: The Japanese Secret to a Long and Happy Life (García and Miralles) 219
    Japanese diet 214
    Japan Gerontological Evaluation Study (JAGES) 234
    Japan Institute for Labour Policy and Training (JILPT) 65
    Kampo medicine 114, 115
    laughter and mortality 235
    National Health Insurance System 71
    One Hundred Year Life Program 219–220
    population doubling in 12
    population problems 63–64
    psychological stress and diseases 230
    quality of life 70–71
    rakugo 232
    regional councils 68
    robots development 266
    shinrin-yoku 219
    social work model 257
    super-ageing society 68
    well-ageing society summit 67–68
    wellness tourism 69–70
Jordan **119**

Kazakhstan
    traditional medicine in 110, **121**, 122, 123
Korea
    Korean medicine health insurance 76–77, 77–78
    Law on Long-Term Care Insurance 16
    National Health Insurance 17
Kuwait
    traditional medicine in 118, **119**
Kyrgyzstan **121**

Laos **112**
Lebanon **119**

Malaysia 25
    age-friendly requires 16
    ageing population in 5, 6, 11, 15–16, 254
    aging and mental health in 151, 210–211
    Annual Report of the Oral Health Programme 13
    Association for Residential Aged Care Operators of Malaysia (AgeCOpe) 40

    crude birth rate 26, *27*
    crude death rate 26, *27*
    demographic ageing 26, *27, 28, 29,* 30, **30,** 31, **31**
    demographic transformation 21
    economic dimension 259
    8th Malaysia Plan (2001–2005) 35
    11th Malaysia Plan (2016–2020) 38
    empowerment in 258–259
    environment dimension 259–260
    Fifth Malaysia Plan (1986–1990) 33
    5th Malaysian Population and Family Survey (MPFS-5) 39
    geriatric services 22, 34
    healthcare system 15
    health dimension 260
    health education programmes 15
    life expectancy in 14
    local training programme 22
    long-term care insurance 17
    The Malaysian Dietary Guidelines 136
    Malaysian Food Pyramid 136
    Malaysian National Cancer Registry Report 2012–2016 142
    Malaysia's vision 57
    modernization and industrialization 45
    national day of older persons 33
    national policy for older persons 13
    national policy for the elderly 33
    older people associations 33
    older person assistance scheme 33
    organ system 22
    our system and challenges 22
    pension programmes 42, *44*
    PLANMalaysia 38
    policy development on ageing in 25–57
    population doubling in 12
    Second Malaya Plan (1961–1965) 33
    7th Malaysia Plan (1996–2000) 34, 35
    6th Development Plan (1991–1995) 33
    social dimension 260–261
    socio-demographic in 12
    spiritual dimension 261–262
    supported decision-making 16
    tai chi and Otago exercise programmes 15
    T&CM regulatory system 18
    technology for health 273, 274
    10th Malaysia Plan (2011–2015) 36
    total fertility rate 26, *27*
    traditional and complementary practices in 15, 109–111, **112,** 113, 114
    12th Malaysian Plan 39
    welfare-centric approach 33
Maldives
    traditional medicine in **116**
Mongolia **112**
Myanmar 273

Index of Countries

303

Nepal **117**
New Zealand 295
North Korea
    traditional medicine in 117, **117**

Oman
    traditional medicine in 118, **120**

Pakistan
    disability-adjusted life years 211
Palestine **120**
Philippines
    technology for health 274
    traditional medicine in 111, **112,** 114
Poland 204

Qatar **120**

Russia
    traditional medicine in 110, 122,
        122, 123

Saudi Arabia 118, **120**
Serbia 246
Singapore
    baby boomer generation 274
    Biofourmis 275
    healthcare system in 258–259, 273, 274
    longer life expectancy 254
    Start-up SG Accelerator 277
    traditional medicine in 111, **113,** 114
Slovenia 246
South Korea
    aging population 73–74, 78–79, 291
    Korean medical institutions 75
    Korean medicine 74–75
        rapid growth in usage of 76
        Western medicine usage and 76, 78
    Korean medicine health insurance 75
        aging benefits 77
        coverage lack of 76–77
    traditional medicine in 117
Spain 204
Sri Lanka **117**

Sweden
    healthcare technologies in 55
    population doublings in 12
Switzerland 204
Syria **120**

Tajikistan **122**
Thailand
    ageing society 179–180
    Centella asiatica in 215
    The Fifth National Health Examination
        Survey 179
    healthcare technology 274, 277
    health promotion activities 185
    herbal medicines 182–183
    hot herbal compress 184–185
    Jivitanamai 182
    Kayanamai 181
    knee herbal poultice 185
    Luk Prakob/hot herbal compress 184–185
    National Innovation Agency 277
    Nuad Thai 183–184
    traditional medicines in 6–7, **117,** 180–182,
        182–183
Timor-Leste **117**
Turkey
    traditional medicine in **122,** 123
Turkmenistan **122**

United Arab Emirates
    complementary and alternative medicine in 118
United Kingdom 82, 266
United States of America
    ageing population in 189
    baby-seal PARO in 266–267
    laughter and life expectancy 234
    population doubling in 12
Uzbekistan **122**

Vietnam
    start-up health tech development 273
    traditional medicine in **113,** 114, 115

Yemen **120**

Index of Policies & Legislation

Note: Bold page numbers refer to tables; *italic* page numbers refer to figures and page numbers followed by "n" denote endnotes.

Action Plan (2010–2020) 36
Afghanistan National Medicines Policy 2019 118
annuity scheme 45, 54
Article 10 of the law on the Protection of the Rights of the Elderly 97
Article 21 of the Marriage Law 97
Australian Trade and Investment Commission (Austrade) 38

British colonial rule 25
The Brunei Darussalam Declaration on Strengthening Family Institution: Caring for the Elderly (2010) 39

Capital Markets and Services Act (CMSA) 2007 38
Care Centres Act 1993 (Act 506) 17, 34, 47
Civil Servant Medical Benefit Scheme (CSMBS) 182
Committee on Ethical Issues of the European Psychiatric Association 210
Committee on the Development of the National Medicine System 182
COVID-19 Strategy Update in April 2020 2–3
Cultural Revolution 88, 91

Decision No. (33) of 2016 Issuing Regulation on the Practice of Alternative and Complementary Medicine 119
The 1978 Declaration of Alma Ata 17, 96
Destitute Persons (Welfare Homes) Rules 1981 34

Elderly-friendly Scheme *(Skim Mesra Usia Emas)* 50
11th Malaysia Plan (2016–2020) 38
Employees' Social Security Act 4, 1969 42
Employment Insurance System (EIS) 42
empowerment strategy 257
EPF Act 452, 1991 42
EPF scheme 42

The Federal Law on the Basis of Protecting the Health of Citizens in the Russian Federation 122, **122**
Fifth Malaysia Plan (1986–1990) 33
The Fifth National Health Examination Survey, Thailand 179

5th Malaysian Population and Family Survey (MPFS-5) 39
first healthcare revolution 86
First (1966–1970) Malaysia Plans 33
the first plan, 2006–2010, Korean Medicine Health Insurance 77

government policies, Japan 64–65

Health and Aging in Malaysia 33
Household Expenditure Survey 45
Household Living Aid *(Bantuan Sara Hidup)* 36, 42
100-Year Life Society/One Hundred Year Life Program 5, 8, 64–65, 68, 70, 219–220

Income Tax (Deduction for Employment of Senior Citizen, Ex-Convict, Parolee, Supervised Person and Ex-Drug Dependant) Rules 2019 40
Institute of Medicine (US) Committee 110

Japan Institute for Labour Policy and Training (JILPT) 65, 115

Korean medical health insurance 5, 74–79
Korean National Healthcare System 115
Kuala Lumpur Declaration on Ageing: Empowering Older Persons 39

Lancet Commission on Dementia (2020) 82
Lancet Commission on Global Mental Health and Sustainable Development 210, 212
The Law Commission Revisions, 2015 114
The Law of the Republic of Kazakhstan N 111-1 **121,** 122
Law on Long-Term Care Insurance for the Senior Citizens in Korea 16–17
Living Longer Better system, England 87
Lotteries Act 1953 32

Madrid International Plan of Action on Ageing (MIPAA) 35
Malaysia National Health Accounts (MNHA) Health Expenditure Report 1997–2017 50
Malaysian National Cancer Registry Report 2012–2016 142

Index of Policies & Legislation

Malaysia's pension programmes *44*
Minimum Retirement Age Act 2012 (Act 756) 37

National Action Plan for Ageing Population
    2021–2025 16
National Coordinating Committee on Food and
    Nutrition 2010 136
National Dementia Plan 51
national development plans in Malaysia 5
National Family Policy 2010 32
the National Health and Morbidity Survey
    2015 109
The 2018 National Health and Morbidity Survey
    (NHMS) 12, 13, 39, 40
national healthcare systems 1, 18, 51, 110, 113
National Health Commission of the People's
    Republic of China 3
National Health Insurance Program
    in Korea 17, 74, 76, 78
    in Malaysia 51
    in Taiwan 123
national health insurance system, Japan 71, 114
National Health Policy 15
National Health Policy for Older Persons 2008
    13, 14, 15, 17, 36, 259
National Health Security Systems 186
National Innovation Agency, Thailand 277
National Key Economic Area (NKEA) 38
national long-term care insurance, Malaysia
    52, 54
National Oral Health Plan 2011-2020 13, 51
National Palliative Care Strategy and Policy 51
National Plan of Action for Health Care of Older
    Person (revised in 2008) 13
National Plan of Action for Nutrition of Malaysia
    III, 2016–2025 51
national policy and plan of action for older
    persons, Malaysia *37*
National Policy for Older Persons in 1995
    (amended 2011) 13, 36, 55, 259–261
National Policy for the Elderly (NPE) 32–36, 48,
    50, 55
National Policy of Traditional and
    Complementary Medicine 113
National Population and Family Development
    Board Malaysia 33
National Social Policy 2003 32
National Social Welfare Policy 1990 32
National Strategic Plan for Active Living,
    2017–2025 51
National Strategic Plan for Non-Communicable
    Diseases, 2016–2025 (2016) 51
National Wages Consultative Council Act 2011
    (Act 732) 37–38
naturally occurring retirement communities
    (NORC) 31

New Cooperative Medical Scheme (NCMS) 96
9th Malaysia Plan (2006–2010) 35

oldage pensions system in Malaysia 42
old-age social welfare assistance scheme 54
Older Person Assistance Scheme (*Skim Bantuan
    Orang Tua* or BOT) 33, 36, 42, 53
The Older Persons' Aid scheme 36
one-child policy 92, 100

Penal Code 17
Pensions Act 1980 17, 53
pension schemes 54
Pensions Trust Fund Act 53
Physical Planning Guideline for Older Persons
    (GP031-A) 38, 48
Plan for New Urbanization (2014–2020),
    China 91
PLANMalaysia 38, 48
Plan of Action for Older Persons 1998 13
Plan of Action (1997–2005), NPE 34–36
Policy development in Malaysia 31
Practice of the Arts of Healing Act B.E. 2542 118
Private Aged Healthcare Facilities and Services
    Act 2018 (Act 802) 38, 52
Private Healthcare Facilities and Services Act
    1998 (Act 586) 34, 47
Private Hospitals Act 1971 (Act 43) 34
Private Retirement Schemes (PRS) 38, 53
Professional Commission of Thai Traditional
    Medicine, 2007 184
Professional Committee 118
Program Cari 36
Protection and Promotion of Thai Traditional
    Medicine Wisdom Act B.E. 2542 in
    1999 115, 118
provisions of Decree Law No. 18 **119**
public pension and health insurance systems 96
Public Service Pension scheme (Act 227, 1980) 42

Rules for the Management of Old Folks Homes
    1983 34
rural healthcare insurance 92
rural pension system 92, 100

second healthcare revolution 86
Second Malaya Plan (1961–1965) 33
Second (1971–1975) Malaysia Plans 33
the second plan, 2011–2015, Korean Medicine
    Health Insurance 77
Securities Commission Malaysia (SC) 38
Senior Citizen Appreciation Programme 50
Senior Citizens' Aid 42
7th Malaysia Plan (1996–2000) 34, 35
Shared Prosperity Vision 2030 (SPV2030) 39, 57
6th Development Plan (1991–1995) 33

Index of Policies & Legislation

social assistance schemes 53
Social Security Scheme 182

T&CM Regulation 2021 18
T&CM regulatory system 18
10th Malaysia Plan (2011–2015) 36
Thai national healthcare system 118
third healthcare revolution 86
the third plan, 2016–2020, Korean Medicine
 Health Insurance 77
"Three TCM prescriptions and three
 medicines" 3
Traditional and Alternative Medicine Act 1997
 112, 114
Traditional Chinese Medicine Practitioners Act
 (Chapter 333A) 2001 **113,** 114
12th Malaysian Plan 39
2016 Population Data Sheet 1

United Nations Economic and Social
 Commission for Asia and the Pacific
 (ESCAP) 1
United Nations Principles for Older Persons
 (UNGA Resolution 46/91) 33
Universal Health Coverage Scheme (UHC) 75,
 80, 110, 125, 182, 185, 299, 300
Universal Two-Child Policy 100n2
University of the Third Age (U3A) programme 48
urban social health insurance 92

Vienna International Plan of Action on Ageing
 (VIPAA) 13, 33
Vision 2020 32, 39

*WHO Policy Framework on Active Ageing
 2002* 14
World Population Prospects 2019 11

Index of Herbal Plants

Note: **Bold** page numbers refer to tables.

Alpinia galanga **139**, 142
Anacardium occidentale 135, 136, **139**, 141–144
Andrographis paniculata 183
Archidendron pauciflorum 136, 137, **139**
Asparagus racemosus 166
Averrhoa bilimbi 138, **139**, 142

Barringtonia racemosa 139, 142, 143
Boerrhavia diffusa 166

Caenorhabditis elegans 135
Carica papaya 136, 137, 139, 142
Centella asiatica (*C. asiatica*) 136, **139**, 143, 144, 166, 215
Cissus quadrangularis 183
Cleome rutidosperma **139**, 142
Clitoria ternatea 137, **139**, 166
Commiphora mukul 166
Cosmos caudatus (*C. caudatus*) 136, **139**, 141, 142, 143, 144
Curcuma longa 136, 138, **139**, 141, 142, 144, 185
Curcuma sp. 185
Curcuma zedoaria **140**, 142
Cymbopogon citratus 138, **140**, 144

Derris scandens 183
Desmodium gangeticum 166
Dioscorea 295–296
Dioscorea alata (*D. alata*) 295, 296
Dioscorea collettii (*D. collettii*) 295, 296
Dioscorea japonica 293
Dioscorea opposita 290, 292
Dioscorea oppositifolia 293, 295, 296
Dioscorea zingiberensis (*D. zingiberensis*) 295, 296

Gynura procumbens 136, 138, 141–143

Leptadenia reticularis 166

Manihot esculenta 142, **140**
Momordica charantia 136, **140**
Morinda citrifolia 143, **140**
Moringa oleifera 137, **140**, 141
Murraya koenigii (*M. koenigii*) 136, 137, **140**, 142, 143, 144
Musa balbisiana 143, **140**
Musa × *paradisiaca* 138, **140**

Ocimum basilicum **140**, 142, 143
Oenanthe javanica 136, 138, **140**, 144

Pachyrhizus erosus **140**, 142
Parkia speciosa 136, **140**, 141
Persicaria hydropiper **140**, 142
Persicaria minor **140**, 143
Persicaria minus 144
Phyllanthus emblica 166, 183
Piper betle **140**, 142
Piper sarmentosum **140**, 143
Plectranthus rotundifolius **139**, 142
Pluchea lanceolata 166

Sauropus androgynus **140**, 142, 143
Senna alexandrina 183
Solanum melongena **140**, 142

Terminalia bellirica 183
Terminalia chebula 166, 183
Tinospora cordifolia 166
Trichosanthes anguina 142

Vitex negundo 138

Zingiber cassumunar (*Z. cassumunar*) 185
Zingiber montanum 183, 185

Index of Practices

Note: Bold page numbers refer to tables; *italic* page numbers refer to figures.

acupuncture 69, 75, 77, 111, **113,** 114, 115, 122, 123, 151, 200, 207
Ahimsa 173
Aparigraha (Yoga) 173
apitherapy 123
Arab-Greek medicine 118
art & art therapy 217–218
Asian diets 215
Astanga Yoga 172, 172–173, 177
  Asana 174–176, *175–176*
  Dharana 177–178
  Dhyana 177–178
  Niyama 173, *174*
  Pranayama 177
  Pratyahara 177
  Samadhi 177–178
  Yama 173, *174*
Asteya 173
Ayurveda 4, 115
  Abhyanga 167–168
  Ahara 166
  aspect 164–165
  Basti 168
  Brahm Muhurta 165
  Dharniya 166
  Gandusha 167
  Karnapoorana 167
  Nasya 167
  Nidra 166
  Padabhyanga 168
  Shiroabhyanga 168
  Snana 166
  Ushnah Pana 165
  Vayasthapana Gana 166–167
  Vyayama 165–166

baguan 123
bone reduction 123
Brahmacharya 173
Buddhist meditation 181

Chinese Daoism 153, 154, 155
Chinese medicine 7, 111, **113,** 118, 122, 157–162, 197, 201, 203, 205, 206, 207, 218
chiropractic 114, 123
Chittanamai 181
cupping therapy 123

Dhammanamai 7, 181, 185

folk medicine **121,** 123, 124
folk therapies 123

Gandusha 167
Georgian traditional medicine **121**

Health Qigong Tuo Five-Animal Play
  (Traditional Chinese medicine) 158
  the bear's stance 159–60
  the crane's stance 160–161
  the deer's stance 159
  the monkey's stance 160
  the tiger's stance 158
herbal therapy 115, 123
homoeopathy **112,** 114, 115, **116,** 122, 123, 124
hormone replacement therapy (HRT) 290
hypnosis 123

India traditional medicine
  Ayurveda 115
  homoeopathy 115
  naturopathy 115
Siddha 115
Sowa-Rigpa (Tibetan medicine) 115
Unani system 115
  yoga 115

Ishwara Pranidhana 173

Japanese diet 214
Jivitanamai 182

Kampo medicine 114
Karnapoorana 167
Kayanamai 181
Khmer traditional medicine 124
Koryo medicine 117

laughter therapy 2, 7, 15, 229–239
leech therapy (hirudotherapy) 123
Luk Pra Kob 7
maggot therapy 123

Malaysian diet 277
Mediterranean diet 214
mesotherapy 123
moxibustion 75, 77, 115, 123
music therapy 4, 7, 123, 217, 241–250

311

312 Index of Practices

naturopathy 115, **116,** 122, 124
Nuad Thai 7, 181, 183–185

osteopathy 114, 122, 123
ozone therapy 123

Padabhyanga 168
phytotherapy 123
prolotherapy 123

qigong 2, 8, 98, 111, 151, 158, 197–204

rational therapy 115
reflexology 123
rejuvenation therapy 6, 166
Ruesi Dadton 181

Santosh 173
Satya 173
Saucha 173
Shiroabhyanga 168
SKT meditation 181
Swadhyaya 173

Tai chi and Otago exercise 15
 Otago exercise program 191

Tai Chi Qigong
 Chui Zi Jue (吹字诀) 202–203
 Hu Ju (虎举) 199–200
 Hu zi Jue (呼字诀) 200–201
 Kai Kuo Xiong Huai (开阔胸怀) 198
 Ma Bu Yun Shou (马步云手) 198
 Ma Bu Zhan Zhuang (马步站桩) 198–199
 Niao Fei (鸟飞) 203–204
 Qi Shi Tiao Xi (起势调息) 197
 San Pan Luo Di (三盘落地) 202
 Ta Bu Pai Qiu (踏步拍球) 198
 Tiao Li Pi Wei Xu Dan Ju
  (调理脾胃须单举) 201
 Zan Quan Nu Mu Zeng Qi Li
  (攒拳怒目增气力) 200
Tapa 173
Thai traditional medicine 180–182
Timorese medicine 124
traditional dislocation treatment 123
traditional fracture treatment 123
traditional trauma treatment 123
tuina 123, 151, 207

Western diet 214

Yangsheng (养生) 98

Subject Index

Note: **Bold** page numbers refer to tables and *italic* page numbers refer to figures.

"able X" 266
activities of daily living (ADL) 13
adult-child migrants
    longer-term migration 94–5
    multi-morbidities 97
    neoliberalism 97
    number of children 94
    responsibilities 95
    rural healthcare role 96–7
    vulnerability differences 95–6
    workload 95
AFC *see* Age-Friendly Cities (AFC)
age differences 230–1
Age-Friendly Cities (AFC) 267
age-friendly environments 267
ageing/aging 210–11
    challenges 50–6
    demography 26, *27,* 28, *29,* 30, **30,**
        31, **31**
    gonadal hormone decline 291
    health challenges 12–13
    healthy ageing 15–17
    Korean medicine health insurance
        measures 77–8
        problems 76–7
    physiological influence 163
    policies 31–40
        1995–2010 34–6
        issues 50–6
        2011 to present 36–40, *37*
    populations 291, 299
    programmes 31–40
        1995–2010 34–6
        finance 42, **43,** *44,* 45, *46*
        healthcare 40–1, **41**
        housing 45, **47,** 47–8
        social programmes 48–9, **49**
        2011 to present 36–40, *37*
        transport and others 50
    recommendations 50–6
    services
        finance 42, **43,** *44,* 45, *46*
        healthcare 40–1, **41**
        housing 45, **47,** 47–8
        social programmes 48–9, **49**
        transport and others 50
    social support 218
    world assembly on 26

ageing/aging in place
    age-friendly environments outside home 267
    digital age, pitfalls of 268
    safe and enabling homes 266–7
ageing populations
    community education 2
    medical health insurance 5
    national healthcare systems 1
AKTA Purifier FPLC system 292
all-cause mortality 235
Alzheimer's disease 82, 143
    medial temporal lobe 214
    music therapy 217
    non-communicable diseases 254
anticancer activity 142–3
antidiabetic activity
    aqueous extract 137, 138
    ethanol extract 137
    ethyl acetate fraction 138
    hypoglycaemic effects 136
anti-GAPDH antibody 295
antihyperlipidaemic activity 141–2
antihypertensive activity 139, **139–41,** 141
anxiety 217
artificial intelligence (AI) 275
average life span 219

baby boomer generation 274
baby-boom generation 64
bathroom 285
BDNF *see* brain-derived neurotrophic factor
    (BDNF)
the bear's stance
    modern medicine 160
    traditional Chinese medicine 159–60
blood pressure 233
BlueChilli 277
body mass index (BMI) 135
brain ageing 214
brain-derived neurotrophic factor (BDNF) 290
brain fog 211

Capital Markets and Services Act (CMSA)
    2007 38
carbohydrate intake 215
cardiovascular diseases 230
Central Welfare Council (CWC) 32
CGR *see* complicated grief reactions (CGR)

313

314 Subject Index

challenges, in empowerment
  economic barrier 262
  healthcare environment barriers 262
  physical accessibility barrier 262
  social barriers 262
China Health and Nutrition Survey (CHNS) 92
China Health and Retirement Longitudinal Study
  (CHARLS) 92
Chinese and western medicines
  integrated management
    advantages 206
    arthritis 207
    chronic obstructive pulmonary disease
     207
    congestive cardiac failure 206–7
    coronary heart disease 206–7
    early-stage hypertension 207
    hypertension complications 208
    idiopathic pulmonary fibrosis 207
    mild diabetes/early-stage diabetes 208
    osteoporosis 207
    principles and strategies 206
    renal failure patients 208
    stroke 207
Chinese Communist Party (CCP) 90
Chinese health guidelines 151
Chinese medicine; *see also* traditional Chinese
  medicine
  theory 197
Chinese yam 292
chronic obstructive pulmonary disease 207
Circulation Risk in Communities Study
  (CIRCS) 233
Civil Servant Medical Benefit Scheme
  (CSMBS) 182
civil service pension 54
cognition 218
collaborative health care 75, 78
collective reflexivity 283–4
comorbidity 244
compassion 8
complementary and alternative medicine
  (CAM) 110
complementary medicine 15, 109, 110
complicated grief (CG) criteria 242, 244
complicated grief reactions (CGR) 242–4
congestive cardiac failure 206–7
consequences, complicated grief 244
contextual behavioral empowerment model 257
continuing bonds theory 242
Cooperative Medical System 75
coping 217
coronary heart disease 206–7
coronavirus disease-2019 (COVID-19) 211–13,
  238, 254, 272
  in elderly 2–4
  priority actions 3

corporate funding 300
the Crane's stance
  modern medicine 161
  traditional Chinese medicine 160–1
critical reflexivity 283–4
'cultural' level concept 256
culture 82–3, 86–8

daily life 237–8
DALYs *see* disability-adjusted life years
  (DALYs)
dance 216–17
Daoism, internal cultivation system 154
Deep Breathing Bathing 69
Deep Breathing Regimen 70
the deer's stance
  modern medicine 159
  traditional Chinese medicine 159
dementia 143–4
dementia-friendly design 279–82
depression 217
Desert Rose House 8, 279–82
Dhammanamai 7, 181, 185
digital age, pitfalls of 268
disability-adjusted life years (DALYs) 211
'disenfranchised grief' concept 245
distress 217
DocDoc, healthcare technology 276
DOI
  bone mineral density and microarchitecture
   294–5
  brain, prefrontal cortex of 295
  characterization of 292–3
  DOI-like proteins 295–6
  estradiol-stimulating effect 293
  FSHR and aromatase *in vivo* 294
  stimulatory effect of 293
  in vitro, estradiol-stimulating effect 293
  in vivo, estradiol-stimulating effect 294
dual-process model 242, 245

early-stage hypertension 207
Eastern Mediterranean Region (EMR) 111
  perspective from 118, **119–20,** 120
eat local, health preservation 153
eat on time, health preservation 153
economic barrier 262
economic dimension 259
Economic Planning Unit (EPU) 32
Economic Transformation Programme
  (ETP), 38
elderly 211–13
employees provident fund (EPF) 38, 259
Employment Insurance System (EIS) 42
empowerment
  challenges in
   economic barrier 262

Subject Index

315

healthcare environment barriers 262
  physical accessibility barrier 262
  social barriers 262
contextual behavioral empowerment
    model 257
definition of 254–5
iterative empowerment process model 258
linear empowerment process model 256
in Malaysia
  economic dimension 259
  environment dimension 259–60
  health dimension 260
  social dimension 260–1
  spiritual dimension 261–2
social work model, empowerment oriented
    practice 257–8
England
  health span 83
  living longer better system 87
  population ageing systems
    aims 83–4, *84, 85*
    drop a decade 84
    evidence base and culture 82–3
    living longer science 81–2, *82*
    network needs 86
    right culture 86–8, *87*
    set objectives 84–6, *85*
    20th century 83
environment dimension 259–60
EPF *see* employees provident fund (EPF)
ER *see* estrogen receptor (ER)
e-skin wearable technology 275
estrogen 291
estrogen receptor (ER) 290
ethical issues 244–5
Europe
  culture of care 87
  population ageing systems
    aims 83–4, *84, 85*
    drop a decade 84
    evidence base and culture 82–3
    living longer science 81–2, *82*
    network needs 86
    right culture 86–8, *87*
    set objectives 84–6, *85*
    20th century 83
European Region (EUR) 111
  perspective from 120, **120–1,** 121–3
exercise 215
  older people
    essential element 190
    falls prevention 193
    prescription 191
    researched intervention approach 192
    research evidence supporting 192
    resistance training programs 190, 192
    walking programs 190

facial expression 230
family unity 283
financial assistance schemes 42, **43,** *44,* 45, *46*
financing, older persons 53–4
follicle-stimulating hormone receptor (FSHR)
    expression 293
Forest Power Walk 69
frozen shoulder 184
FSHR expression *see* follicle-stimulating
    hormone receptor (FSHR)
    expression
functional disability 234–5

Galen Growth report 273
G7 countries 64
gene–environment interaction effect 244
Global Wellness Institute 216
good conjugal love, health preservation 153–5
good sleep quality, health preservation 152
government policies, Japan 64–5

healthcare 40–1, **41**
  older persons 50–2
  technologies 55, 276
healthcare environment barriers 262
health connotation
  modern medicine
    the bear's stance 160
    the crane's stance 161
    the deer's stance 159
    the monkey's stance 160
    the tiger's stance 159
  traditional Chinese medicine
    the bear's stance 159–60
    the crane's stance 160–1
    the deer's stance 159
    the monkey's stance 160
    the tiger's stance 158
health dimension 260
health education programmes 15
health preservation
  eat local 153
  eat on time 153
  good conjugal love 153–5
  good sleep quality 152
  seasonal foods 153
  sufficient sleep time 152
health prevention and wellness 277–8
  enrolment 278
  interessement 278
  mobilization 279
  problematization 278
health promotion
  activities 185
  concepts 300
  and prevention programs 190
health technology 272–4

316 Subject Index

healthy ageing/aging 14, 265, 291, 299
   comprehensive public health action 17
   long-term plan 16
healthy ageing start-ups
   accelerators and incubators 276
   Asia, accelerators/incubators in 277
   Asian start-ups tackling 274–6
   bathroom 285
   collective reflexivity 283–4
   critical reflexivity 283–4
   dementia-friendly design 279–82
   Desert Rose House 279–82
   health prevention and wellness 277–8
      enrolment 278
      interessement 278
      mobilization 279
      problematization 278
   health technology 272–4
   iAccelerate 279–82
   kitchen 285–6
   master bedroom 285
   methodology 282
   privacy 284
   social and technological change 274
healthy life span 65, 219–20
herbal medicines 182–3
HICs *see* high-income countries (HICs)
high-income countries (HICs) 272
Homage 274, 275
housing 45, **47,** 47–8
Huashi Baidu Formula 3
Hua Tuo Five-Animal Play
   modern medicine
      the bear's stance 160
      the crane's stance 161
      the deer's stance 159
      the monkey's stance 160
      the tiger's stance 159
   practising essentials 161–2
   step-by-step exercise requirement 161
   traditional Chinese medicine
      the bear's stance 159–60
      the crane's stance 160–1
      the deer's stance 159
      the monkey's stance 160
      the tiger's stance 158
The Hukou System 91–2
human epidermal growth factor receptor-2
     (HER2) 290
hypertension complications 208

iAccelerate 279–82
iCarbonX 275
idiopathic pulmonary fibrosis 207
Ikigai: The Japanese Secret to a Long
     and Happy Life (García and
     Miralles) 219

income security, older persons 53–4
Indian traditional systems 111
innovation 8, 32, 55, 67–70
integrated management
   elderly patients
      advantages 206
      arthritis 207
      chronic obstructive pulmonary
         disease 207
      congestive cardiac failure 206–7
      coronary heart disease 206–7
      early-stage hypertension 207
      hypertension complications 208
      idiopathic pulmonary fibrosis 207
      mild diabetes/early-stage diabetes 208
      osteoporosis 207
      principles and strategies 206
      renal failure patients 208
      stroke 207
integration approach
   age-friendly requires 16
   healthcare system 15
   health education programmes 15
   long-term care insurance 17
   supported decision-making 16
   tai chi and Otago exercise programmes 15
   traditional and complementary medicine 15
ischemic heart disease 230
iterative empowerment process model 258

Jean Woo 7
Jinhua Qinggan Granule 3
Jivitanamai 182
Journal of Ayurveda and Integrative Medicine
     (J-AIM) 4

Khmer traditional medicine 124
kitchen 285–6
knee herbal poultice 185
Korean medicine 76, 115
   benefits 77
   vs. Cooperative Medical System 75
   duplicate medical treatment 76
   growth in 76
   systems 5
Korean medicine health insurance
   measures
      benefits 77
      collaborative health care 78
      other future 78
   problems
      duplicate medical treatment 76
      insurance coverage 76–7
      medical use and medical expenses 76
   status 75
Korean traditional medicine 74–5; *see also*
     Korean medicine

Subject Index

The Lancet Psychiatry (Sarris) 214
late-life depression (LLD) 211
laughing face 230
laughter
   age differences 230–1
   daily life *231,* 237–8
   functional disability 234–5
   lifestyle-related diseases 232–4
   mortality 234–5
   pain 231–2
   physical health 235–6
   psychological health 235–6
   psychological stress and diseases 230
   sex differences 230–1
left-behind elderly health
   adult-child migrants
      longer-term migration 94–5
      multi-morbidities 97
      neoliberalism 97
      number of children 94
      responsibilities 95
      rural healthcare role 96–7
      vulnerability differences 95–6
      workload 95
   agency role 98–100
   factors impacting
      The Hukou System 91–2
      one-child policy 92
      rapid urbanization 91
      rural pension system 92
      wealth inequality 90–1
   rural migration impacts 92–4
   social capital 98–100
   social cohesion 98–100
   understand recuperation 98–100
Lianhua Qingwen Capsule 3
lifelong learning 48, 265
lifestyle-related diseases 229–30, 232–4
light reflective values (LRVs) 284
linear empowerment process model 256
LLD *see* late-life depression (LLD)
LMICs *see* low-to-middle-income countries
      (LMICs)
Longevity Prescription for the 21st Century 83
long-term care 50–2
low-to-middle-income countries (LMICs) 272
LRVs *see* light reflective values (LRVs)
Luk Prakob/hot herbal compress 184–5
lyric substitution 241

major depressive disorders (MDD) 211
master bedroom 285
mClinica 275
MCM-TS *see* musical choice method-therapeutic
      singing (MCM-TS)
MDD *see* major depressive disorders (MDD)
medial temporal lobe 214

medical health insurance 5
meditation 2, 6, 177–178
Mediterranean diet 214
menopausal syndrome 290
mental health
   and aging 210–11
   art & art therapy 217–18
   dance 216–17
   definition of 210
   and elderly 211–13
   exercise 215
   healthy life span 219–20
   Japan, ikigai 219
   music therapy 217
   nature and environment 218–19
   nutrition 213–15
   social support 218
   Tai chi 216
   wellness pathways 213
   Yoga 215–16
Mental Health Atlas 209
mental well-being 100, 213, 218
mental wellness 216
methodology 282
   music therapy 244–6
mobile health (mHealth) 272–3
modern medicine
   health connotation
      the bear's stance 160
      the crane's stance 161
      the deer's stance 159
      the monkey's stance 160
      the tiger's stance 159
the monkey's stance
   modern medicine 160
   traditional Chinese medicine 160
mood 217
morbidity 254
mortality 234–5
movement 7, 8, 33, 55, 91, 158
multivariable-adjusted diabetes 233
musical choice method-therapeutic singing
      (MCM-TS) 244, 245
myofascial pain syndrome 184
The MyRapid Senior Citizen Concession Card 50

naturally occurring retirement communities
      (NORC) 31
nature and environment 218–19
naturopathy 115
NCDs *see* non-communicable diseases (NCDs)
New England Journal of Medicine 216
NGOs *see* non-governmental organizations
      (NGOs)
non-cardiovascular mortality 215
non-communicable diseases (NCDs) 210, 211,
      254, 272

318   Subject Index

non-governmental organizations (NGOs) 16,
    49, 263
nutrition and ageing 213–15

older persons
    assistive technology 54–5, *56*
    built and social environments 54–5, *56*
    financing 53–4
    health care 50–2
    income security 53–4
    long-term care 50–2
    mobile/home-based nursing regulations 52
    programmes and services
        finance 42, **43,** *44,* 45, *46*
        healthcare 40–1, **41**
        housing 45, **47,** 47–8
        social programmes 48–9, **49**
        transport and others 50
    social care 50–2
older populations
    exercise
        essential element 190
        falls prevention 193
        health promotion and prevention
            approaches 190
        planning and resourcing changes 189
        prescription 191
        researched intervention approach 192
        research evidence supporting 192
        resistance training 192
        resistance training programs 190, 192
        walking programs 190
'ongoing' attachment theory 245
osteoporosis 207

pain 231–2
Parkinson's disease/rheumatoid arthritis 82, 216
PCBD *see* prolonged complex bereavement
    disorder (PCBD)
people with dementia (PWD) 243
'personal, cultural and structural' (PCS)
    levels 255
'personal' level concept 256
PGD *see* prolonged grief disorder (PGD)
physical health 235–6
physiotherapy (PT) 184
Ping An Good Doctor 275
place of safety 283
policy development
    1995–2010 34–6
    challenges 50–6
    importance 32
    policy issues 50–6
    pre-independence to 1994 32–3
    programmes and services
        finance 42, **43,** *44,* 45, *46*
        healthcare 40–1, **41**

        housing 45, **47,** 47–8
        social programmes 48–9, **49**
        transport and others 50
    recommendations 50–6
    2011 to present 36–40, *37*
policy on ageing 31–40
population ageing systems
    aims 83–4, *84, 85*
    drop a decade 84
    evidence base and culture 82–3
    living longer science 81–2, *82*
    network needs 86
    right culture 86–8, *87*
    set objectives 84–6, *85*
    20th century 83
post-COVID era 2
post-partum care 184
premature ageing 163
prevalence 242–3
prevention 190, 193, 277–8
privacy 284
problems, music therapy
    aim and methodology 244–6
    comorbidity 244
    consequences 244
    ethical issues 244–5
    prevalence 242–3
    terminology issues 242
    treatment issues 244–5
progesterone receptors (PRs) 290
programmes and services
    older persons
        finance 42, **43,** *44,* 45, *46*
        healthcare 40–1, **41**
        housing 45, **47,** 47–8
        social programmes 48–9, **49**
        transport and others 50
prolonged complex bereavement disorder
    (PCBD) 242
prolonged grief disorder (PGD) 242
Prospective Urban Rural Epidemiology study 215
PRs *see* progesterone receptors (PRs)
psychological health 235–6
psychological stress 230
    and diseases 230
Puraka-Kumbhaka-Rechaka 177
    physiology 177
PWD *see* people with dementia (PWD)

Qingfei Paidu Decoction 3, 4
quality of life 70–1, 217, 299

rakugo, traditional comedy 232
reactive oxygen species (ROS) 143
receptive music-based counselling 241
renal failure 208
rural healthcare

Subject Index

access 96–7
multi-morbidity 97
quality 96–7
rural pension system 92

safe and enabling homes 266–7
SARS-CoV-2 2, 212; *see also* coronavirus
disease-2019
scapulocostal pain syndrome 184
SCH *see* schizophrenia (SCH)
schizophrenia (SCH) 256
SDGs *see* Sustainable Development Goals
(SDGs)
seasonal foods, health preservation 153
second lumbar vertebra (L2) 295
self-esteem 218
senior citizens clubs 48
Serbian folk songs 246
severe acute respiratory syndrome (SARS) 3
sex differences 230–1
Shinzo Abe 64
silver-hair economy 49
social and technological change 274
social care 50–2
social dimension 260–1
social programmes 48–9, **49**
social protection system
redistribution 54
risk pooling 54
social support 218
social work model, empowerment oriented
practice 257–8
socioeconomic status (SES) 212
Solar Decathlon 279
"sources of laughter" 237
South-East Asia Region (SEAR) 111
perspective from 115, **116–17,** 117–18
spiritual dimension 261–2
Sprague-Dawley rats 293
stage grief theory 245
StAR expression *see* steroidogenic acute
regulatory protein (StAR)
expression
steroidogenic acute regulatory protein (StAR)
expression 296
stroke 207
'structural' level concept 256
sufficient sleep time, health preservation 152
Sun Simiao 218
super-ageing society 11
superoxide dismutase activity (SOD) 144
Sustainable Development Goals (SDGs) 299
systemic hormone estrogen therapy 290

Taeuigam 117
Tao Qian 218
TCM treatment 3

tension headache 184
terminology issues 242
Thai national healthcare system 118
the tiger's stance
modern medicine 159
traditional Chinese medicine 158
Tomonori Maruyama 5, 219
traditional and complementary medicine
(T&CM) 109
traditional Chinese Daoist Health
preservation 151
traditional Chinese medicine (TCM) 3, 111
Daoism's cultivation 6
health connotation
the bear's stance 159–60
the Crane's stance 160–1
the deer's stance 159
the monkey's stance 160
the tiger's stance 158
traditional healthcare 2, 3, 158
traditional Indian medicine 6
traditional Indian system, Yoga 171
traditional Malay Ulam
anticancer activity 142–3
antidiabetic activity 136–8
antihyperlipidaemic activity 141–2
antihypertensive activity 139, **139–41,** 141
dementia 143–4
recommendation 144
traditional medicine (TM) 4
anaesthesiology 113
definition 110–11
pain-free clinic 113
perspective
from Eastern Mediterranean Region
(EMR) 118, **119–20,** 120
from European Region (EUR) 120,
120–1, 121–3
from South-East Asia Region (SEAR) 115,
116–17, 117–18
from Taiwan 123
from Western Pacific Region (WPR) 111,
112–13, 113–15
from World Health Organization
(WHO) 111
Philippines 114
in Singapore 114
traditional Thai medicine (TTM) 6
traditional/tradition *see specific entries*
trauma 217
treatment issues 244–5
TTM health-promotion approach 181

ulam *see* traditional Malay Ulam
Unani 115

vulnerable populations 101, 272

wealth inequality 90–1
wearable technology 275
wellness pathways 213
wellness tourism 69–70
Western blotting analysis 293
Western medicine 3, 76
    duplicate medical treatment 76
Western Pacific Region (WPR) 110, 258
    perspective from 111, **112–13,** 113–15
WHO *see* World Health Organization (WHO)
WHO Health System Framework 272
World Health Organization (WHO) 2, 21, 209,
    213, 254

    perspective from 111
The World Health Organization (WHO) 12
The World Values Survey 48
WPR *see* Western Pacific Region (WPR)

Xenoma 275
Xie 7
Xuanfei Baidu Formula 3
Xuebijing Injection 3

Yale Bereavement Study 242
100-Year Life Society 64–5
years lived with disability (YLD) 272

Index of Name

Note: *Italic* page numbers refer to figures and page numbers followed by "n" denote endnotes.

Abdul Khalid, M. 42
Abdullah, R. 33
Abel, E. L. 234
Adams, T. 176
Adulyadej, B. 118
Aekplakorn, W. 180
Afshar, S. 17, 254
Aizenstein, H. J. 211
Akiyama, H. 11, 267
Al-Ajmi, S. 120
Al-Hashel, J. Y. 118
Ali, A. M. 143
Al-Kindi, R. 118
Al-Rowais, N. 118
Al Thiab Al Kendi, A. 118
Amalia, L. 138
Anad, P. 171
Andawurlan, N. 137
Angelidis, P. 273
Ang, J. Y. 113
Antman, F. 94
Arizmendi, B. 244
Ashari, A. 191
Atarodi, S. 55
Averbuch, E. 122
Awad, A. I. 120
Azhar, M. E. 144

Babykutty, S. 142
Barcella, C. A. 212
Barker, A. 193
Barton, H. 55, *56*
Baskaran, A. 276
Bauer, K. R. 290
Beckwée, D. 191
Begg, M. D. 272
Belyea, N. 255
Beynon, M. 272
Bhandari, H. 99
Bharti, S. K. 138
Bhixavatimath, P. 137
Black, K. 55
Blake, H. 192
Blomberg, S. 16
Bodeker, G. 8, 214, 216
Boden-Albala, B. 211
Böhme, M. H. 94
Boonruab, J. 185
Borikar, S. P. 137
Boss, G. R. 163

Bowman, G. L. 214
Brayne, C. 279
Brem, A. 274
Brooks, S. J. 212
Bujnowska-Fedak, M. M. 268
Burton, E. 191, 192
Buttagat, V. 184
Buys, N. 191
Byrow, Y. 211
Byun, S. J. 77

Cameron, I. D. 193
Carter, J. 272
Casarini, L. 294
Cattaneo, L. B. 258n4
Chae, J. M. 75, 76, 77
Chai, S. T. 36, 41, 42
Chander, R. 26
Chandran, V. G. R. 276
Chan, E. 98
Chang, F. 93, 94, 95
Chan, J. 98
Chapman, A. 258n4
Chartsuwan, J. 184
Chau, P. H. 267
Chayaratanasin, P. 137
Chen, A. J. 26
Chen, C. Y. P. 33
Chen, K. H. 99, 141
Chen, M. 96
Cheung, J. T. K. 265
Chiranthanut, N. 184
Chitirabaib, S. 185
Cho, J. K. 78
Chokevivat, V. 118
Cho, K. S. 76
Chong, S. A. 211
Chou, Y.-J. 109
Chuan-li, L. 138
Chusak, C. 137
Chuthaputti, A. 118
Clare, L. 135
Coburn, D. 99
Cohen, S. 276
Conger, J. A. 254n1, 256
Corburn, J. 272
Coulmas, F. 26
Cousins, N. 231
Cowen, V. 176
Cowgill, D. O. 26

321

Index of Name

Cox, E. O. 257, 257n3
Cozza, S. J. 242
Crapo, L. M. 83
Crawford Shearer, N. B. 254
Crépieux, P. 294
Crosette, B. 114
Crunfli, F. 2, 211

Daisy, P. 137
Dai, Y. 218
de La Rubia Ortí, J. E. 217
Demir Doğan, M. 236
DeSantis, L. 245
Dhippayom, T. 184
DiMaio, L. P. 242
Dinesh, D. 143
Doka, K. J. 245
Donabedian, A. 86
Do, S. R. 78
Douaud, G. 214
Duangjan, C. 135
Dufner, M. 234
Dunér, A. 16
Dwira, S. 143
Dwyer, D. 33

Echeverria, V. 290
Economos, A. 242
Eisma, M. C. 242
El Batran, S. A. E. S. 136
Eriksson, M. 283
Everett, B. 94

Faber, R. 217
Fargher, S. 272
Farrier, K. 192
Fasullo, L. 216
Fawcett, S. B. 257, 257n2
Fernández-Alcántara, M. 244
Fields, G. 91
Fleury, J. G. 254
Fotoukian, Z. 254
Frandsen, B. 22
Frankl, V. 67
Frederiksen, D. L. 274
Fries, J. F. 83
Fujikawa, Y. 114
Fujimori, J. 232
Fujiwara, Y. 236
Fu, S. 109

Gajula, D. 143
Gan, C. Y. 141
García, H. 219
Garg, G. 172, 173
Ghasemzadeh, A. 142, 143
Ghesquiere, A. 244

Ghodsbin, F. 236
Giangregorio, L. M. 192
Gillespie, L. 192
Goodkind, D. 190
Goto, S. 267
Grant, M. 55, *56*
Grata-Borkowska, U. 268
Gupta, R. 171

Hadira, O. 136
Hafiz, Z. Z. 144
Hamid, T. A. 5, 34, 36, 41, 42, 48
Hanprasertpong, N. 184
Hansa Jayadeva, S. 115
Haron, L. 48
Hasenoehrl, T. 192
Hashim, S. M. 243
Hasmuk, K. 45
Hassan, Z. 138
Hasson, H. 16
Hayashi, K. 232
Helbing, D. 99
Hernandez, A. 216
He, W. 28, 190
Hewitt, J. 193
He, Y. 90
Hildebrand, C. 272
Hill, K. D. 191
Hioki, A. 238
Hirosaki, M. 230
Hirschman, C. 26
Hisham, N. 5
Ho, B. K. 40
Hogan, N. 245
Ho, H. C. 267
Ho, I. Y. M. 143
Holmes, L. D. 26
Holzmann, R. 42, 44
Horstman, A. M. 290, 291
Hougaard, R. 272
Hou, R. 142
Howard, G. 244
Huang, B. 92
Huang, C. 90, 99
Huang, N. 109
Huang, Y. 191, 216
Huang, Z. 191
Huda-Faujan, N. 144
Hughes, K. J. 192
Huizingh, E. K. R. E. 274
Husna, F. 137
Hu, Y. 92
Hwang, N. H. 77

Iampornchai, S. 183
Ibrahim, I. 47, 120
Ichikawa, H. 236

Index of Name

Ikeda, S. 233
Ikehara, S. 230
Iliya, Y. A. 242
Imai, Y. 237
Imano, H. 230
Inaba, R. 238
Iso, H. 230

Jacob, A. 185
Jaidee, S. 183
Jaiswal, D. 137
Jaiswal, Y. 115
James, S. L. 272
Jamia, A. J. 6
Jansons, P. S. 193
Jee, D. 290
Jeong, H. S. 76
Jeon, H. S. 78
Jester, D. J. 55
Jiang, D. 90, 92
Jones, G. 26
Jones, G. W. 33
Juárez-Rojop, I. E. 136, 137, 142

Kadetz, P. 5, 99, 100
Kalil, A. 4
Kamontum, T. 185
Kamtchouing, P. 136
Kang, E. J. 78
Kang, F. J. 78
Kang, S. K. 78
Kanungo, R. N. 254n1, 256
Kariippanon, K. 8
Katarina, Madan Dr. 238
Kavadar, G. 123
Kawachi, I. 99
Kaweekorn, P. 182
Kersting, A. 243
Keshet, Y. 120, 122
Khalaf, A. J. 118
Kickbusch, I. 255
Kim, C. Y. 17
Kim, J. S. 78
Kim, K. H. 76
Kim, M. J. 141
Kim, Y. J. 76, 77
Kim, Y. M. 78
Kinsella, K. 28
Klass, D. 245
Kohda, M. 232
Ko, H. J. 236
Kok, R. N. 236
Koris, R. 41
Kowal, P. 190
Krinski, K. 192
Kronenberg, F. 214
Kruapanich, C. 184

Kruger, M. L. 234
Kuhn, R. 94
Kumar, A. 192
Kumnerddee, W. 184
Kuptniratsaikul, V. 185
Kurup, S. B. 138
Kwok, K. K. 26
Kwon, S. 17
Kwon, Y. K. 74

Lai, M. 55
Lai S. L. 30
Lam, F. M. 193
Lam, S. 266
Langås-Larsen, A. 274
Latham, N. 190
Lauber, C. 211
Lee, C. 31
Lee, D. W. Y. 3, 5
Lee, H. J. 77
Lee, H. S. 75
Lee, M. S. 74
Lee, P. S. 78
Lee, S. Y. 76
Leete, R. 26
Lee, T. J. 17
Lei, X. 95
Lei, Y. 95, 212
Lekshmi, P. C. 138, 141
Levinger, P. 192
Lewin, G. 192
Lhamo, N. 115
Liao, W. H. 192
Li, C. 4, 90, 91n1, 93, 95, 96, 101
Lindström, B. 283
Lingaraju, S. M. 142
Ling, T. L. 243, 244
Li, T. 96
Liu, C. 91n1, 96, 190
Liu, F. 243
Liu, X. 7, 191, 216
Li, Y. 90, 99, 192
Logue, J. K. 212
Loh, S. P. 136
Lo, V. 98
Lu, J. 296
Luo, H. 3
Lupton, D. 277

Maciejewski, P. K. 242
Mahwish Saeed, F. 136
Maniyar, Y. 137
Maple, M. 244
Masferrer, L. 244
Mathias, M. 272
Mat Zin, R. 42
Mauss, M. 99

Index of Name

Ma, X. 90, 93, 94, 95, 96, 97
Ma, Z. 91, 93, 94, 95, 96, 101
McPhate, L. 193
Mehta, K. 141
Meli, M. A. A. 143
Mendenhall, E. 272
Mervin, M. C. 267
Michael, N. 241
Milic, J. 244
Miller, V. 215
Minton, S. 216
Miralles, F. 219
Mofredj, A. 217
Mohanty, S. 4
Mohd Nor, H. S. 15
Mohd. Yatim, M. 33
Mokhtar, N. F. 143
Molina, N. 244
Moon, K. H. 76
Moreno, C. 212, 213
Morgan, F. 192
Morley, J. 21, 265
Murakami, A. 142
Muramatsu, N. 11
Muto, K. 212

Nadareishvili, I. 123
Nagasu, M. 212
Nebel, S. 115
Netchanok, S. 183
Newson, R. S. 243
Ng, B. K. 276
Nielsen, J. A. 278
Nimit-arnun, N. 185
Noolu, B. 143
Nugroho, A. E. 141
Nurhayati, B. 143
Nurulita, N. A. 142, 143
Nutbeam, D. 255

O'Callaghan, C. 241, 242
O'Connor, M. F. 244
Ogbo, F. A. 211
Ohira, T. 7, 230, 232, 238
Oh, Y. H. 78
Okamura, H. 236
Oktem, O. 294
Olson, K. R. 272
O'Mullan, A. 135
Onaya, T. 55
Ong, F. S. 34, 42
Ozer, O. 123

Pala, J. 26
Pang, W. 3
Pan, H. 243
Park, B. J. 74, 219

Parkes, C. M. 245
Park, H. 117
Parsons, R. J. 257, 257n3
Pattamadilok, D. 142
Pebriana, R. B. 143
Pejovic, M. 242
Perez-Breva, L. 274
Perrow, C. 83
Persian, R. 94
Peungsuwan, P. 184
Pickett, J. 279
Pizzo, P. A. 83
Pokpermdee, P. 180
Pongprayoon, U. 185
Poonsuk, P. 185
Popper-Giveon, A. 120, 122
Prasanna, R. P. 138
Prigerson, H. J. 242
Putnam, R. 99, 100
Puttarak, P. 144

Quach, A. 135

Radulovic, R. 7, 242, 244, 245
Rafat, A. 144
Rahmat, A. 143
Rajamanickam, M. 137
Rajathi, M. 137
Ramasay, A. 138
Ramely, A. 259n6
Ravishankar, B. 115
Ray, B. 176
Reihani, S. F. S. 144
Revadigar, V. 143
Reyburn, S. 118
Robertson, M. C. 191
Robinson, H. 267
Roca, C. P. 99
Rogerson, M. 192
Rössler, W. 211
Ruangritchankul, S. 180

Saavedra Pérez, H. C. 244
Sakurada, K. 234, 235
Sales, M. 192
Santaş, F. 123
Scheffel, J. 92, 93, 95, 100
Schein, E. 86
Schein E. H. 86
Schiele, M. A. 244
Schut, H. 242, 245
Seegmiller, J. E. 163
Sen, G. 176, 177
Seo, D. Y. 136
Shahidi, M. 236, 238
Sharma, G. 4
Sharma, M. 171

Index of Name

Sharma, P. 4
Shear, K. M. 242, 243, 244
Shengelia, R. 123
Sherrington, C. 190, 192
Shih, C. C. 123
Shi, N. 4
Shirai, K. 234
Shi, X. 92
Shrestha, L. 28, 40
Shukla, V. J. 115
Shukri, R. 138
Shuval, J. T. 122
Sia, Y. S. 143
Silvey, R. 94
Sims, J. 190
Singh, R. 172
Siow, H. L. 141
Sitthitanyakij, K. 182, 183, 185
Song, L. 191, 216
Song, Y. 91, 93
Son, N. K. 15
Sooktho, S. 184
Soon, G. C. 6
Spillane, A. 242
Spiteri, K. 192
Srithupthai, K. 184
Srividya, A. R. 142
Steffen, E. M. 245
Stickley, A. 122
Stocco, C. 294
Stöhr, T. 94
Stott, N. 274
Stroebe, M. 242, 245
Subcharoen, P. 180, 181, 182, 185
Subramanian, S. V. 99
Sugawara, J. 236
Sun, J. 191
Sushama, P. C. 33
Suttanon, P. 191
Sze, S. C. W. 296

Taiwo, B. J. 143
Tamada, Y. 235
Tanaka, H. 236
Tanasilangkoon, B. 182, 183, 185
Tankitjanon, P. 184
Tan, M. P. 41
Tan, P. C. 33
Tantipidok, Y. 183
Tao Qian 218
Tarumi, T. 236
Teekachunhatean, S. 184
Tey, N. P. 30
Thanakiatpinyo, T. 184
Thas, J. J. 115
Theou, O. 191
Thepsongwatt, J. 183

Thomas, C. 136
Thompson, N. 255
Thompson, S. 255
Tiemeier, H. 211
Toda, M. 236
To, H. P. 98
Tomonori, M. 5
Tracey, P. 274
Triamchaisri, S. 181, 182
Tse, C. 90, 93, 94, 95, 97
Tuorkey, M. J. 137

Uttley, L. 217
Uzir Mahidin, Datuk Seri Dr Mohd 110

Valtorta, N. K. 211
van Barele, M. 290
van der Wal, C. N. 236
Vanoh, D. 40
Velagapudi, R. 144
Verghese, J. 216
Vilhena, R. O. 138
Viña, J. 190
Visvanathan, R. 267
Voukelatos, A. 190

Waerass, A. 278
Waheedi, M. A. 120
Walia, S. 11
Wang, H. 99, 100
Wanthong, P. 185
Watanabe, K. 114
Wen, M. 99
Whitford, D. L. 118
Williams, L. 115
Wilms, S. 98
Won, C. W. 17
Wong, K. 296
Wong, K. M. 291
Wong, M. 267
Wongwan, S. 185
Woods, R. 244
Woo, J. 7, 267

Xiang, A. 90, 92, 93, 95, 96
Xie-fen, L. 138
Xie, Y. 7
Xu, J. 90
Xu, X. 135

Yaakob, U. 31
Yahaya, N. 34
Yamamoto, I. 212
Yamaoka, K. 99
Yang, D. 98
Yang, X. J. 191
Yardley, L. 193

Index of Name

Yasunobu, K. 99
Yazdani, M. 236
Yeung, M. 291
Yildirim, H. H. 123
Yim, J. 15
Yip, W. 99, 101
Yoon, K. J. 76, 78
Yoshino, S. 232
Youn, C. H. 236
You, Y. X. 143

Yunus, N. M. 22
Yu, R. 266, 267

Zhang, L. 91, 296
Zhang, Y. 4, 6, 91, 92, 93, 95, 100
Zhao, J. 236
Zhao, K. 4
Zhao, Z. 90, 92
Zhong, Y. 99
Zhou, G. 91, 93, 94, 95, 96, 101

Ingram Content Group UK Ltd.
Milton Keynes UK
UKHW022115040523
421267UK00019B/187